Wolfgang Harth • Uwe Gieler • Daniel Kusnir • Francisco A. Tausk

Clinical Management in Psychodermatology

Wolfgang Harth
Uwe Gieler
Daniel Kusnir
Francisco A. Tausk

Clinical Management in Psychodermatology

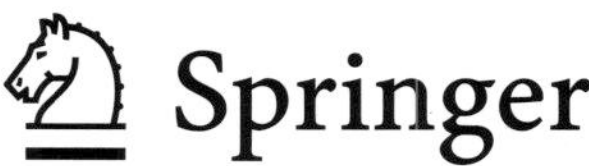

PD Dr. Wolfgang Harth
Vivantes Klinikum im Friedrichshain
Klinik für Dermatologie und Phlebologie
Landsberger Allee 49
10249 Berlin
Germany

Prof. Dr. Uwe Gieler
Universitätsklinikum Gießen
Klinik für Psychosomatik und Psychotherapie
Ludwigstr. 76
35392 Gießen
Germany

Daniel Kusnir
The Multi-Cultural Psychotherapy Training
and Research Institute
26081 Mocine Avenue
Hayward, CA 94544
USA

Prof. Francisco A. Tausk
University of Rochester
School of Medicine
Department of Dermatology
601 Elmwood Ave., Box 697
Rochester NY 14642
USA

ISBN 978-3-540-34718-7
e-ISBN 978-3-540-34719-4
DOI 10.1007/978-3-540-34719-4
Library of Congress Control Number: 2008931000

Cover design: eStudio Calamar, Spain
Production & Typesetting: le-tex publishing services oHG, Leipzig, Germany

Printed on acid-free paper

9 8 7 6 5 4 3 2 1

springer.com

Foreword

Every doctor and certainly every dermatologist knows that chronic skin diseases located on visible areas of the skin may lead to considerable emotional and psychosocial stress in the affected patients, especially if the course is disfiguring or tends to heal with scars. In the same way, as we know, emotional or psychovegetative disorders may trigger skin events.

Emotional or sociocultural factors of influence have dramatically changed the morbidity, pathogenetic understanding of causality, and therapy concepts in dermatology over the past decades; the relationship between the skin and the psyche or between the psyche and the skin is being given increasing attention.

There is a circular and complementary relationship between the skin and the psyche that becomes more evident during mental or skin disease. Not only is the skin part of the perception, but it is also a relational organ. The understanding of this multilevel relationship will help physicians understand the psychic and skin changes during disease.

This book is dedicated to such relationships. The picture atlas offers the morphologically trained dermatologist a summarizing presentation of diseases in psychosomatic dermatology for the first time.

The objective of this publication is to depict the relationships between skin diseases and psychiatric disorders to make the diagnostic vantage point for such disorders more clear. This affects, for example, the systematization of body dysmorphic changes, factitious disorder patients, little-known borderline disorders, and special psychosomatic dermatoses that have received little attention to date. Patients with skin or hair diseases that are rather insignificant from an objective point of view, such as diffuse effluvium, can endure great subjective suffering.

The present clinical atlas should help physicians recognize masked emotional disorders more quickly in patients with skin diseases and thus initiate adequate therapies promptly. This informative textbook has been admirably written by authors with much experience in the area of psychosomatic disorders in dermatology and venereology, and it provides many insights and aids from a psychosomatic perspective that, for various reasons, were not infrequently all but ignored.

This publication can be recommended to all doctors working in the areas of practical dermatology and psychosomatics, since it deals not only with the diseased skin but takes into account the suffering human in his or her physical and emotional entirety.

O. Braun-Falco
Munich, October 2007

Preface

The present textbook offers for the first time a summarizing overview of special clinical patterns in psychosomatic dermatology. The specialty is considered from an expanded biopsychosocial point of view.

Thus, both common and rare patterns of disease are presented for doctors and psychologists as an aid in recognizing and dealing with special psychosocial traits in dermatology.

Dealing with and treating skin diseases involves special features. While the skin and central nervous system are ectodermal derivatives, a good part of an individual's perception takes place through the skin. This experience is expressed in characteristic patient quotes and expressions such as "He's thin-skinned" or "My scaly shell protects me," or, increasingly, "I'm ugly and can't stand myself."

In recent years, psychosomatic medicine has developed, out of the limited corner of collections of personal experiences and individual case reports, into evidence-based medicine.

Cluster analyses and current psychosomatic research demonstrate that in addition to parainfectious, paraneoplastic, and allergic causes, psychosocial trigger factors can also cause disease in subgroups of multifactorial skin diseases.

In the present atlas, the psychosomatic subgroup will receive equal consideration and systematic presentation with the biomedical focal points, in order to facilitate diagnostics with clear diagnosis criteria for the somatization patient and to point out the good possibilities and rich experiences that exist today with adequate psychotherapy and psychopharmaceutical therapy.

The authors hope to reduce the fear of contact and encourage incorporation of the biopsychosocial concept in human medicine. Moreover, the sometimes varying language of doctors and psychologists is to be made more understandable and uniform. For this reason, the classification codes of the ICD-10 and current evidence-based guidelines are especially used in this reference work.

We wish to express particular thanks to Asst. Prof. Dr. Volker Niemeier, who contributed extensively and constructively to discussions in preparation of the manuscript, and to Asst. Prof. Dr. Hermes for providing numerous images. To our patients, who contributed the clinical descriptions and images in this book, we also express our thanks, since we were always impressed that their sometimes very problematic and difficult life histories helped us understand their world. Additional thanks are due to the editors at Springer, who, from the beginning of this book project, shared our enthusiasm and supported us in finishing it.

Last but not least, the authors wish the readers pleasure in reading this picture atlas of psychosomatic dermatology.

Wolfgang Harth, Uwe Gieler, Daniel Kusnir,
Francisco A. Tausk
Spring 2008

Contents

Part IV From the Practice for the Practice

Part V Appendix

Part I

General

Introduction

The basis of a successful strategy for combating a skin disease is elucidation of the various factors leading to the onset, course, and healing process of dermatoses.

The psychodermatology practice includes modifications to the regular dermatological practice, not targeting the patient's underlying psychiatric disease in general but specifically geared to overcome his or her psychiatric/psychological difficulties to obtain a good diagnosis and promote the endurance needed for compliance with treatment, dealing with the inherent stress and the psychosocial context.

Dermatoses, by their localization on the border (Schaller 1997) between internal and external, body and environment, visual exposition and stigmatization (Anzieu 1991), present with distinctive features in the objective assessment as well as in the individual's subjective assessment and in interpersonal communication.

Although many pathogenetic causalities have been revealed by medical advances, it has been found that the influence of individual psychic disposition and sociocultural factors can play an important role in the genesis and chronification of cutaneous diseases, in the transmission of infectious diseases, and as promoters of carcinogenesis. Historically, psychosomatic dermatology can only have existed since the term "psychosomatic" was introduced in 1818 by Heinroth (Heinroth 1818). The interactions between the patient and his or her disease and those conditions (or the context) in which the patient perceives a disease are related to the individual character and the circumstances configuring the context.

Psychosomatic dermatology addresses skin diseases in which psychogenic causes, consequences, or concomitant circumstances have an essential and therapeutically important influence.

In this respect, dermatoses are viewed as a unit in a biopsychosocial model.

Psychosomatic dermatology in the narrower sense encompasses every aspect of intrapersonal and interpersonal problems triggered by skin diseases and the psychosomatic mechanisms of eliciting or coping with dermatoses. Emotional disorders are present in one-third of all patients in dermatology. In addition, there are negative influences in coping with disease. The coping process (coined by Lazarus in 1966) is often equated with overcoming stress. The stress factor plays an important role, especially in chronic dermatoses (Consoli 1996).

Patients with emotional disorders are hospitalized for medical reasons two to four times more often than those without emotional disorders (Fink 1990). When associations with psychological and psychiatric disorders are initially concealed, the resulting physical symptoms often cannot be cured without adequate psychodermatologic intervention. In general, consequences of undiscovered psychiatric/psychological disorders in hospitalizations lead to

- Considerably longer in-hospital treatment episodes
- Greater use of posthospitalization care and readmissions

Moreover, patients with psychiatric disorders undergo surgery more frequently than patients with only organic diseases; however, they receive comparable somatic treatment without treatment of the psychiatric condition (Fink 1992).

In light of such basic data, the purely biomechanistic model of disease is being continually expanded with psychosocial concepts in all medical specialties (Niemeier and Gieler 2002).

The biopsychosocial model (Engel 1977) enjoys broad recognition these days and serves as one of the modern approaches to a dermatosis/disease. The patient is increasingly viewed as a holistic individual in whom lifestyle, perception, interpretation of the perceived, reality testing, past experiences and psychosocial context are decisive in the development of disease.

Thus, disorders may begin at the biological, psychological, or social system level and be offset by another or may also be negatively influenced by another (see Table 1).

Among the frequent problem areas in psychosomatic dermatology are the psychosomatic skin diseases, in which psychiatric factors play a basic role. Dermatitis artefacta is a psychiatric illness with skin reference, somatoform disorders, and sexual disorders, including problems in reproductive medicine and problems in coping with disease.

The problem of suicide among dermatologic patients (Gupta and Gupta 1998), especially in dermatoses such as acne vulgaris, has received little attention and has been underestimated in the past. One of the most serious and often concealed disorders in psychosomatic dermatology concerns the group of dermatitis artefacta patients. Patients with this group of diseases often have a borderline (or psychotic) disorder (Moffaert 1991).

Interpersonal contact difficulties are often in the foreground for many patients with skin diseases and result in a proximity–distance conflict. Feelings of shame and disgust are especially elicited by the patients' real or imagined perception of their skin disease.

The visibility of the skin and its changes makes it easy for patients to charge their diseased skin with psychological contents, thus reinforcing the splitting defense of their conflicts and often recruiting the aid of somatically oriented dermatologists. Overcoming this splitting may be very difficult in light of the concurrent proximity–distance problem that often exists (Gieler and Detig-Kohler 1994).

In dermatology, the question also arises as to the primary causality and reaction onset with respect to psyche or soma. If the genesis or the difficulties for successfully treating the disease lies in a psychiatric disorder, we speak of a psychosomatic disorder. If the somatic disorders are primary, we speak of a somatopsychic disorder. Thus, clear categorization and systematization are more important than ever in dermatology, not least for understanding the pathogenesis of a biopsychosocial disease that for planning therapy. Based on research results now available and on practical experience, classification in psychosomatic dermatology can now be differentiated in the following way:

- Dermatoses of primarily psychological/psychiatric genesis
- Dermatoses with a multifactorial basis, whose course is subject to emotional influences (psychosomatic diseases)
- Psychiatric disorders secondary to serious or disfiguring dermatoses (somatopsychic illnesses)

This division is used in the present book as a systematization and structuring of psychosomatic medicine in dermatology.

Table 1 Biopsychosocial resources (adapted from Becker 1992)

	Internal	External
Physical	Bodily disposition (genetics)	Healthy environment
		Healthy diet
		Safe working conditions
Psychosocial	Emotional health	Constitutional country
	Healthy living habits	Family ties
		Adequate workplace
		Material livelihood
		Established health network

References

Anzieu D (1991) Das Haut-Ich. Suhrkamp, Frankfurt/Main

Becker P (1992) Die Bedeutung integrativer Modelle von Gesundheit und Krankheit für die Prävention und Gesundheitsförderung. In: Paulus P (Hrsg) Prävention und Gesundheitsförderung. GwG-Verlag, Köln

Consoli S (1996) Skin and stress. Pathol Biol (Paris) 44: 875–881

Engel GL (1977) The need for a new medical model: a challenge for biomedicine. Science 196: 129–136

Fink P (1990) Physical disorders associated with mental illness. A register investigation. Psychol Med 20: 829–834

Gieler U, Detig-Kohler C (1994) Nähe und Distanz bei Hautkranken. Psychotherapeut 39: 259–263

Gupta MA, Gupta AK (1998) Depression and suicidal ideation in dermatology patients with acne, alopecia areata, atopic dermatitis and psoriasis. Br J Dermatol 139: 846–850

Heinroth J (1818) Lehrbuch der Störungen des Seelenlebens oder der Seelenstörung und ihre Behandlung, Teil II. Vogel, Leipzig

Lazarus RS (1966) Psychological stress and the coping process. McGraw-Hill, New York

Moffaert VM (1991) Localization of self-inflicted dermatological lesions: what do they tell the dermatologist? Acta Derm Venereol Suppl (Stockh) 156: 23–27

Niemeier V, Gieler U (2002) Psychosomatische Dermatologie. In: Altmeyer P (Hrsg) Leitfaden Klinische Dermatologie, 2. Aufl. Jungjohann, Neckarsulm, S 161–168

Schaller C (1997) Die Haut als Grenzorgan und Beziehungsfeld. In: Tress, W (Hrsg) Psychosomatische Grundversorgung, 2. Aufl. Schattauer, Stuttgart, S 94–96

1) want to convey? - genre -

2) theasaurus for words

3) Google search

4) Domain available

target market

end of name
ooo books, publishi
publications,

baby - academ
hat

Prevalence of Somatic and Emotional Disorders

A representative cohort study showed that about 40% of the normal population can be considered emotionally healthy with no need for psychotherapeutic treatment, whereas 23% require psychosomatic primary care, 10% require short-term psychotherapy, 15% would benefit from long-term psychotherapy, 4% require in-hospital psychotherapeutic treatment, and 8% cannot be treated, despite the indication (Franz et al. 1999).

Overall, data are scarce on the prevalence of emotional disorders in the individual somatic specialties, including dermatology, and these differ greatly depending on their focus.

The frequency of emotional disorders in the general medical practice has been found to range between 28.7% (Martucci et al. 1999) and 32% (Dilling et al. 1978); in the dermatological practice it has been reported to be 25.2% (Picardi et al. 2000), 30% (Hughes et al. 1983), and 33.4% (Aktan et al. 1998). In various dermatology inpatient services, this incidence has varied between 9% (Pulimood et al. 1996), 21% (Schaller et al. 1998), 31% (Windemuth et al. 1999), and even 60% (Hughes et al. 1983). The prevalence of psychosomatic disorders among dermatological patients is three times that for somatically healthy control cohorts (Hughes et al. 1983; Windemuth et al. 1999). The prevalence among dermatological patients is slightly higher than that of neurological, oncological, and cardiac patients combined.

Looking more closely at the specific somatic and emotional symptoms, there are studies on the prevalence and incidence of dermatological skin symptoms and the occurrence of dermatological diseases in a representative cross-section of the total population. In a study of 2,001 persons age 14–92 years, 54.6% of those questioned reported that they were presently suffering from at least a mild skin symptom; 24.1% of those questioned stated that they presently had at least one skin symptom of moderate to severe intensity, corresponding to about 75 million persons in the recorded age group in the United States. Women rated their skin symptoms as more severe than men did (Kupfer et al.). This difference is usually explained as greater attention being paid by women to their bodies, not as a greater susceptibility to disease. Whereas problems of seborrhea comedones and inflammatory papules decrease markedly with age, concerns with other skin changes, erythema, and dysesthesias increase with more advanced age. In reviewing the frequency of individual complaints in Germany, it becomes apparent that two of the most frequent bothersome complaints stem from more cosmetic aspects (seborrheic dermatitis of the scalp, 6.1 million; bromhidrosis, 3.5 million), and 19.9% presently have symptomatic acne or comedones. Another significant symptom area is pruritus; 30% of the general population suffers from some form of itching, 16.9% from generalized pruritus and 23.1% from pruritus localized to the scalp.

In a university outpatient clinic, 26.2% (n=195) of the patients presented with psychosomatic alterations. Somatoform disorder (18,5%) was the most frequent, and among the specific dermatological symptoms, pruritus was classified especially often (10.3%) as somatoform (Table 1).

The results confirm a high prevalence of somatoform disorders in dermatological patients, who represent one of the most difficult groups of patients to treat (see Sect. 1.3). The proportion of patients with increased depressive complaints was 17.3% in the group examined.

A survey of 69 dermatology clinics in Germany performed in 1999 (Gieler et al. 2001) documented the in-

Table 1 Frequency of complaints and dermatological somatoform symptoms (total sample, n=195; from Stangier et al. 2003)

	Dermatological symptoms		Dermatological somatoform symptoms	
Dermatological complaints	**Frequency (n)**	**% of total sample**	**Frequency (n)**	**% of total sample**
Itching	106	54.4	20	10.3
Burning	53	27.2	15	7.7
Cutaneous pain	40	20.5	15	7.7
Hair loss	15	12.8	3	2.5
Disfigurement	60	30.8	17	8.7
Total	126	66.2	36	18.5

creasing importance of psychosomatic medicine within dermatology. A clear trend to include psychosomatic aspects in the treatment of dermatological patients was observed. Among the dermatology clinics that returned the questionnaire, about 80% stated that psychosomatic aspects are taken into account in the therapy of dermatological patients; on average, they were of the opinion that offering psychosomatic therapy is necessary in nearly one-quarter of patients with skin diseases.

References

Aktan S, Ozmen E, Sanli B (1998) Psychiatric disorders in patients attending a dermatology outpatient clinic. Dermatology 197: 230–234

Dilling H, Weyerer S, Enders I (1978) Patienten mit psychischen Störungen in der Allgemeinpraxis und ihre psychiatrische Behandlungsbedürftigkeit. In: Häfner H (Hrsg) Psychiatrische Epidemiologie. Springer, Berlin, S 135–160

Franz M, Lieberz K, Schmitz N, Schepank (1999) A decade of spontaneous long-term course of psychogenic impairment in a community population sample. Soc Psychiatry Psychiatr Epidemiol 34: 651–656

Gieler U, Niemeier V, Kupfer J, Brosig B, Schill WB (2001) Psychosomatische Dermatologie in Deutschland. Eine Umfrage an 69 Hautkliniken. Hautarzt 52: 104–110

Hughes J, Barraclough B, Hamblin L, White J (1983) Psychiatric symptoms in dermatology patients. Br J Psychiatry 143: 51–54

Kupfer J, Niemeier V, Seikowski K, Gieler U, Brähler E (2008) Prevalence of skin complaints in a representative sample. Br J Psychol, in press

Martucci M, Balestrieri M, Bisoffi G, Bonizzato P, Covre MG, Cunico L, De Francesco M, Marinoni MG, Mosciaro C, Piccinelli M, Vaccari L, Tansella M (1999) Evaluating psychiatric morbidity in a general hospital: a two-phase epidemiological survey. Psychol Med 29: 823–832

Picardi A, Abeni D, Melchi CF, Puddu P, Pasquini P (2000) Psychiatric morbidity in dermatological outpatients: an issue to be recognized. Br J Dermatol 143: 983–991

Pulimood S, Rajagopalan B, Rajagopalan M, Jacob M, John JK (1996) Psychiatric morbidity among dermatology inpatients. Natl Med J India 9: 208–210

Schaller CM, Alberti L, Pott G, Ruzicka T, Tress W (1998) Psychosomatische Störungen in der Dermatologie–Häufigkeiten und psychosomatischer Mitbehandlungsbedarf. Hautarzt 49: 276–279

Stangier U, Gieler U, Köhnlein B (2003) Somatoforme Störungen bei ambulanten dermatologischen Patienten. Psychotherapeut 48: 321–328

Windemuth D, Stücker M, Hoffmann K, Altmeyer P (1999) Prävalenz psychischer Auffälligkeiten bei dermatologischen Patienten in einer Akutklinik. Hautarzt 50: 338–343

Part II

Specific Patterns of Disease

In classic dermatology, psychiatric and psychological factors either play a primary role or occur secondarily in a number of skin diseases.

The differentiation in primary and secondary disorders is critical for understanding the etiopathogenesis and deciding on the treatment. In classifying psychosomatic dermatoses, particular attention was paid to practical aspects to enable better understanding of the differentiation between those that are associated with psychiatric disorders and those that underlie a primary, purely psychiatric disorder. Three main groups can be differentiated.

Classification of Biopsychosocial Disorders in Dermatology

1. Dermatoses of primary psychiatric genesis (emotional/psychiatric disorders):
   Dermatitis artefacta, trichotillomania, delusion of parasitosis, somatoform disorders (glossodynia), body dysmorphic disorder (dysmorphophobia), etc.
2. Dermatoses with a multifactorial basis, of which the course is subject to psychiatric influences (psychosomatic diseases):
   Psoriasis, atopic dermatitis, acne, chronic forms of urticaria, lichen simplex chronicus, hyperhidrosis, etc.
3. Secondary psychiatric disorders due to serious or disfiguring dermatoses (somatopsychic diseases):
   Adjustment disorders with depression, anxiety, or delusional symptoms

Ad 1: To date, primary psychiatric disorders have been treated almost exclusively by psychiatrists and psychologists. However, patients with psychiatric disorders frequently first consult a dermatologist because of assumed somatic diseases and then often show no motivation for psychosomatic approaches.

Ad 2: The large group of diseases of multifactorial genesis is being given increasing attention; their importance has long been underestimated. Here, the dermatosis may be triggered by psychosocial factors, and corresponding disease groups (subgroups) of patients (clusters), such as stress responders and nonstress responders, can be differentiated. These subgroups with psychosomatic causality were often not given sufficient attention in the past, but they can be adequately identified. Therapy of the emotional trigger factors can decisively improve the quality of treatment.

Ad 3: Secondary psychiatric disorders due to serious or disfiguring dermatoses (somatopsychic diseases) are usually adjustment disorders with depression and/or anxiety, which may complicate the course of the disease. Supplementary nonpharmacological therapy is necessary and may achieve decisive improvement, especially in quality of life, compliance, and coping with the disease.

It is not always possible to adequately separate primary and secondary psychiatric disorders in biological systems, but independent of their genesis, the psychiatric disorders must be diagnosed and treated, when required, in both cases.

1

Primarily Psychogenic Dermatoses

In purely psychogenic dermatoses, the psychiatric disorder is the primary aspect, and somatic findings arise secondarily. These are the direct consequences of psychological or psychiatric disorders.

In dermatology, there are four main disorders with primarily psychiatric genesis.

Disorders of Primarily Psychiatric Genesis

1. Self-inflicted dermatitis: dermatitis artefacta syndrome, dermatitis paraartefacta syndrome (disorder of impulse control), malingering
2. Dermatoses due to delusional disorders and hallucinations, such as delusions of parasitosis
3. Somatoform disorders
4. Dermatoses due to compulsive disorders

Note: Self-inflicted dermatitis reflects a variety of conditions that share the common finding of automutilating behavior resulting in trauma to the skin. They represent a spectrum that spans from conscious manipulation of skin and appendages all the way to a delusional psychosis. The degree of severity is mostly determined by the progressive loss of awareness of the process. Although we classify these as distinct entities, the differences among them may be blurred. For example, a subject who has been repeatedly infested with mites may at some point be convinced that he or she is still infected.

1.1 Self-Inflicted Dermatitis: Factitious Disorders

Definition. Factitious disorder refers to the creation or simulation of physical or psychiatric symptoms in oneself or other reference persons. Factitious disorders (ICD-10: F68.1, L98.1) is the term used to describe self-mutilating actions (DSM-IV 300.16/ 300.19) that lead directly or indirectly to clinically relevant damage to the organism, without the direct intention of committing suicide.

The current division differentiates three groups as follows.

> **Categorization of Factitious Disorders**
>
> 1. Dermatitis Artefacta Syndrome: dissociated (not conscious) self-injury behavior
> 2. Dermatitis Paraartefacta Syndrome: disorders of impulse control, often as manipulation of an existing specific dermatosis (often semiconscious, admitted self-injury)
> 3. Malingering: consciously simulated injuries and diseases to obtain material gain

This categorization is helpful in understanding the different pathogenic mechanisms and the psychodynamics involved, as well as in developing various therapeutic avenues and determining prognosis.

Additionally, other special forms exist, such as the Münchhausen syndrome and Münchhausen-by-proxy syndrome (Sect. 1.1.4).

Even though factitious disorder is the most common cause for dermatitis artefacta syndrome (DAS), several psychiatric conditions can cause the syndrome (refer to the list, "Frequent Psychiatric Disorders in Self-Inflicted Dermatosis"). The skin presentation will vary depending on the genesis of the lesions or artefacts (see list of genesis of dermatitis artefacta).

Factitious disorders are caused by conscious or dissociated self-injury. The patient may be unable or unwilling to integrate the dissociated action of self injury; this functioning is often present in factitious disorder and/or in borderline personality disorder in which several varieties of dissociative defenses are typically present. With less frequency, other psychiatric conditions may cause the syndrome.

To make the diagnosis, the clinician explores the type of benefit or gain produced by the symptom. If the gain is to be treated as a patient in the absence of suicidal symptoms, it suggests a dermatitis artefacta syndrome; if the secondary gain is economic or if the patient is avoiding work or receiving other material rewards, it indicates malingering.

Prevalence/incidence. The prevalence of factitious disorders is estimated at 0.05–0.4% in the population (AWMF 2003). With the exception of malingering, often observed as part of fraudulent behavior, which occurs more often in men, self-injurious behavior is observed mostly in women (5–8:1), usually beginning during puberty or early adulthood.

Pathogenesis. Frequently there are mechanical injuries, self-inflicted infections with impaired wound healing, and other toxic damage to the skin. Hematological symptoms may occur by occluding the extremities, creating petechiae, and by covert intake of additional pharmaceuticals or injection of anticoagulants.

> **Genesis of Dermatitis Artefacta**
>
> - Mechanical
>   - Pressure
>   - Friction
>   - Occlusion
>   - Biting
>   - Cutting
>   - Stabbing
>   - Mutilation
> - Toxic damage
>   - Acids
>   - Alkali
>   - Thermal (burns, scalding)
> - Self-inflicted infections
>   - Wound-healing impairments
>   - Abscesses
> - Medications (covert taking of pharmaceuticals)
>   - Heparin injections
>   - Insulin

1.1.1 Dermatitis Artefacta Syndrome (DAS)

Clinical findings. The clinical appearance of dermatitis artefacta syndrome (ICD-10: F68.1, unintentional L98.1; DSM-IV-TR 300.16 and 19) is characterized by self-manipulation. Basically, the morphology of these can imitate most cutaneous diseases (Figs. 1.1–1.9).

"Typical is what is atypical."

This means that dermatitis artefacta syndrome must be suspected in clinical patterns with atypical localization, morphology, histology, or unclear therapeutic responses. Effort should be directed to detect foreign, infectious, or toxic materials.

The consequences are particularly dangerous when the patient delegates the body-damaging action to the

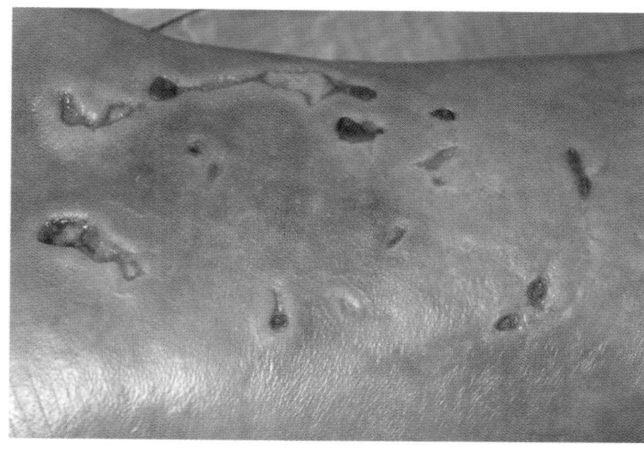

Fig. 1.3 Dermatitis artefacta syndrome: 58-year-old woman with skin defects on the lower calf in acute psychosis and hospital-wandering in Germany. She had had admission to four hospitals (three dermatology services) and outpatient consultation of three dermatology specialists within the previous 14 days

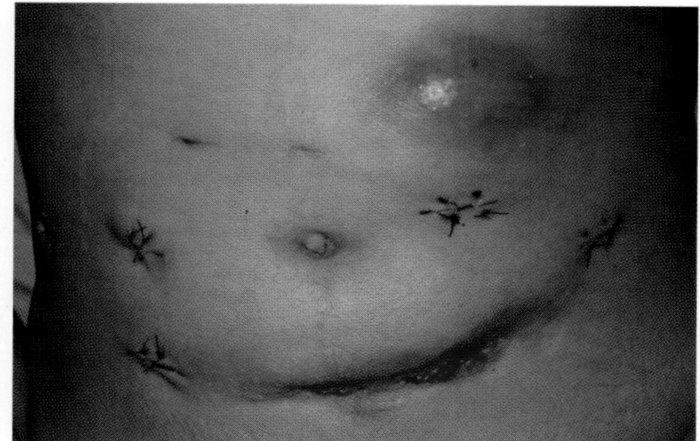

Fig. 1.1 Multiple foreign-body granulomas, partly with abscessing after self-injection. Occurrence of new lesions and artefacts after surgical treatment

Fig. 1.2 Same patient as in Fig. 1.1 with punched-out, self-induced skin defects

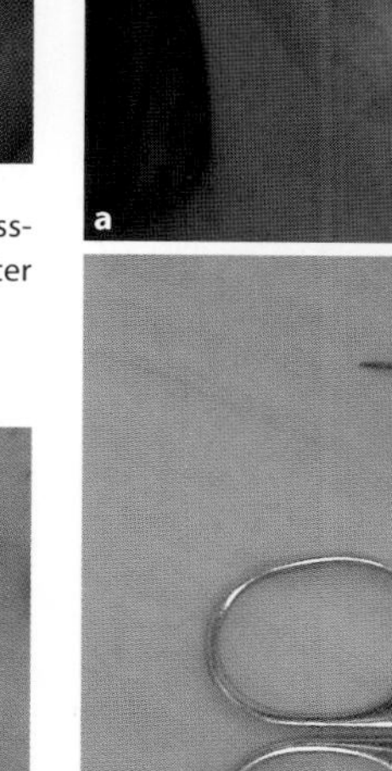

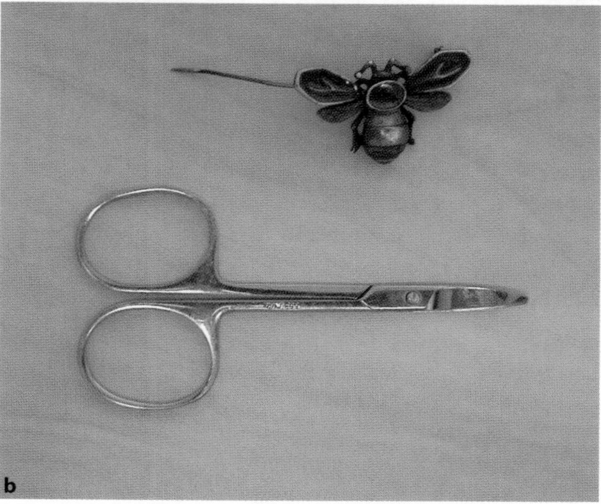

Fig. 1.4 **a** Extensive scarred dermatitis artefacta syndrome in the face. **b** Corresponding instruments for self-manipulation

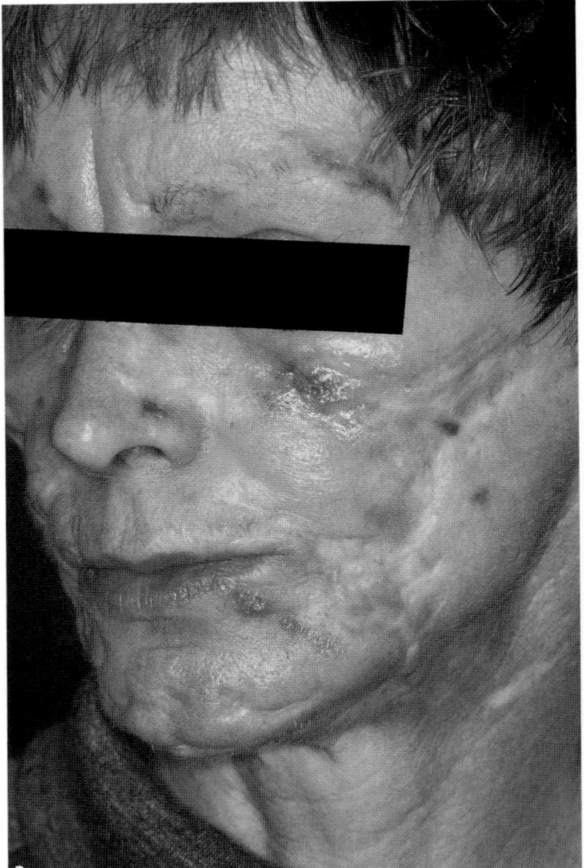

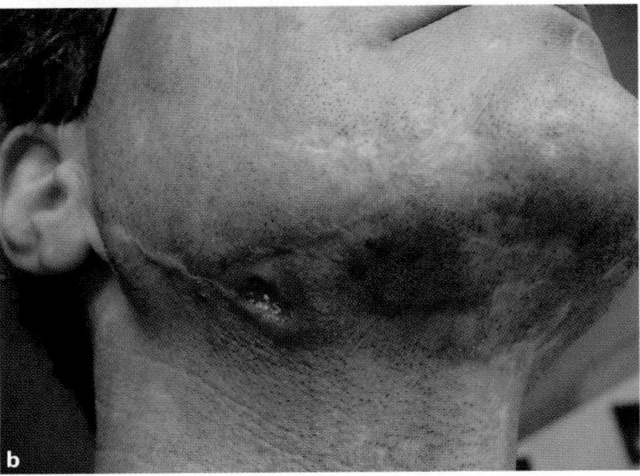

Fig. 1.5 **a** Extensive scarred dermatitis artefacta syndrome in the face. **b** Severe artefacts are also seen in males

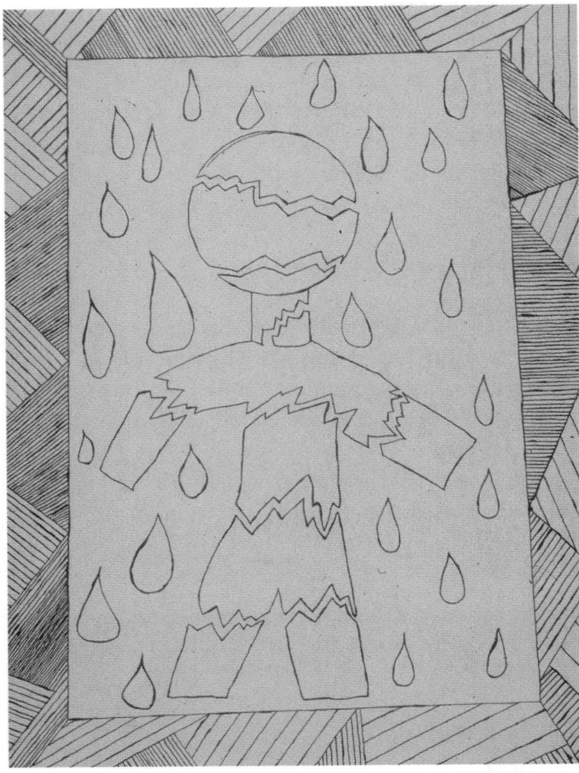

Fig. 1.6 Signs of body mutilation in a patient with dermatitis artefacta syndrome

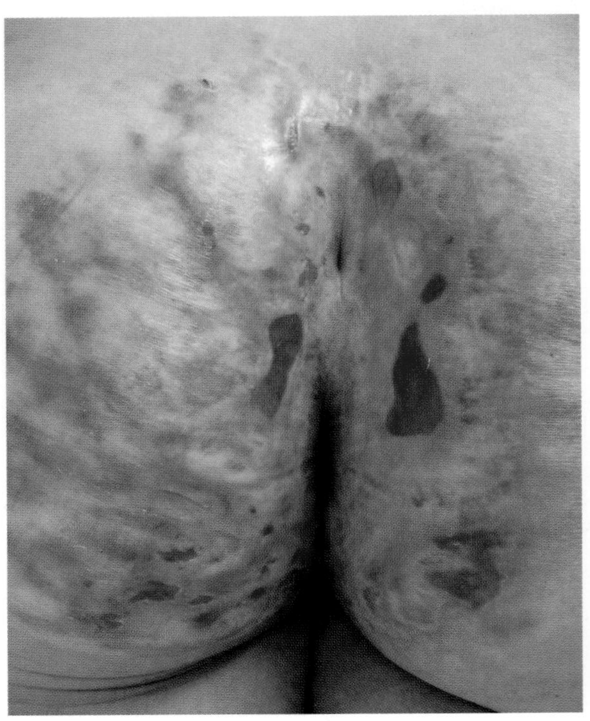

Fig. 1.7 Unconscious artefacts: 55-year-old woman with mesh-like skin defects in the perianal area and compulsive personality disorder

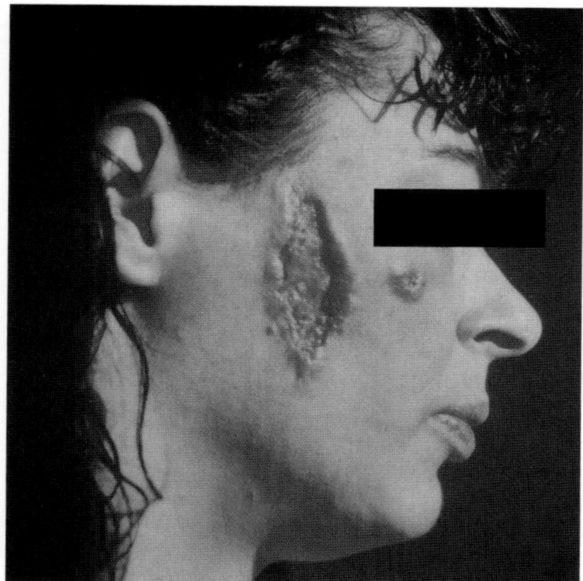

Fig. 1.8 Differential diagnosis: pyoderma gangrenosum in the face; clinical presentation of dermatitis artefacta syndrome could not be confirmed. Healing under immunosuppression

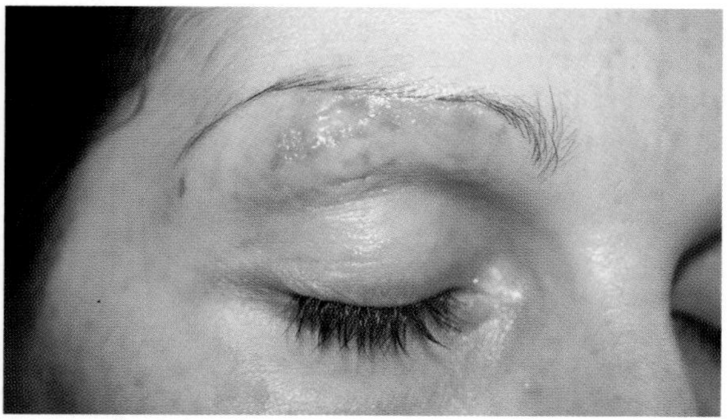

Fig. 1.9 Artefact in a patient with immigration problems

physician or when simulated complaints result in invasive or damaging medical treatment measures such as surgical interventions (Sect. 1.1.4).

Psychological symptomatics. DAS as dissociated self-injury may express a reactivation of injuries suffered in childhood based on a serious psychiatric disorder from earlier times, and may contain a nonverbal connotation.

The damaging behavior usually occurs covertly, often in dissociative states, without the patient's being able to remember or emotionally comprehend the event.

The so-called hollow history (van Moffaert 2003) is characteristically often found when taking the history of patients with DAS. This refers to the fact that unclear, vague statements are made about the onset of disease, which appeared suddenly with no warning or symptoms.

Typically, the patients themselves appear astonished by the skin changes and cannot give clear statements or details about the first occurrence or appearance and course of development. The history remains unclear. The patients are conspicuously emotionally uninvolved while they relate the history of their disease, as though they were not affected themselves when details of the often disfiguring lesions are related. Pain that would be medically expected to result from the lesions is also often not reported. The family, on the other hand, is often enraged and accusatory, complaining of the physician's incompetence at reaching an appropriate diagnosis and treatment.

A heterogeneous psychopathological spectrum exists among patients with DAS. There are often serious personality disorders (mainly emotionally unstable personality disorders of the borderline type, ICD-10: F60.31; DSM-IV-TR: 301.83 borderline personality disorder) or other disorders as described below.

Frequent Psychiatric Disorders in Self-Inflicted Dermatosis

- Early personality disorders
- Emotionally unstable personality disorders of the borderline type
- Narcissistic personality disorders
- Histrionic personality disorders
- Antisocial personality disorders
- Dependency personality disorders
- Depressive disorders
- Anxiety disorders
- Compulsive disorders
- Posttraumatic stress disorders

In the anamnesis, two-thirds of patients report traumatizing experiences such as sexual and physical abuse and situations of deprivation.

Mild forms of self-inflicted dematosis result from conflicts of adolescence or from alcohol, medication, or drug abuse.

In addition, DAS can occur as a comorbidity in depressive, anxiety, and compulsive disorders, as well as in posttraumatic stress disorders. Dissociative amnesias and serious depersonalization states may occur in connection with self-mutilating behavior.

The autoaggressive behavior of DAS patients manifests in other conspicuous incidents, so the connection between artefacts and suicidal behavior should be emphasized, a point that is highlighted in the literature to the extent that dermatitis artefacta syndrome may represent a masked suicidal behavior.

Very often, the patients report being under great pressure and tension prior to self-injury and feel relieved following it, which releases tension and acts as a form of "tranquilizer" (Janus 1972; Paar and Eckhardt 1987; Eckhardt 1992).

Overt self-damaging behavior or conscious DAS may represent the desire for secondary gain from illness, or it may show blurred transitions to dermatitis paraartefacta syndrome.

Differential diagnosis in the group of self-inflicted dermatoses. At the time of the self-damaging acts, manifest psychotic illness or other psychiatric conditions may be present, within the framework of which the self-injury occurs. The illnesses listed in the following overview belong in this category.

The underlying co-occurring psychiatric conditions need to be enumerated as well as other medical conditions triggering or co-occurring with the skin condition or generating additional psychiatric/psychological burden.

Differential Diagnosis in Dermatitis Artefacta Syndrome (AWMF Guideline 2003)

- Emotionally unstable personality disorders of the borderline type
- Schizophrenias, schizotypal and delusional disorders
- Affective disorders with psychotic symptoms, juvenile autism
- Hypochondriacal delusion
- Parasitosis
- Monosymptomatic psychosis
- Acute intoxications, psychotropic substances, withdrawal syndrome
- Brain-organic psychosyndrome
- Seizures
- Cultural or religious acts
- Sexual acts
- Suicidal intent
- Comorbidity with organic diseases
  - Lesch–Nyhan syndrome
  - Cornelia de Lange syndrome
  - Rett syndrome
  - Chronic encephalitis, neurosyphilis, temporal lobe epilepsy
  - Oligophrenia
  - Dementia syndrome (F00-F04)

References

AWMF (2003) Leitlinie Artifizielle Störungen. http://www.AWMF-Leitlinien.de

Eckhardt A (1992) Artificial diseases (self-induced diseases) – a review. Nervenarzt 63(7): 409–415

Janus L (1972) Personality structure and psychodynamics in dermatological artefacts. Z Psychosom Med Psychoanal 18(1): 21–28

Moffaert M van (2003) The spectrum of dermatological self mutilation and self destruction including dermatitis artefacta and neurotic excoriations. In: Koo J, Lee C-S (eds) Psychocutaneous medicine. Dekker, New York

Paar GH, Eckhardt A (1987) Chronic factitious disorders with physical symptoms – review of the literature. Psychother Psychosom Med Psychol 37(6): 197–204

1.1.2 Dermatitis Paraartefacta Syndrome (DPS)

In dermatitis paraartefacta syndrome (DPS), the most common underlying psychiatric condition is an impairment of impulse control (ICD-10:F63.9; DSM-IV-TR: 312.30 impulse-control disorder NOS), but other psychiatric conditions may underlie this syndrome. The patients have lost control over the manipulation of their skin. In dermatology, a minimal primary lesion is often characteristically excessively traumatized, leading to pronounced, serious clinical findings.

The patterns of disease listed in the following summary belong to DPS.

Dermatitis Paraartefacta Syndrome (DPS)

- Skin/mucosa
  - Skin-picking syndrome (epidermotillomania, neurotic excoriations)
  - Acne excoriée
  - Pseudoknuckle pads
  - Morsicatio buccarum
  - Cheilitis factitia
- Integument
  - Onychophagia, onychotillomania, onychotemnomania
  - Trichotillomania, trichotemnomania, trichoteiromania

The differential diagnosis should also consider DPS in the Köbner phenomenon.

Table 1.1 Overview of skin-picking syndrome/neurotic excoriations

Group	Self inflicted dermatoses	
Subgroup	Dermatitis paraartefacta/impaired impulse control	
Diagnosis	Skin-picking syndrome (usually acute course)	
Localization	Face	Acne excoriée
	Body	Skin-picking syndrome
Differential diagnosis	Compulsive disorders/lichen simplex chronicus	
	Atopic eczema/neurodermatitis circumscripta	
	Prurigo group	

Clinical presentation. The clinical presentation of DPS is characterized by the following specifically defined dermatoses.

Skin-Picking Syndrome (Neurotic Excoriations)

One of the greatest confusions of terms in psychosomatic dermatology is the definition of the skin-picking syndrome, which largely corresponds to the skin lesions formerly called neurotic excoriations (ICD-10: F68.1, L98.1, F63.9; F68.1; DSM-IV-TR 312.30), partly because the terms "neurosis" and "psychosis" have mostly been abandoned in the modern classification systems and have been replaced generically by the term "disorder" (Table 1.1).

Generally this is a single nosological entity; however, a variety of synonyms have been used: skin-picking syndrome, emotional excoriations, nervous scratching artefact, neurotic excoriations, paraartificial excoriations, epidermotillomania, dermatotillomania, and acne excoriée or acne urticata.

The term "neurotic excoriations" corresponds to skin-picking syndrome.

Our recommendation for the definition is as follows:

> **Skin-picking syndrome is a DPS most often facilitated by impaired impulse control, resulting in self-injury to the skin or mucosa and usually serving to reduce underlying emotional tension.**

Clinical findings. Skin-picking syndrome (neurotic excoriations; ICD-10: F63.9; DSM-IV-TR 312.30) is characterized by excoriations, erosions, and crusting in addition to atrophic and hyperpigmented scarring secondary to self-inflicted trauma (Figs. 1.10, 1.11).

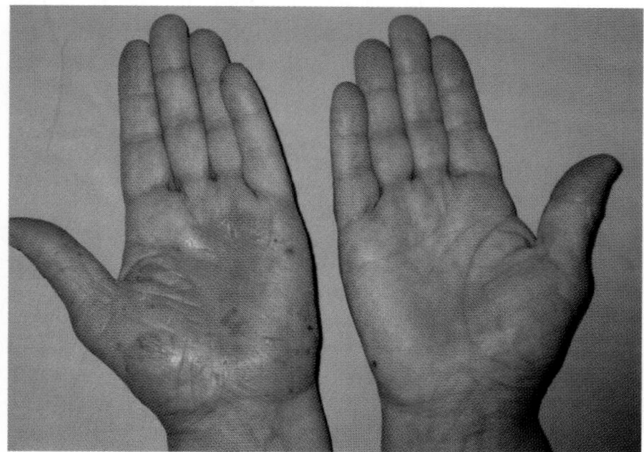

Fig. 1.10 Skin picking in a 62-year-old right-handed woman with impaired impulse control in combination with rage affects

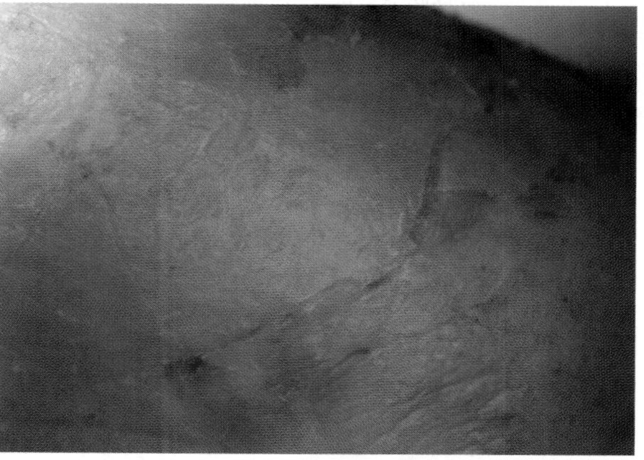

Fig. 1.11 Close-up of a 62-year-old, right-handed woman with typical triangular skin defects

Table 1.2 Differential diagnosis: skin-picking syndrome and lichen simplex chronicus

	Skin-picking syndrome	Lichen simplex chronicus
Clinical presentation	Primary disorder, intensive itching, discrete papules	Chronic, lichenified, severely pruritic dermatitis
Psychiatric disorder	Disorder of impulse control, psychovegetative lability, and adjustment disorders, which in part occur in episodes under stress and are associated with loss of control	Compulsive disorders, chronic stress, or conflict problematics, whereby the subjectively unalterable compulsive act of scratching the skin predominates

Most commonly localized on arms and legs, the skin-picking syndrome may also occur in the face, where it is frequently referred to as acne excoriée (see the following section).

Psychiatric symptoms. The psychiatric disorder is characterized by an impairment of impulse control with repeated inability to resist the impulse to scratch. In some cases, there is an urgency to suppress or destroy a skin lesion perceived as disfiguring. In the skin-picking syndrome (neurotic excoriations) and acne excoriée, some relief of the patient's conflict-related tension is obtained through the skin in a circular process of lack of impulse control, picking, and progressive concern and guilt about the new lesion created.

At the beginning of the skin-picking behavior, there is a progressive buildup of a feeling of tension, which may or may not be accompanied by itching, followed by excoriation of the skin in the second phase, and subsequently a third phase of satisfaction or a feeling of relief after this act. The syndrome is often accompanied by comorbid depressive and anxiety disorders.

Some authors believe this behavior has a correlate of sexual satisfaction (see Chap. 5) due to the comparable staged course and possible symbolic content.

Differential diagnosis. The psychiatric and somatic differential diagnosis includes lichen simplex chronicus (Table 1.2), in which most compulsive disorders (Sect. 1.4) are in the foreground of the psychiatric symptoms. Clinically, there are chronically lichenified areas.

Therapy. Therapy for skin-picking syndrome is based on the treatment measures and guidelines for DPS and is summarized in that section.

In mild cases, therapy may be achieved by psychoeducation or supportive psychosomatic primary care. In individual cases, medication therapy with benzodiazepines or selective serotonin reuptake inhibitors (SSRIs) is indicated and justified.

Acne Excoriée (Special Form)

A special form of skin-picking syndrome is acne excoriée (ICD-10:F68.1,L70.5;F68.1;DSM-IV-TR312.30), which is characterized and defined by its localization in the face.

Acne excoriée is the special form of skin-picking syndrome in the face in which there is minimal acne (maximal picking with minimal acne) and significant scarring.

In this, usually minimal lesions are extensively manipulated by squeezing and pressing, usually with the fingernails or sharp instruments. Often the patients cannot resist the impulse to perform these acts but justify the manipulations with the argument that they are removing infectious material. This results in excoriations, erosions, or even ulcerations that heal with stellate discolored scarring (Figs. 1.12, 1.13).

The therapeutic approach is similar to that for DPS, although questions of disease coping may be more urgent due to the stigmatization in the face.

Further Reading

Arnold LM, Auchenbach MB, McElroy SL (2001) Psychogenic excoriation. Clinical features, proposed diagnostic criteria, epidemiology and approaches to treatment. CNS Drugs 15(5): 351–359

Bach M, Bach D (1993) Psychiatric and psychometric issues in acne excoriée. Psychother Psychosom 60(3–4): 207–210

Fruensgaard K (1991) Psychotherapeutic strategy and neurotic excoriations. Int J Dermatol 30(3): 198–203

Gupta MA, Gupta AK, Haberman HF (1986) Neurotic excoriations: a review and some new perspectives. Compr Psychiatry 27: 381–386

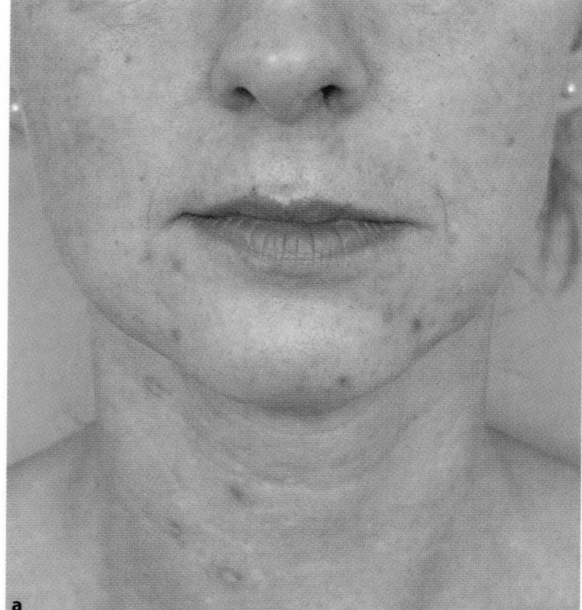

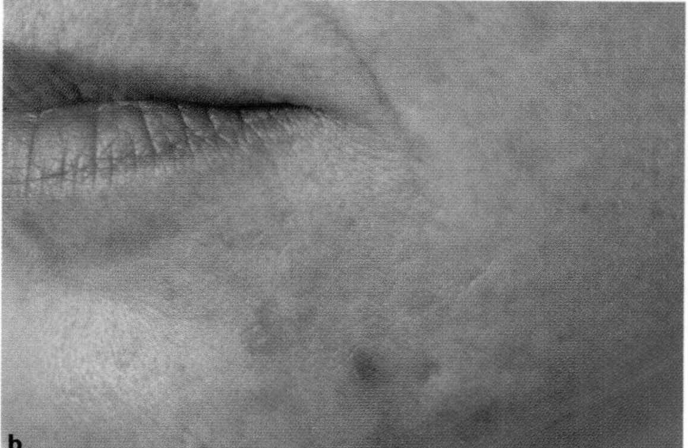

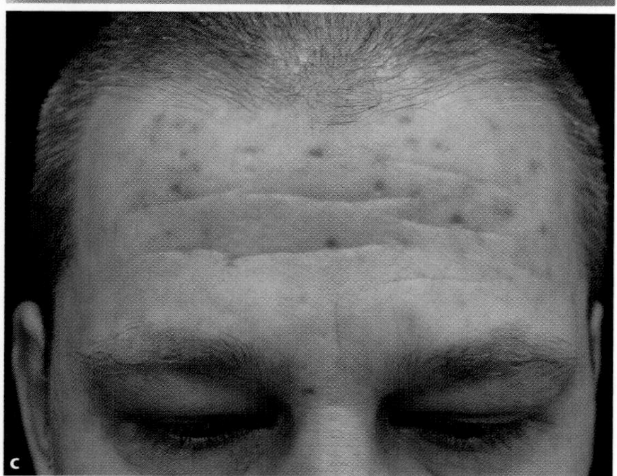

Fig. 1.12a–c Minimal form skin-picking syndrome (acne excoriée) with minimal preexisting acne and a manipulation urge for more than 20 years. **a** Overview. **b** Close-up of patient in **a**. **c** Skin picking in a male

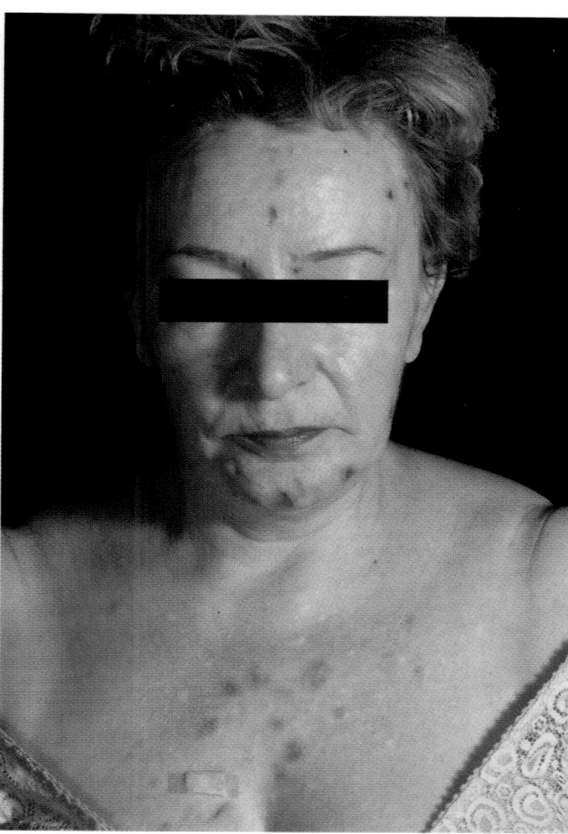

Fig. 1.13 Maximal form skin-picking syndrome (acne excoriée) with manipulation urge for several years and now acute exacerbation during a life crisis

Morsicatio Buccarum

Morsicatio buccarum (ICD-10: F68.1, K13.1; F68.1; DSM-IV-TR 312.30) are benign, sharply demarcated, usually leukodermic lesions around the tooth base and buccal mucosa. These may result from continuous, unconscious sucking and chewing on the oral mucosa. The diagnostic criteria of impaired impulse control are in the foreground of the psychiatric symptoms (Fig. 1.14).

Compulsive disorders may also be present in the underlying psychiatric condition.

Morsicatio buccarum is found more often among denture wearers without other psychiatric symptoms. Lichen planus can be ruled out by a biopsy in cases of doubt.

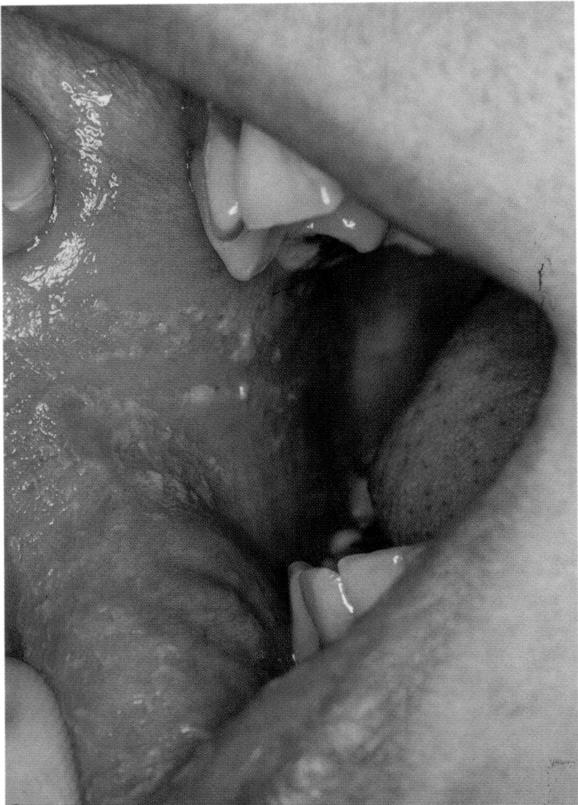

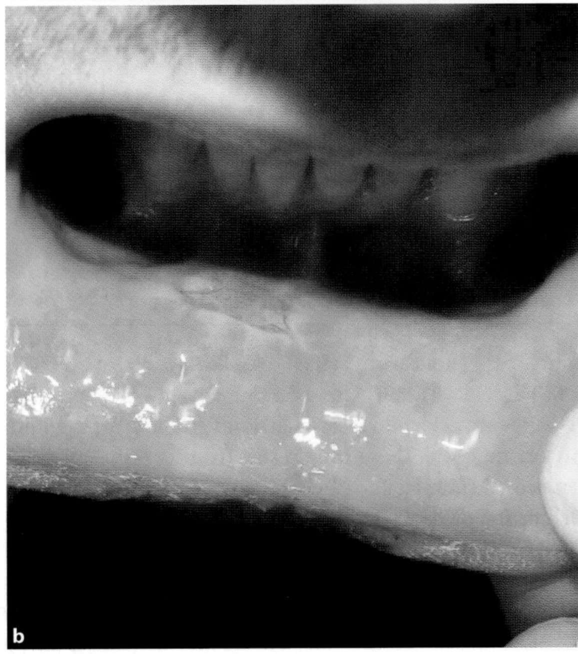

Fig. 1.14 **a** Morsicatio buccarum (linea alba buccalis) with constantly changing sucking of the cheek mucosa in situations of tension. **b** Ulcer from biting in a patient with disturbance of impulse control

Cheilitis Factitia

Cheilitis factitia (ICD-10: F68.1, K13.0; F68.1; DSM-IV-TR 312.30) is compulsive licking (lip-licker's dermatitis) and the basis of the pathogenesis. It results in an irritant contact dermatitis, leading to eczematous skin changes and a predisposition to secondary impetiginization. The licking usually affects discrete, symmetric, sharply delineated areas beyond the outline of the lips, frequently associated with traumatizing lip chewing (Fig. 1.15).

Psychopathologically, impaired impulse control is in the foreground, which often goes unnoticed. Frequently the patients are children, and following diagnosis and careful explanation of the causes to parents and patients, full healing is achieved by controlling the eliciting mechanism.

Pseudoknuckle Pads

Pseudoknuckle pads (ICD-10: F68.1, M72.1; F68.1; DSM-IV-TR 312.30) occur due to trauma (rubbing, massaging, chewing, sucking) to the finger joints and are clinically characterized by hypertrophic, padlike, rough, slightly scaly skin lesions. Mental retardation in these patients may be common (Fig. 1.16).

Real knuckle pads are due to a form of genodermatosis without mechanical trauma and are characterized histologically by cell-rich fibrosis. Explanatory discussions of pseudoknuckle pads in the sense of psychoeducation with the worried parents, subsequent observation, and increased attention may reveal the mechanism. Healing may be promoted by suppression with supportive skin-care measures as a replacement act. Lack of response may require a subsequent referral

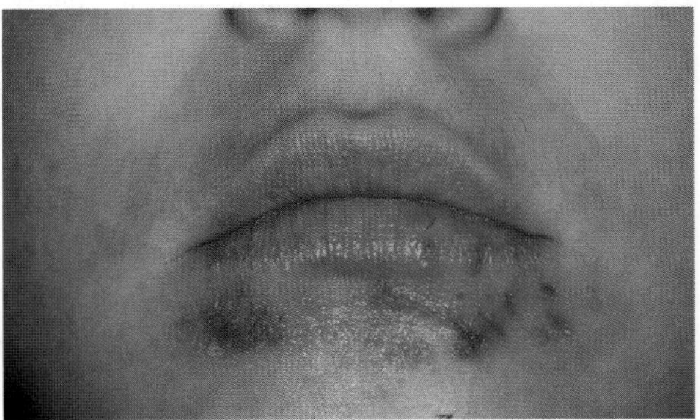

Fig. 1.15 Cheilitis factitia (lip-licking dermatitis) in impaired impulse control, with secondary superinfection

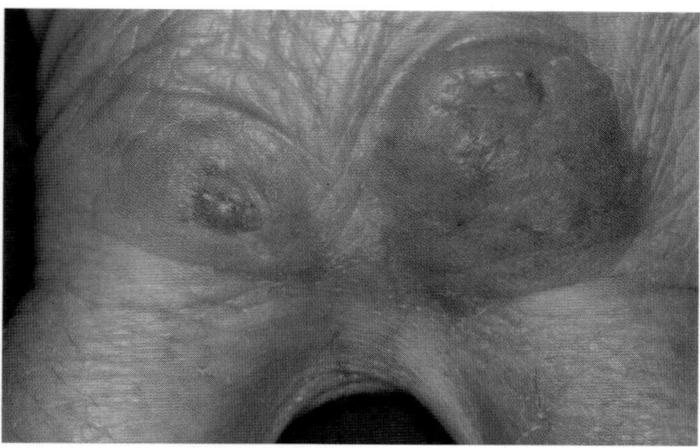

Fig. 1.16 Pseudoknuckle pads due to constant rubbing, especially under stress

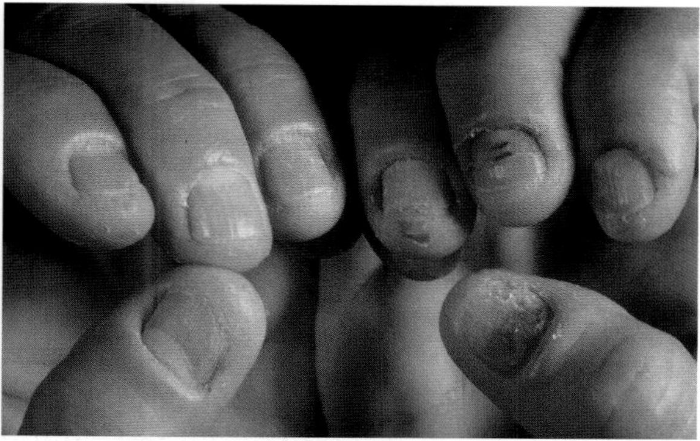

Fig. 1.17 Significant onychophagia in adolescent conflict

for psychotherapy, including behavior therapy modalities aimed at alternative coping strategies and stress reduction techniques.

Further Reading

Meigel WN, Plewig G (1976) Kauschwielen, eine Variante der Fingerknöchelpolster. Hautarzt 27(8): 391–395

Onychophagia, Onychotillomania, Onychotemnomania

Onychophagia

Onychophagia (ICD-10: F68.1, F98.8; DSM-IV-TR 312.30) is nail biting or nail chewing, usually with swallowing of the nail fragments. A combination with thumb sucking is also frequent. Both conditions are considered not relevant as clinical entities from a public health perspective and so are excluded from the ICD-10 and DSM-IV-TR as disorders of impulse control. Currently they are considered as symptoms or behaviors. Nevertheless, bacterial or fungal infections, inflammation, bleeding, and malformations may arise or be triggered by the repeated trauma, with shortening of the distal nail plate. Onychophagia usually occurs as part of unresolved conflicts or tension and is especially observed in adolescence (Fig. 1.17).

The frequency cited is up to 45% of adolescents, so certainly not every patient with onychophagia has a serious personality disorder or urgently requires psychotherapy.

The central causality factor is inappropriate dealing with stressful situations.

Onychotillomania

In onychotillomania, trauma of the paronychium or constant manipulation, picking, and removal of the cuticle and/or nail is seen as the elicitor of self-induced nail diseases. These may range from onychodystrophy to serious paronychias.

Onychotemnomania

Cutting nails too short leads to traumatization of the nail body or nail fold.

Further Reading

Hamann K (1982) Onychotillomania treatment with pimozide. Acta Derm Venereol 62: 364–366

Koo JY, Smith LL (1991) Obsessive-compulsive disorders in the pediatric dermatology practice. Pediatr Dermatol 8(2): 107–113

Leonhard HL, Lenane MC, Swedo SE, Rettew DC, Rapoport JL (1991) A double-blind comparison of clomipramine and desipramine treatment of severe onychophagia. Arch Gen Psychiatry 48(9): 821–827

Leung AK, Robson WL (1990) Nailbiting. Clin Pediatr (Phila) 29(12): 690–692

Trichotillomania, Trichotemnomania, Trichoteiromania

Trichotillomania

Trichotillomania is the best-investigated DPS disorder. Women are thought to be especially affected, with a prevalence of up to 3.5% (Christenson et al. 1991). The disease occurs often at younger ages.

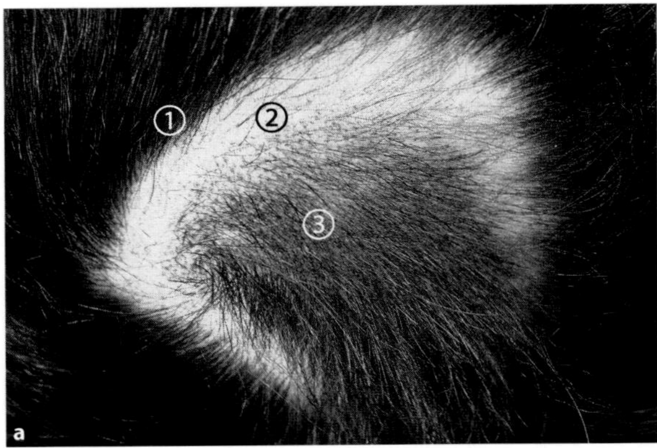

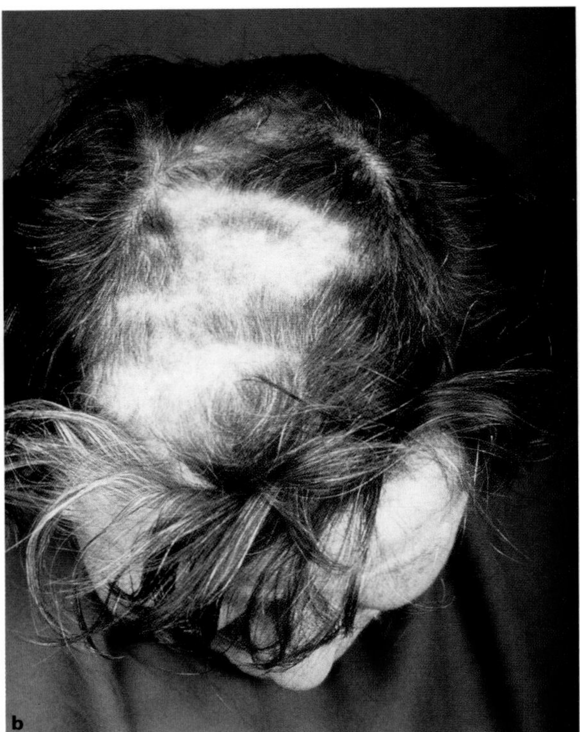

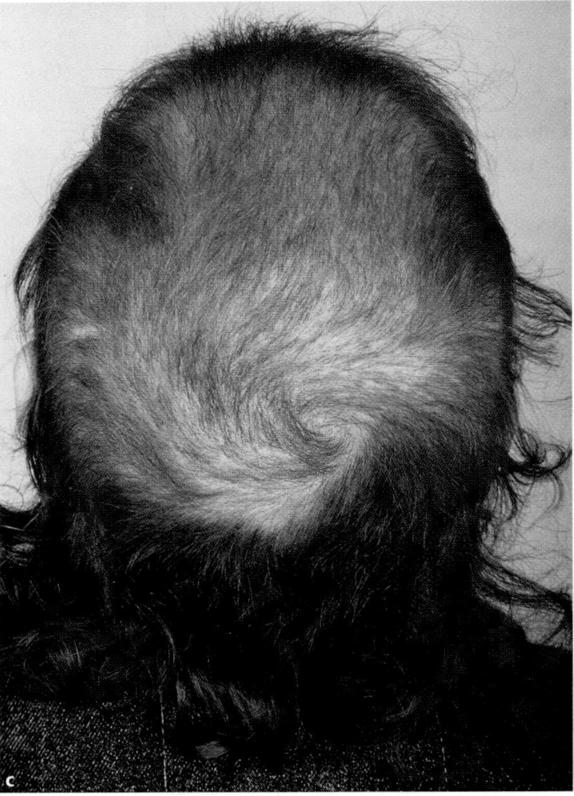

Fig. 1.18a–c Dermatitis paraartefacta syndrome. **a** Close-up: student with trichotillomania and adjustment disorder in a psychosocial stress situation at examination time. The three-zone arrangement is clearly recognizable. **b,c** Other views of patients with trichotillomania

Clinical presentation and pathogenesis. Trichotillomania (ICD-10: F63.3, F68.1; DSM-IV-TR 312.30) is based on pulling out of the hair, resulting in marked hair loss.

Clinically, there is a typical three-phase zone presentation:

- Zone 1: Long hair (unremarkable, not affected, normal hair/haircut)
- Zone 2: Missing hair (recent alopecia due to pulling)
- Zone 3: Regrowth of hair, shorter and less regular than the normal hair (older, former alopecia areas with irregular hair regrowth after intermittent pulling)

As to the cause of the three-zone presentation, healthy long hair (zone 1) can be easily grasped and then pulled (Fig. 1.18).

Around the torn hair is a hairless zone 2. Isolated hemorrhages can be found in the area of the pulled-out hair in the fresh tear area.

In addition, the older areas show regrowth (zone 3) with shorter hair that cannot be grasped and pulled yet, which explains the third zone of shorter hair. If such a three-zone presentation is found, the diagnosis of trichotillomania is confirmed.

Transient tearing of hair in early childhood can be viewed as a nonmalignant habit that will spontaneously resolve. The diagnosis of trichotillomania should be made only with pronounced findings and persistence of the disorder over a period of months. However, the symptoms, especially in adulthood, may last for decades, and anamneses show a high proportion of episodes in childhood or adolescence.

Special psychiatric symptoms. Trichotillomania is based psychopathologically on impairment of impulse control characterized by a buildup of tension prior to pulling, often followed by a feeling of pleasure, satisfaction, or relaxation upon the removal of the hair.

Many people twist and manipulate their hair due to increased anxiety or stress in certain situations without suffering trichotillomania. In the differential diagnosis, some authors discuss or prefer to classify trichotillomania among the compulsive disorders. In compulsive disorders, repeated acts are performed as rituals that must be rigidly followed. The further psychopathology of impaired impulse control is presented in the section on psychiatric disorders of DPS (Sect. 1.4).

Tearing out of hair as a stereotype (ICD-10: F98.4) must also be delineated, whereby this is a psychiatric illness with skin reference.

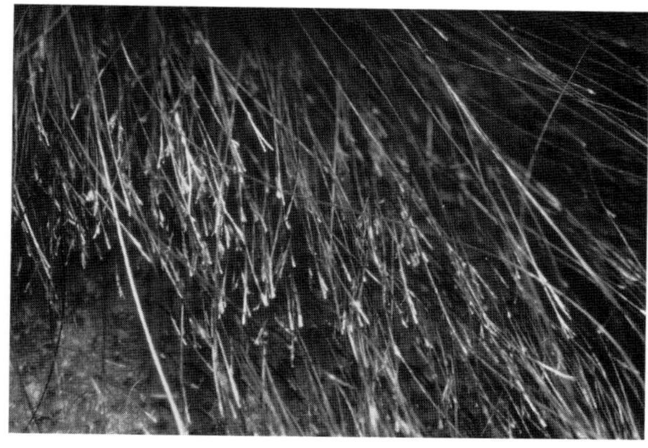

Fig. 1.19 Trichoteiromania: clearly distended whitish terminal hair ends due to mechanical-abrasive traumatization. Dermatitis paraartefacta syndrome with impaired impulse control in a 31-year-old woman

Trichotemnomania

Trichotemnomania is a rare form of hair damage in which the hair is intentionally cut off. This form of hair damage is classified as an artefact/malingering.

Trichoteiromania

In this variant of self-inflicted hair loss, there is physical damage to the hair by rubbing and scratching the scalp, resulting in pseudoalopecia. In trichoteiromania (Greek *teiro*, "I scratch"), macroscopic, whitish hair tips with split ends are seen, corresponding under the light microscope to brushlike hair breaks or trichoptilosis (Fig. 1.19).

Casuistic case reports of trichoteiromania state that the patients additionally complain of trichodynia with dysesthesias and pruritus.

The differences between the three paraartefacts affecting the hair are presented in Table 1.3.

Therapy. In pediatric cases, a session of psychoeducation with the parents is often successful. This condition is frequently a psychoreactive disorder, and a self-limiting course with spontaneous healing can be achieved by attentive observation of the impaired impulse control and appropriate support in the environment.

In older children or adolescents, behavior therapy in the form of habit reversal (see Chap. 13 for different techniques) and having the patient keep a "pulling" diary may be helpful. This is supplemented by relaxation training and replacement of hair pulling by other motor acts to reduce tension, such as the use of stress squeeze balls.

Over a course of several years, the acts of the paraartefacts such as hair pulling may be conditioned to a significant degree. Healing among young patients is thus often easier to achieve than among older patients. In serious cases of trichotillomania, there may be isolated serious psychiatric disorders such as borderline personality disorder, for which inpatient psychotherapy may be indicated and therapeutic success cannot be achieved without concurrent use of neuroleptics.

Table 1.3 Trichotillomania, trichotemnomania, trichoteiromania (Reich and Trüeb 2003)

	Trichotillomania	Trichotemnomania	Trichoteiromania
Injury pattern	Pulling out the hair	Cutting off the hair	Breaking off the hair by scratching
Clinical findings	Typical three-phase configuration with long, missing, and regrowing hair	Pseudoalopecia with hair stubble that appears shaved	Pseudoalopecia with broken hair of normal thickness; hair stubble with whitish-looking ragged ends
Trichogram	Telogen rate reduced	Normal hair root pattern	Dystrophic hair root pattern; sometimes reduced telogen proportion

Fluoxetine and clomipramine have been successfully used in recalcitrant forms of trichotillomania, taking comorbidities into account (Swedo et al. 1989; Wichel et al. 1992).

Psychotherapy and guidelines for paraartefacts are presented below.

References

Christenson GA, Mackenzie TB, Mitchell JE (1991) Characteristics of 60 adult chronic hair pullers. Am J Psychiatry 148: 365–370

Swedo SE, Leonard HL, Rapoport JL, Lenane MC, Goldberger EL, Cheslow DL (1989) A double-blind comparison of clomipramine and desipramine in the treatment of trichotillomania (hair pulling). N Engl J Med 321: 497–501

Winchel RM, Jones JS, Stanley B, Molcho A, Stanley M (1992) Clinical characteristics of trichotillomania and its response to fluoxetine. J Clin Psychiatry 53: 304–308

Further Reading

Kind J (1993) Beitrag zur Psychodynmaik der Trichotillomanie. Prax Kinderpsychol Kinderpsychiatr 32: 53–57

Muller SA, Winkelmann RK (1972) Trichotillomania. A clinicopathologic study of 24 cases. Arch Dermatol 105: 535–540

Pioneer Clinic St. Paul, MN (1993) Trichotillomania: compulsive hair pulling. Obsessive Compulsive Foundation, Milford, CT

Pollard CA, Ibe IO, Krojanker DN, Kitchen AD, Bronson SS, Flynn TM (1991) Clomipramine treatment of trichotillomania: a follow up report on four cases. J Clin Psychiatry 52(3): 128–130

Reich S, Trüeb RM (2003) Trichoteiromanie. JDDG 1: 22–28.

Stanley MA, Swann AC, Bowers TC, Davis ML, Taylor DJ (1992) A comparison of clinical features in trichotillomania and obsessive-compulsive disorder. Behav Res Ther 30: 39–44

Vitulano LA, King RA, Scahill L, Cohen DJ (1992) Behavioral treatment of children and adolescents with trichotillomania. J Am Acad Child Adolesc Psychiatry 31: 139–146

Summary

Psychiatric symptoms of DPS. In DPS, impulse control is impaired.

In the ICD-10, kleptomania, pyromania, pathological gambling, and intermittent explosive disorders also belong to the group of impaired impulse control along with the paraartefacts, whereby patients cannot resist aggressive impulses, responding with violence or destruction.

Impairment of Impulse Control

> **The main characteristic of paraartefacts is impairment of impulse control and thus the failure to resist impulsive urges or temptations to perform a repeated act without reasonable motivation, which is damaging to the person or to others. In questioning, however, the patient can often admit the manipulation, denoting the presence of a semiconscious impairment.**

Diagnostic Criteria of Paraartefacts (DSM IV)

- Repeated inability to resist impulses
- Increasing feeling of tension prior to the act
- Pleasure, satisfaction, or feeling of relaxation during the act
- No causal relationship to other somatic or psychiatric diseases
- The impairment is accompanied by clinically significant suffering

Often, a minimal primary lesion is excessively manipulated, which only then leads to a pronounced, serious finding. A classic example is manipulation of acne in the morning in front of the mirror, at which time the urge to manipulate cannot be resisted. Emotionally tense situations or unresolved conflicts and an ungovernable urge to self-manipulation may be present as the cause. Compulsive disorders often play a causal role.

The Köbner phenomenon can also be considered among the mild DPS; it is frequently observed in psoriasis and lichen planus.

1.1.3 Malingering

Clinical findings. Malingering (ICD-10: Z76.5) (V65.2 in DSM-IV-TR) is defined as intentional and conscious creation and elicitation of physical or psychiatric symptoms, in order to obtain benefit.

In malingerings, too, mechanical injuries from pressing, rubbing, biting, cutting, stabbing, or burning, or self-inflicted infections with wound-healing impairments, abscesses, mutilations, acid burns, or other toxic damages to the skin are in the foreground. Hematological symptoms may occur because of occlusion of extremities, creation of petechiae, and additional covert taking of pharmaceuticals, as well as by heparin injections.

Malingerings provide another focus in dermatology in the framework of expert opinions of occupational illnesses and disability procedures (Fig. 1.20). Additionally, there are manipulations of epicutaneous tests during evaluation procedures and simulation (malingering) of serious symptoms to obtain workman's compensation

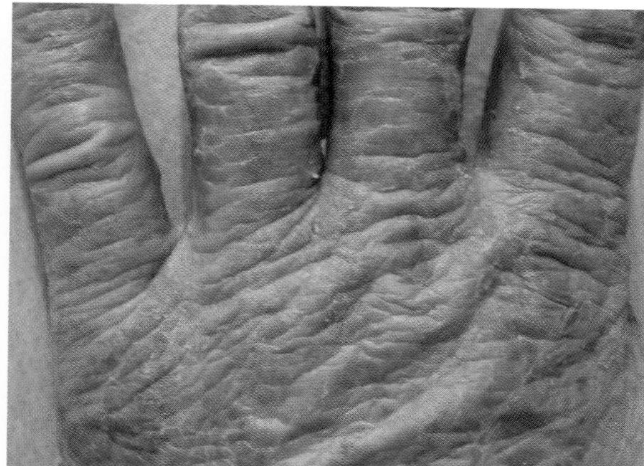

Fig. 1.20 Malingering: 44-year-old construction worker with skin lesions due to constant intentional immersion of the hands in liquid cement without protective gloves. Numerous periods of disability were certified by various doctors, and patient had desire for disability

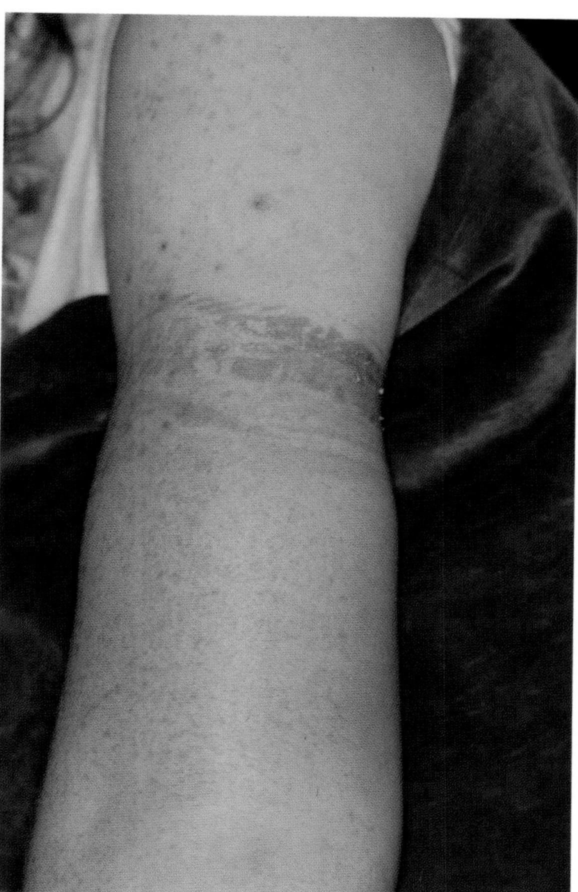

Fig. 1.21 Malingering as constriction dermatitis artefacta syndrome in the left shoulder/upper left arm in order to establish contact with the doctor (secondary profit from illness)

certification. In intentional provocation of contact allergies, the patient is usually familiar with the causative allergen but does not admit this to the doctor.

Psychiatric symptoms. Malingerings are conscious, intentional self-injurious behavior by the patient in order to obtain material advantage from the illness (V65.2 Malingering in DSM-IV-TR). They may also be characterized by another social advantage, such as another secondary gain by eliciting attention and care by the family, as in factitious disorder (300.10 and 300.19 DSM-IV-TR, ICD-10 F68.1), in which the physician is intentionally deceived (Fig. 1.21).

Among the psychosocial motivations for malingerings are to avoid criminal prosecution, obtain narcotics, avoid military service, or obtain financial advantages. The advantage may lie in a higher disability pension and other financial compensations. Intentional and conscious malingerings are hardly amenable to psychotherapeutic measures because there is no patient motivation for therapy.

Therapy

Therapy for self-inflicted dematosis. Compared with other dermatological diseases, therapy of this group is one of the greatest challenges for the dermatologist, especially when the patient comes to the specialist primarily with purely somatic concepts and expectations without insight (Table 1.4).

DAS is especially therapy-resistant because these conditions either arise unconsciously and cannot be recalled by the patient or is malingering created by the patient with intentional calculation. So on the one hand, clear delineation must be drawn in malingering, whereas on the other hand, confronting the patient too soon about the dissociated artificial genesis may lead to termination of the doctor–patient relationship and even end in suicide or attempted suicide (Table 1.5).

DAS. Somatic or monocausal therapy alone often does not achieve healing in DAS patients and may lead to frustration and even to bilateral open aggression in treatment. The therapy of DAS is usually long term, lasting for years.

Cautious (nonaccusatory) creation of a therapeutic relationship is the foundation of the approach in the early stages of therapy. This can begin with local therapy

1

Table 1.4 Psychocutaneous diseases

	Disease entity		Insight 0 to ++++
Primary psychiatric diseases	Delusion of parasitosis		0
	Illusion of parasitosis (formication)		++
	Body dysmorphic disorder		0
	Factitious disorders (Dermatitis artefacta syndrome and Dermatitis paraartefacta syndrome)	Dermatitis artefacta	+
		Trichotillomania	Variable: 0 to ++
		Neurotic excoriations	+++ to ++++
Primary dermatological diseases	Eczema, psoriasis, urticaria, vitiligo, seborrheic dermatitis, etc.		++++

Table 1.5 Therapy of artificial disorders (*DAS* dermatitis artefacta syndrome, *DPS* dermatitis paraartefacta syndrome)

Therapy	DAS	DPS	Malingering
Psychosomatic primary care (complaint diary)	+++	+++	+
Psychoeducation	+++	+++	+
Behavior therapy	+	+++	–
Deep-psychological/psycho-dynamic psychotherapy	+++	+	–
Psychopharmaceuticals	++	+	–
Confrontation	––	+/-	+++

directed at wound healing with topical medications and occlusive bandaging with zinc oxide (Unna boot).

In DAS illnesses in the narrower sense, the patient rarely can perceive or acknowledge the self-manipulations because these are often coupled with a dissociative amnesia, rendering the patient relatively unaware of the act.

Premature confrontation by the physician is contraindicated because it often leads to severing of the doctor–patient relationship and to renewed autoaggressive acts, up to suicidal impulses or a doctor–shopping odyssey.

Most important is the creation of a trusting relationship that the patient experiences as helpful and not a threat to his or her self-esteem. One possible access is often achieved through keeping a complaint diary, since the patient can slowly recognize psychosocial components in the somatic course.

Psychotherapy is usually indicated. Long-term therapy with psychodynamic approaches to stabilize the personality has proven beneficial. However, in the majority of cases, healing of the hidden DAS requires the combination of long-term psychotherapy with psychopharmaceuticals.

Stepwise Plan for DAS Therapy

1. Bland local therapy
2. Complaint diary
3. Psychosomatic primary care
4. Psychoeducation (no confrontation)

5. Relaxation therapy
6. Deep-psychological therapy (analysis of past conflicts) with the inclusion of behavior therapy concepts
7. Psychopharmaceuticals (low-strength neuroleptics, SSRI's)

The treatment of covert long-term consequences of early traumatization is often a nearly impossible task for the dermatologist. At the beginning, the doctor can often only initiate a prephase of problem recognition in the patient by introducing a thinking-through of the problems and checking for motivation to undergo psychotherapy.

The patient should not be confronted with the need of psychiatric or psychotherapeutic approaches until a stable, trusting relationship has been established between the doctor and the patient.

The treating physician should support the patient in therapy until he or she can be motivated to accept a specific therapy, such as treatment in a psychosomatic clinic or even psychotropic medication.

Patience is often important here because the motivation phase may extend over a long period of time. In dermatological practice, regular appointments, such as every 14 days, have proven beneficial in this phase.

DPS. The prognosis in DPS is generally better because the disorder is "semiconscious." Behavior therapy measures for impulse control are particularly indicated and successful in this condition, including methods to improve self-management with promotion of self-observation, cognitive restructuring, and relaxation techniques.

Stepwise Plan for Paraartefacts

1. Psychosomatic primary care (creating awareness)
2. Psychoeducation (taking the environment into account)
3. Relaxation therapy
4. Tension reduction (object displacement)
5. Behavioral therapy for impulse control (manipulation diary)
6. Inclusion of psychodynamic concepts
7. Psychopharmaceuticals (SSRIs)

An explanatory consultation (psychoeducation) with the patient (or parents in the case of children) may be the first step toward making the offending mechanism apparent, laying the foundation for regaining impulse control. Subsequent self-observation or outsider observations and control of the action can often achieve healing. If this is not sufficient, keeping a pulling diary (trichotillomania) or manipulation diary (skin picking) may enable better analysis and control. In addition to the date, time of day, and duration of the manipulation, the place and emotions associated with the situation, as well as any special features, should be recorded.

Moreover, psychoeducation that takes the environment (family) into account is helpful from the perspective of psychosomatic primary care. For example, in pediatric trichotillomania, clarification of the biopsychosocial aspects of the disease (the patient is not alone) may bring relief and contribute to the analysis to enable impulse control of the semiconscious disorder.

Measures to divert tension by replacing pulling of the hair or skin picking with other motor acts, such as clutching and squeezing stress balls, may be successfully used in the next step and are well accepted by patients, as are relaxation measures (Fig. 1.22).

In longer courses, introduction of a behavioral therapy is important. The habit-reversal technique has proven valuable as a behavioral therapeutic measure (see Chap. 13).

The basis begins with the conscious recognition of the impulse to self-injury, followed by interruption of the acts with internal warning signals, and finally achieving and remaining in a relaxation phase.

In courses lasting several years, high-grade conditioning of the actions, or additional serious personality disorders, in-hospital psychotherapy may be indicated along with the use of neuroleptics. Initiation of psychotherapy is determined by the comorbidities.

Malingerings. Due to a lack of motivation for therapy, malingering is difficult or impossible to treat psychotherapeutically. Structuring of the doctor–patient relationship is primary, with clear, often purely somatic reports and confrontation, also in cooperation with health insurance. Special attention should, however, also be paid to depressive or suicidal tendencies, which may be in the foreground in emotionally conspicuous patients with malingerings and thus easily overlooked if the clinical presentation changes.

Psychopharmacotherapy. Psychopharmaceuticals have proven valuable in stabilizing the usually massive affects and must be applied with appropriate expert knowledge. Symptomatic therapy with low-strength neuroleptics to relieve states of tension or antidepressants to relieve con-

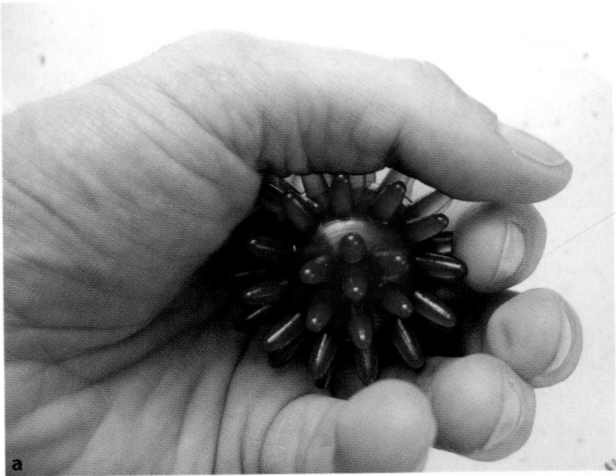

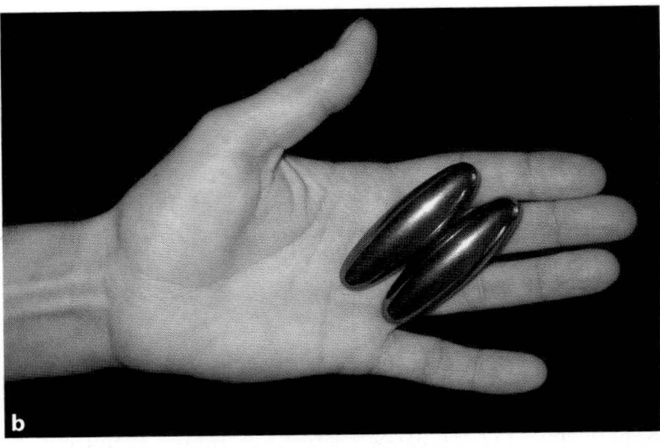

Fig. 1.22a,b Patient with self-manipulation under stress. **a** Ball, **b** Magnet stones (magnetites) to reduce tension

current psychopathological symptoms, such as depressive disorders, may be helpful.

In DPS conditions such as trichotillomania, therapy with SSRIs may be indicated under the aspect of impaired impulse control. For dissociative artefacts, low-strength neuroleptics are usually more effective and are preferred.

In DPS, a combination therapy with drugs and behavioral therapy has been found beneficial.

Prognosis. The prognosis for patients with self-injuries depends on the severity of the symptoms. It is good for mild forms, but even with appropriate treatment it is moderate to poor in serious forms, and patients with Münchhausen syndrome particularly have a bad prognosis.

If there is acute danger to the patient – or to others – and at the same time a lack of treatment motivation, a legal intervention may be necessary for admission to a psychiatric hospital in cooperation with a psychiatrist.

Further Reading

Gieler U (2004) Leitlinien in der psychotherapeutischen Medizin: Artifizielle Störungen. JDDG 2(1): 66–73

Gieler U, Effendy I, Stangier U (1987) Kutane Artefakte: Möglichkeiten der Behandlung und ihre Grenzen. Z Hautkr 62(11): 882–890

Gupta MA, Gupta AK, Habermann HF (1987) The self-inflicted dermatoses: a critical review. Gen Hosp Psychiatry 9(1): 45–52

Harth W, Linse R (2000) Dermatological symptoms and sexual abuse: a review and case reports. J Eur Acad Dermatol Venereol 14(6): 489–494

Herpertz S, Saß H (1994) Offene Selbstschädigung. Nervenarzt 65: 296–306

Koblenzer CS (1996) Neurotic excoriations and dermatitis artefacta. Dermatol Clin 14(3): 447–455

Koblenzer CS (2000) Dermatitis artefacta. Clinical features and approaches to treatment. Am J Clin Dermatol 1: 47–55

Koo J, Lee CS (2003) Psychocutaneous medicine. Dekker, New York

Plassmann R (1995) Psychoanalysis of self injury. Schweiz Rundsch Med Prax 84: 859–865

Sachse U (1994) Selbstverletzendes Verhalten. Vandenhoeck & Ruprecht, Göttingen

Schneider G, Gieler U (2001) Psychosomatic dermatology – state of the art. Z Psychosom Med Psychother 47(4): 307–331

Willenberg H, Eckhardt A, Freyberger H, Sachsse U, Gast U (1997) Selbstschädigende Handlungen: Klassifikation und Basisdokumentation. Psychotherapeut 42: 211–217

1.1.4 Special Forms

Gardner–Diamond Syndrome

Definition. Gardner–Diamond syndrome (ICD-10: F68.1; F68.1) is characterized by periodically occurring painful infiltrated blue patches, multiple physical complaints, and characteristic psychiatric symptoms.

Synonyms are painful ecchymoses syndrome, psychogenic purpura, and painful bruising syndrome.

Occurrence. Gardner–Diamond syndrome mostly occurs in young women.

Pathogenesis. Initially, the first descriptions supported the assumption of an autoimmune process after injection of autologous blood, in the sense of an autoerythrocytic

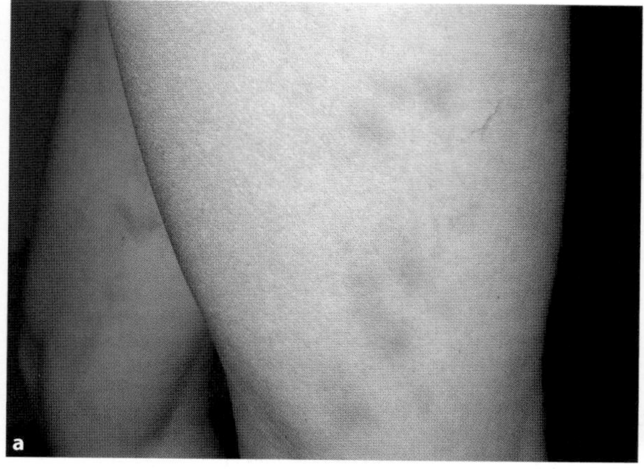

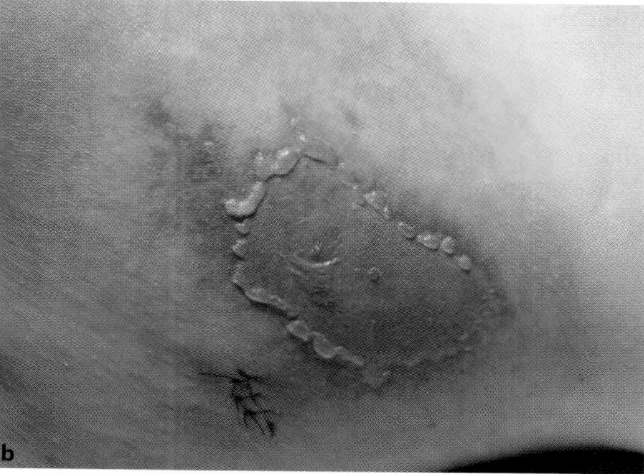

Fig. 1.23 **a** Gardner–Diamond syndrome in a 29-year-old woman. **b** Severe Gardner–Diamond syndrome

sensitization syndrome. Currently, an artificial genesis is accepted as most likely.

Clinical findings. As prodrome, there is initially itching, a feeling of tension, or burning pain, usually in the extremities and most often the legs. Then edematous erythematous plaques develop with ecchymoses, which heal within 1–2 weeks (Fig. 1.23). Characteristically, the course is of periodic episodes and healing without scarring.

Systemic symptoms include episodes of abdominal pain, nausea, vomiting, diarrhea, weight loss, headache, blurred vision, paresthesias, and other neurological symptoms, as well as hematuria, hematemesis, metrorrhagias, and amenorrhea.

Psychiatric symptoms. The personality structure of the patients presents classical features of dissociative disorders, including conversion disorders, masochism, depressiveness, anxiety, and inhibition in emotional expression of feelings (aggression inhibition).

Differential diagnosis. The differential diagnosis includes the spectrum of artefact diseases.

Therapy, course, and prognosis. To date, successful family therapy has been reported in isolated cases.

Further Reading

Behrendt C, Goos M, Thiel H, Hengge UR (2001) Painful-Bruising-Syndrom. Hautarzt 52: 634–637

Frantzen E, Voigtländer V, Gerhardt H (1990) Gardner-Diamond-Syndrom. Hautarzt 41: 168–170

Gardner FH, Diamond LK (1955) Auto-erythrocyte sensitization. A form of purpura producing painful bruising following autosensitization to red blood cells in certain women. Blood 10: 675–690

Vakilzadeh F, Bröcker EB (1981) Syndrom der blauen Flecken. Hautarzt 32: 309–312

Münchhausen's Syndrome

Definition. The Münchhausen syndrome (ICD10: F68.1; DSM-IV-TR 300.16 and 19) is characterized by the triad of hospital wandering, pathological lying, and self-injury (Oostendorp and Rakoski 1993).

In 1951 Richard Asher reported the first cases and features of three female patients with self-induced disease, coining the term Münchhausen syndrome (Asher 1951) in reference to Baron Karl Friedrich Hieronymus von Münchhausen (1720–1797). This disease denotes malingering/simulation of acute diseases with demonstrative dramatic description of complaints and false information in the anamnesis. It includes numerous hospitalizations and surgical procedures, sometimes with visible multiple scars. Frequently it is based on a borderline disorder.

Characteristically, patients often display splitting of the environment into good and bad in the same fashion as seen in subjects with borderline personality disorder.

A pathological doctor–patient relationship is frequently present, making these subjects the most difficult problem patients to treat in medicine.

1

Münchhausen-by-Proxy Syndrome

In the Münchhausen-by-proxy syndrome (ICD-10: F74.8; DSM-IV-TR 300.16 and 19), it is usually children who are injured by their primary caretakers in order to establish contact with medical caregivers. Thus, the Münchhausen-by-proxy syndrome is a special form of child abuse.

Two cases of Münchhausen-by-proxy syndrome were published for the first time in 1977 by an English pediatrician (Meadow 1977). The term was coined because the mothers systematically deceived the doctors with fictitious stories about the disease, but instead of their own bodies, they were abusing their children's (by proxy). This observation was followed by numerous publications of case reports.

In most cases, a "detectivesque" elucidation is necessary. In 98% of cases, women are the perpetrators, and of these, 90% are the biological mother, with the rest being stepmothers or daycare providers.

Bleeding, seizures, clouding of consciousness up to and including respiratory arrest, diarrhea, vomiting, fever, and skin changes with scratching, acid burns, or occlusions may be caused (Fig. 1.24).

Based on individual case reports, from the psychodynamic point of view there appears to be a bizarre split in the mothers in relation to their children. On the one hand, the child is experienced as a threat, with the mother thinking the child will take from her everything she herself needs to live (Plassmann 1995).

By injury or abuse, the child is placed in a completely dependent situation in which the mother devotes herself to the illusion of being a perfect, caring, ideal mother. Characteristically, the mothers appear to the nursing personnel as particularly zealous and engaged.

Breaking through the vicious cycle of violence is primary in the psychotherapeutic process, since the violence will be repeated until it can be made conscious, worked through, verbalized, and thus integrated in the therapeutic process.

References

Meadow R (1977) Munchhausen syndrome by proxy: the hinterland of child abuse. Lancet 2: 343–345

Oostendorp I, Rakoski J (1993) Münchhausen's Syndrom. Artefakte in der Dermatologie. Hautarzt 44: 86–90

Plassmann R (1995) Psychoanalysis of self injury. Schweiz Rundsch Med Prax 84: 859–865

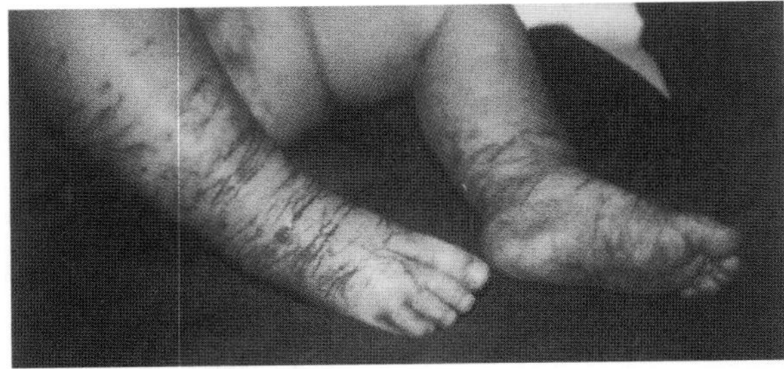

Fig. 1.24 Münchhausen-by-proxy syndrome

Further Reading

Asher R (1951) Munchhausen's syndrome. Lancet 1: 339–341

Gattaz WF, Dressing H, Hewer W (1990) Munchhausen syndrome: psychopathology and management. Psychopathology 23: 33–39

Kapfhammer HP, Rothenhausler HB, Dietrich E, Dobmeier P, Mayer C (1998) Artefactual disorders – between deception and self-mutilation. Experiences in consultation psychiatry at a university clinic. Nervenarzt 69: 401–409

Koblenzer CS (1996) Neurotic excoriations and dermatitis artefacta. Dermatol Clin 14(3): 447–455

Koblenzer CS (2000) Dermatitis artefacta. Clinical features and approaches to treatment. Am J Clin Dermatol 1: 47–55

Rothenhausler HB, Kapfhammer HP (2002) Munchhausen patients in general hospitals – clinical features and treatment approaches in C-L psychiatry settings. Psychiatr Prax 29(7): 381–387

Smith K, Killam P (1994) Munchausen syndrome by proxy. MCN Am J Matern Child Nurs 19: 214–221

Thomas K (2003) Munchausen syndrome by proxy: identification and diagnosis. J Pediatr Nurs 18: 174–180

Wojaczynska-Stanek K, Skubacz M, Marszal E (2000) Munchausen's syndrome by proxy – a malignant form of child abuse. Pol Merkuriusz Lek 9: 799–802

1.2 Dermatoses as a Result of Delusional Illnesses and Hallucinations

Patients with delusions appear in the dermatological practice with clear somatic complaints and denial of psychopathological issues. Characteristically, the dermatologist is confronted mostly with patients presenting with monosymptomatic delusions. This is usually an encapsulated idea, while the rest of the character structure and personality appears unchanged.

Often, the symptoms are characterized by the development of a single or several related delusional ideas, without presenting the degree of or a definite relationship to schizophrenia. This is a heterogeneous series of clinical disorder presentations.

Definition. The most conspicuous clinical characteristic of the group of persistent delusional disorders in dermatology (ICD-10: F22.0; DSM-IV-TR 297.1 somatic type) is the impossibility of the delusion.

A delusion is generally characterized by
- **The patient's great subjective certainty**
- **Unshakeability of the patient's belief**
- **Clear evidence to the contrary**

Categorization. Delusions involving the skin appear commonly in the form of perceived parasitosis, body dysmorphic delusions, and other body-related delusional disorders such as bromhidrosis and chromhidrosis, as well as olfactory and tactile hallucinations. Although these diseases have a psychiatric etiology, they are still dermatological conditions.

Presentations of Delusional Disease in Dermatology

- Parasitosis F22.8 DSM-IV-TR 297.1 somatic type (coenesthetic delusion, body hallucinations, delusion of infestation)
- Body odor delusion F22.8; DSM-IV-TR 297.1 somatic type (olfactory hallucinations): bromhidrosis [(usually with presumed chromhidrosis (sweat discoloration)]
- Hypochondriacal delusions F22.0; DSM-IV-TR 297.1 somatic type (syphilis delusion, AIDS delusion)
- Body dysmorphic delusion F22.8; DSM-IV-TR 297.1 somatic type (delusional dysmorphophobia)

Frequency. Delusional disorders are generally very rare and are estimated at a prevalence of less than 0.05% in the general population.

Differential diagnosis. Serious organically caused, schizophrenic, or affective disorders need to be ruled out. Schizophrenia is the most common and important differential diagnosis of the monosymptomatic delusional disorders. Differentiation is often difficult to make clinically, especially in the early stages of the disorder.

Differential Diagnosis: Main Symptoms of Schizophrenia

- Delusions (so-called contentual thought disorder):
  - Delusional ideas
  - Delusional moods
  - Delusional perceptions
  - Systematized delusions
- Hallucinations:
  - Acoustic
  - Optical
  - Olfactory
  - Taste
  - Tactile
  - Body hallucinations (coenesthesias)
- Alogia
- Affect flattening
- Anhedonia
- Asociality
- Ego disorders
- Formal thought disorders
- Affective disorders
- Catatonia
- Impaired drive and social behavior

Pathogenesis. The onset of delusional disorders is determined by multicausal factors, and its development is promoted by an interaction of various biological and psychosocial factors.

One possible model for explanation is the vulnerability–stress model, according to which a subclinical, congenital, or acquired multifactorially mediated disposition to illness (susceptibility) is present, and the disorder crosses the manifestation threshold when additional factors (stress/conflicts or biological stressors) are present.

Other hypotheses include a polygenic hereditary disposition with incomplete penetrance, and the dopamine hypothesis, which assumes that hyperactivity of certain messenger systems in certain regions of the brain, especially in the limbic system, is essential to the onset of psychotic symptoms. This is also an important foundation of modern psychopharmacological treatment.

Further Reading

AWMF (2003) Wahnstörungen http://www.AWMF-Leitlinien.de

Musalek M (1991) Der Dermatozoenwahn. Thieme, Stuttgart

Weltgesundheitsorganisation (1995): ICD-10 Internationale statistische Klassifikation der Krankheiten und verwandter Gesundheitsprobleme. 10. Revision, Bd 1. Deutscher Ärzte Verlag, Köln

Delusion of Parasitosis

Delusion of parasitosis is the most frequent delusional disorder with which the dermatologist is confronted.

Definition. In delusion of parasitosis (ICD-10: F22.8 delusional; DSM-IV-TR 297.1 delusional vs. somatic type, or F06.0 in organic hallucinosis), there is a skin-related delusional assumption of parasitic invasion.

Although they are now considered antiquated, we mention here the terms coenesthesia (body hallucinosis) and tactile hallucinosis, which are sometimes used.

Occurrence. These are rare cases among the overall patient population in dermatology. Elderly, socially isolated women are typically the ones affected by a delusional fixation.

Pathogenesis. An elicitor is reported in the history of some patients. Thus, when the complaints begin, there may be an actually experienced parasitic infestation or observation in the environment (such as pediculosis in a granddaughter) so that the delusional disorder occurs for the first time according to the vulnerability–stress model.

Clinical findings. Symptomatically, the patient complains of itching, tingling, pain, or formication, coupled with the subjective certainty that the symptoms are being caused by insects, mites, worms, or other parasites.

Manipulations of the skin in the sense of self-damage are intended to remove the assumed parasites, whereby dermatitis artefacta may be created. Many times, the patient brings the removed assumed pathogen to the health provider in jars and boxes, requesting further diagnostic procedures. Microscopically and macroscopically, these are usually skin scales, fibers, or foreign matter without pathogens (Figs. 1.25, 1.26).

The clinical presentation of self-induced damage occurs to various degrees and depends on the type of manipulation or the applied substances. Clinically, there are usually excoriations, erosions, cuts, or burns on the upper arms, legs, and easily reached areas of the trunk.

Self-therapy can thus lead to pronounced irritation of the skin, for example, by numerous courses of antiparasitic substances such as lindane. Often during self-therapy, aggressive chemical substances, sometimes from veterinary medicine, are applied to the skin in order to destroy the perceived parasites. The skin of the afflicted person is often significantly damaged by frequent brushing, cleansing procedures, and the application of caustic substances.

Psychiatric symptoms. Delusion of parasitosis is characterized by the delusional ideation of skin infestation with insects, mites, worms, or other organisms, which is uncorrectable and presents with high subjective certainty as well as symptoms that are objectively absent.

The delusional assumption leads to great suffering and massive limitations in quality of life. The constant preoccupation with the delusion leads to detriment in various social areas and numerous visits to health providers.

The body-related delusional disorder occurs mainly within paranoid (20%) and depressive disorders (50%) and is often isolated monosymptomatically, as well as under the effects of delirium and after noxae (Hornstein et al. 1989).

Three forms are differentiated in the literature (Musalek 1991):

1. Hypochondriacal parasitosis as a monosymptomatic hypochondriacal psychosis
2. Infestation delusion with paranoid symptoms
3. Mixed patterns of 1 and 2

This differentiation is important when deciding upon the appropriate pharmacological intervention (antidepressants vs. neuroleptics).

Five to 15% of those individuals close to patients with delusional parasitosis develop an associated delusion (refer to the below section on folie à deux; Trabert 1999). Recently, a considerable number of patients have complained of the appearance of eroded mucocutaneous lesions with the extrusion of multicolored fibers and filaments. The skin manifestations are associated with complaints of formication, fibromyalgia-like symptoms, arthralgias, altered cognitive function, and extreme fatigue. These symptoms have been termed Morgellons disease, and although its etiology remains unclear and is currently been studied by the Centers for Disease Control, many of these patients have symptoms similar to those with delusions of parasitosis. (Fig. 1.26). This disease has gained notoriety in the media as well as on the Internet, and some have referred to it as "folie à Internet."

Differential diagnosis. Differentiation must be made from other purely psychiatric diseases as well as brain-organic diseases, particularly schizophrenia, brain-organic psychosyndromes, and cerebral arteriosclerosis. The delusion must be further differentiated from pure anxiety and compulsive disorders (Sect. 1.4).

Differential diagnosis must include somatoform disorders including sensory complaints with burning and itching, dermatitis artefacta and neurotic excoriations, as well as pruritic diseases, since these at times may also take on delusional features. The differential diagnosis is important in order to select the appropriate therapeutic approach, including the target symptomatics of psychopharmaceuticals.

Therapy. Delusion of parasitosis has become more amenable to treatment with the advent of the atypical antipsychotics.

Bland local therapy with wound-healing dermatological treatments can usually be attempted. Detailed medical discussions about a psychiatric genesis of the

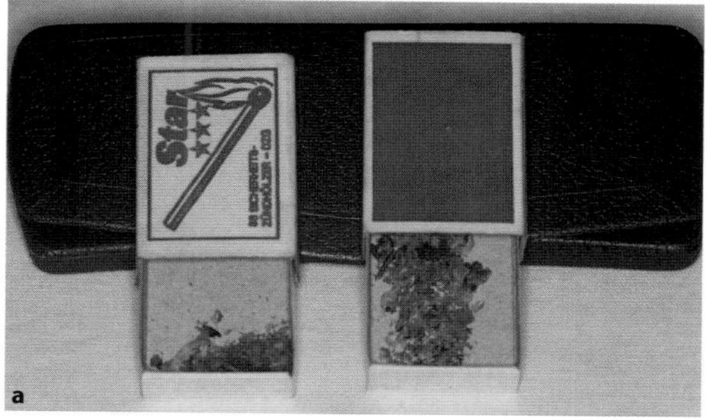

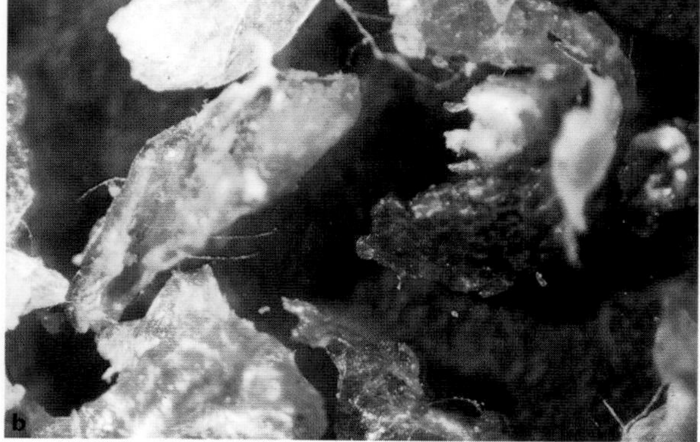

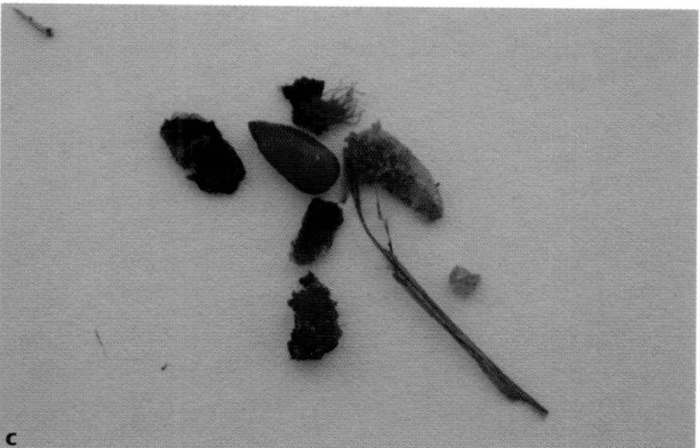

Fig. 1.25 **a** Delusion of parasitosis in a 71-year-old woman: containers in which the presumed parasites were collected. **b** Magnification of presumed parasites, which consisted of skin particles. **c** A 52-year-old man with delusion of parasitosis presented crumbs as presumed parasites in the dermatological office

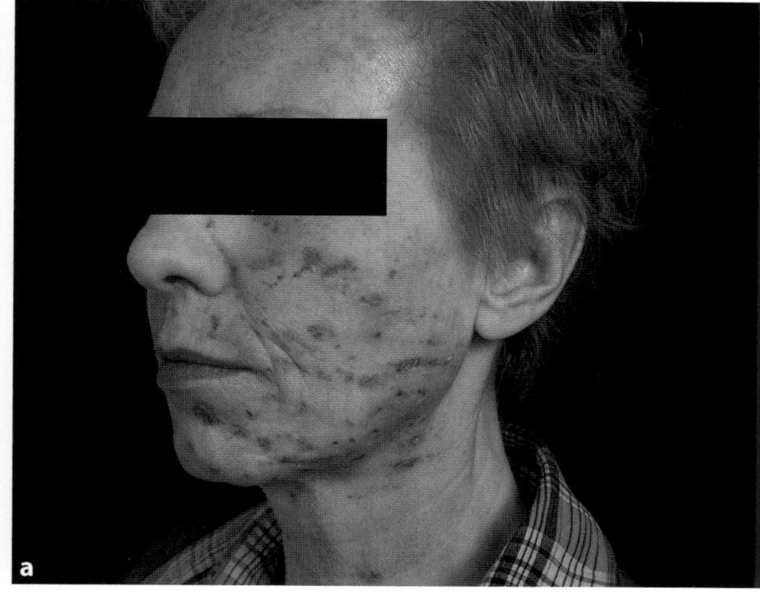

Fig. 1.26 **a–g** Morgellons disease. A 53-year old woman (**a**) complained of eroded mucocutaneous lesions (**a, b**) with the extrusion by tweezers (**c**) of multicolored fibers and filaments (**d**). The patient's drawings of the assumed mechanism (**e**) included histological pictures (**f**). (**g**) skin biopsy of patient with regular histological findings

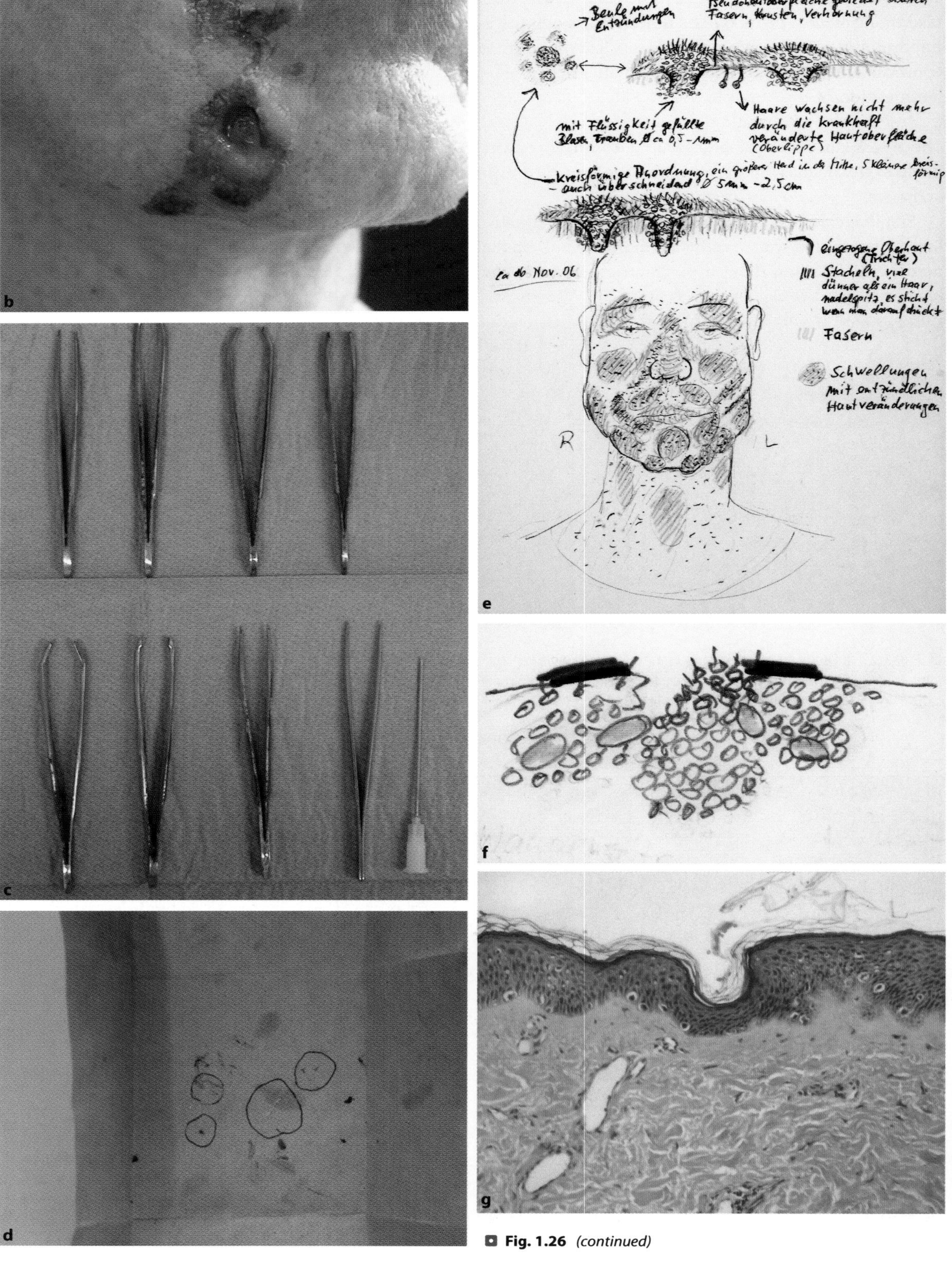

Fig. 1.26 *(continued)*

symptoms, as well as discussion addressing the negative results and findings of the histological or microbiological diagnostic tests, rarely result in relief or abating of the complaints and symptoms.

Initiation of a psychopharmacological therapy with neuroleptics in cooperation with the psychiatrist is of critical importance. The pathological character of the misinterpretation is usually not accepted by the patient, and a referral to a psychiatrist is often refused.

Treatment of delusion of parasitosis as part of the liaison service within the dermatology clinic, including the dermatologist, psychiatrist, and patient, has been found beneficial. But because of organizational aspects, this is usually possible only in tertiary medical centers.

If a liaison consultation cannot be held, the dermatologist often has to initiate the treatment with psychopharmaceuticals. For this, it is necessary that he or she acquire appropriate experience and postgraduate training in their use.

Treatment with neuroleptics has been successful (see below); however, very few studies with significant numbers of patients are available.

It is important to gain the patient's confidence to be able to treat the disease adequately. Initially, slow establishing of a trusting doctor–patient relationship over several consultations is necessary. Experience has shown that patients are more likely to accept this therapy if the explanation given is the necessity to "calm the skin's superficial nervous system" and decrease the distress suffered by the patient. Psychotherapy is additionally useful.

Psychopharmaceuticals. In addition to haloperidol, the spectrum of psychopharmaceuticals has undergone marked expansion in recent years on the basis of new research results. Therapy with modern psychopharmaceuticals has achieved a decisive improvement in the prognosis of patients with delusion of parasitosis. Delusional disorders can usually be approached with lower doses of neuroleptics than are usually prescribed for patients with other psychiatric illnesses.

The choice of psychopharmaceutical depends on the underlying psychiatric disorder and the target symptoms to be treated. If a depressive disorder is in the foreground, an antidepressant may be used. In the case of paranoid symptoms, neuroleptics are the drugs of first choice (Musalek 1991).

Currently, the following medications are primarily used in delusional disorders in dermatology (see Chap. 15): risperidone (Risperdal), olanzapine (Zyprexa), quetiapine (Seroquel), aripiprazole (Abilify), and pimozide (Orap).

The most experience is with pimozide, reported in case reports in the United States. Although still widely used, it has a significant broad spectrum of untoward effects and is losing adepts since the advent of atypical neuroleptics, which have considerably fewer side effects.

In our experience, a combination therapy of a neuroleptic with an SSRI or an anxiolytic is often necessary when monotherapy does not bring decisive improvement in the complaints, or if psychiatric mixed symptoms are present.

It is noteworthy that no significant skin-specific studies have been performed using modern neuroleptics and that initiation of therapy must usually be preceded by a precise psychiatric diagnosis.

Suffering can often be relieved under psychopharmacological therapy, the self-injurious behavior can be considerably improved, and psychosocial integration of the patient can be restored. However, complete eradication of the disease cannot be achieved in most cases, even with long-term therapy. The delusional disorder usually becomes "silent," which can be considered a good therapeutic result.

References

Hornstein OP, Hofmann P, Joraschky P (1989) Delusions of parasitic skin infestation in elderly dermatologic patients. Z Hautkr 64(11): 981–982, 985–989

Musalek M (1991) Der Dermatozoenwahn. Thieme, Stuttgart

Trabert W (1999) Shared psychotic disorder in delusional parasitosis. Psychopathology 32(1): 30–34

Further Reading

Damiani JT, Flowers FP, Pierce DK (1990) Pimozide in delusions of parasitosis. J Am Acad Dermatol 22: 312–313

Evans P, Merskey H (1972) Shared beliefs of dermal parasitosis: folie partagee. Br J Med Psychol 45(1): 19–26

Gieler U, Knoll M (1990) Delusional parasitosis as "folie à trois." Dermatologica 181(2): 122–125

Koo J, Lee CS (2001) Delusions of parasitosis. A dermatologist's guide to diagnosis and treatment. Am J Clin Dermatol 2(5): 285–290

Lee M, Koo J (2004) Pimozide: the opiate antagonist hypothesis and use in delusions of parasitosis. Dermatol Psychosom 5: 184–186

Raulin C, Rauh J, Togel B (2001) "Folie à deux" in the age of lasers. Hautarzt 52(12): 1094–1097

Body Odor Delusion (Bromhidrosis)

Many publications address the disease complex of body odor delusion (ICD-10: F22.8, DSM-IV-TR-297.1 delu-

1

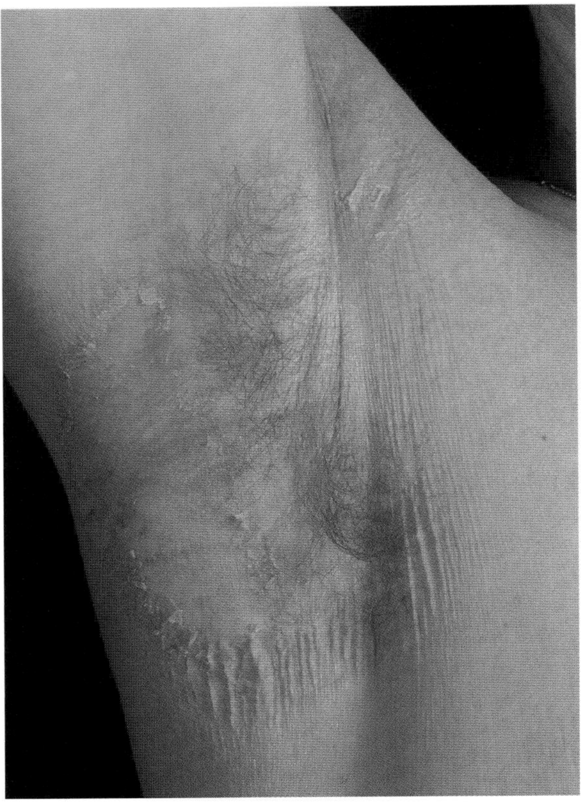

Fig. 1.27 Eczema due to continuous washing in body odor delusion

sional disorder, somatic type), but in everyday practice, it is a rare disease entity (Fig. 1.27).

Bromhidrosis is the subjective unpleasant odor resulting from physiological sweat, and chromhidrosis is the secretion of subjectively colored sweat.

In a delusional disorder, an attempt can first be made to educate the patient in the sense of psychoeducational measures about the physiological variation of his or her "disease." By these means, any delusional components that may be present can be exposed.

In stubborn cases, the use of a low-strength neuroleptic (Chap. 15) may be indicated.

Hypochondriacal Delusions

In hypochondriacal delusions (ICD-10: F22.0; DSM-IV-TR 297.1 somatic type), there is persistent, uncorrectable delusional preoccupation with the fear or conviction of suffering from a serious physical disease (Fig. 1.28).

The delusional contents must be viewed in light of the patient's social background with regard to biopsychosocial aspects and are influenced by his or her degree of knowledge as well as by social and cultural factors. Hypochondriacal delusion has undergone repeated changes in recent years. Whereas syphilis was in the foreground of venereology in the past, this has been replaced more frequently by a delusion of having contracted AIDS.

Delusional themes and delusional contents (Sect. 1.3.2) refer these days mainly to infections or neoplasias (cancerophobia, melanoma phobia).

Differential diagnosis. Differentiation must be made from psychoses with hypochondriacal content or hypochondriacal comorbidity. An important differentiation of delusional disorder from anxiety disorder must be made (Sect. 3.3.2).

Therapy. Characteristically, delusional diseases are almost exclusively disorders that cannot be corrected by discussions with the physician.

In delusional cutaneous hypochondriasis, atypical neuroleptics are the therapy of first choice (for example, risperidone and olanzapine or aripiprazole). Treatment with SSRIs may be successful in the blurred transition to somatoform disorders. Psychotherapy can have significant adjunct results.

Body Dysmorphic Delusions

Body dysmorphic delusions (ICD10: F22.; DSM-IV-TR 297.1 somatic type) consist of an excessive preoccupation with an uncorrectable, imagined deficiency or disfigurement in the outward appearance, which takes on delusional proportions. The excessive preoccupation causes massive detriment to social, professional, or other important functional areas.

In this disorder, there is often a blurred transition between phases of insight and the delusional fixation on the conviction of being disfigured. The difference between dysmorphophobic disorder and body dysmorphic delusions is also important with respect to the necessity of indicating psychopharmaceuticals in the latter diagnosis, even if it is not easy to distinguish between the two in individual cases. The differentiation may involve considerable difficulties. Often there are blurred transitions between body dysmorphic delusions (delusional dysmorphophobia) and somatoform disorders, including body dysmorphic disorder, whereby the delusional

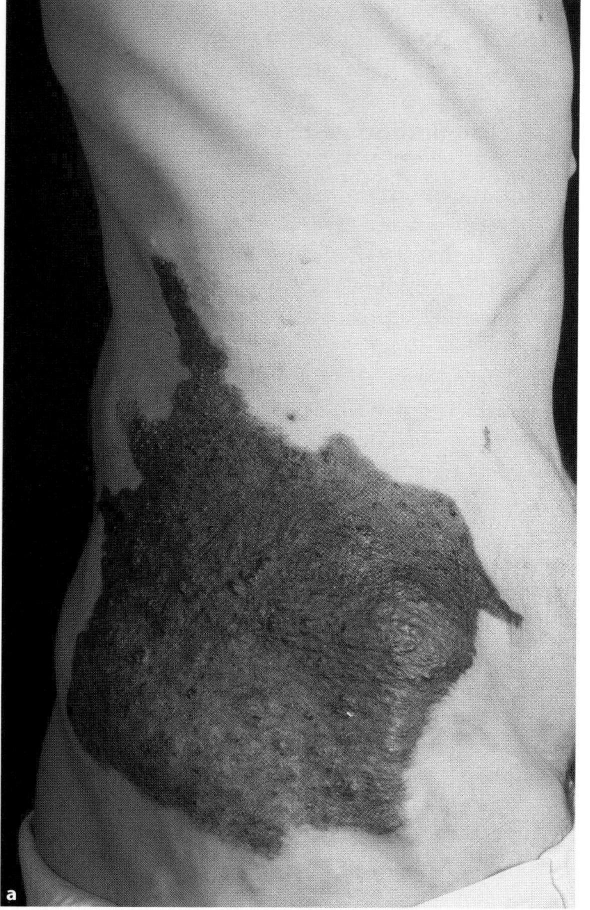

Tag	früh	nachmittags	abends
12.12.	36,7	36,9	37,7
13.12.	36,9	36,8	38,2
14.12.	36,8	36,9	38,1
15.12.	36,4	36,8	38,0
16.12	36,2	36,9	37,5
17.12.	36,8	37,7	38,3
18.12.	37,0	36,9	38,0
19.12.	36.3	36,7	37,4
20.12.	36,0		

Entwicklung der Temperatur (C°)
Christa Jablonski

Tag	früh	nachmittags	abends	spät abends
7.11.05	.	38,6	38,7	.
8.11	.	37,9	37,4	.
9.11	38,1	38,2	38,0	37,3
10.11	36,0	37,1	.	37,2
11.11	37,3	37,7	37,3	36,7
12.11	37,2	37,2	37,6	37,2
13.11	37,0	37,3	37,1	37,2
14.11	37,3	37,1	36,7	37,1
15.11	37,1	36,6	37,1	37,3
16.11	37,0	37,0	37,3	37,2
17.11	36,9	36,7	36,9	36,9
18.11	36,9	37,0	37,2	37,7
19.11	37,0	37,4	37,6	37,0
20.11.	36,7	36,9	37,4	37,4
21.11	36,9		37,2	37,4
22.11.	36,9	37,1	37,9	37,1
23.11.	37,0	37,3	37,3	37,2
24.11.	36,7	37,2	37,2	37,2

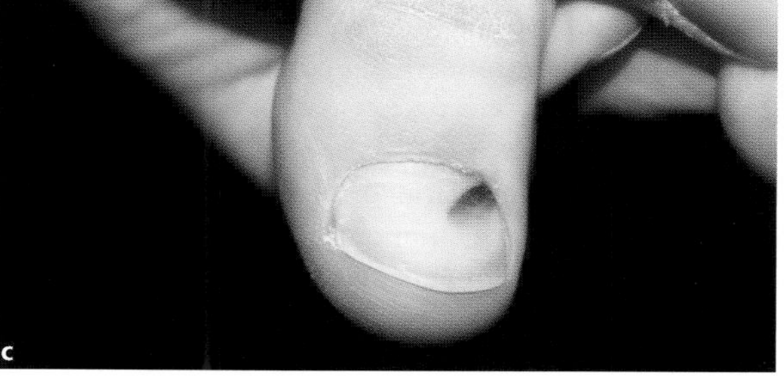

Fig. 1.28 a Hypochondriacal delusion in patient with pronounced nevus teleangiectaticus (Klippel–Trenaunay syndrome). Patient displays weight loss due to the delusional misinterpretation that fasting can prevent bleeding into the nevus. **b** Hypochondrial disturbance; 54-year-old patient measuring temperature three times a day in fear of a fungus infection. **c** Melanoma phobia

form is characterized by the uncorrectability of the disorder. Schizophrenia must also be ruled out in the case of bizarre delusions.

Further Reading

Bishop ER Jr (1983) Monosymptomatic hypochondriacal syndromes in dermatology. J Am Acad Dermatol 9(1): 152–158

Musalek M (1991) Der Dermatozoenwahn. Thieme, Stuttgart

Special Form: Folie à Deux

In folie à deux (ICD10: F24.0), a delusional disorder is shared by two or more people who are in close relationship. Usually, it is an induced delusional disorder whereby the partner or family members take on the delusions (folie partagee, shared delusion), which disappear upon separation from the patient.

The authors have observed this induced delusion especially in the delusional forms of the ecosyndrome (for example, mycophobia). This disorder is rare, and there are few individual case reports in the dermatological literature.

Further Reading

Musalek, M (1991) Der Dermatozoenwahn. Thieme, Stuttgart

Raulin C, Rauh J, Togel B (2001) "Folie à deux" in the age of lasers. Hautarzt 52(12): 1094–1097

1.3 Somatoform Disorders

In dermatological practice, it is not only clearly defined dermatoses that are diagnosed in the patients, but there are also patients in whom categorization to a dermatological entity is not successful, in whom no objectifiable symptoms can be found, or who complain of a number of symptoms that cannot be explained. The dermatological symptoms usually consist of pruritus (itching), pain, dysesthesias, formication, feeling of disfiguration, or nonobjectifiable hair loss.

Dermatology has recently been confronted with patients who think they have acquired skin changes due to environmental toxins or detergents or who suffer from nondetectable *Candida* infections or undetectable "covert" food allergies. This group of dermatological patients is often classified with diagnoses like "nihilodermia," "clinical ecosyndrome" (Ring et al. 1999), or, as Cotterill (1996) termed it, "dermatological nondisease," sometimes exacerbated by a physician's temptation to diagnose a very rare syndrome or entity.

Somatoform disorders are disorders that are common in everyday dermatological practice and which confront the treating physician with serious problems, but they have received very scarce attention thus far, considering the frequency of their occurrence.

Definition. The characteristic of somatoform disorders (ICD-10: F45; DSM-IV-TR: 300.82) is repeated presentation of physical symptoms not caused intentionally, suggesting a medical condition coupled with the stubborn demand for medical examination, despite repeated negative findings and assurance by the health provider that the symptoms cannot be explained physically.

Classification of somatoform disorders in dermatology. Somatoform disorders in dermatology comprise a heterogeneous presentation of completely different clinical entities, with an underlying comparable psychiatric disorder.

The essential somatoform disorders are somatization disorders; hypochondriacal disorders, including body dysmorphic disorders; autonomic somatoform function disorders; somatoform pain syndromes of the skin; somatoform itching; and skin-related somatoform burning (Table 1.6).

Occurrence. In studies in Marburg, Germany, 18.5% of skin patients at the routine outpatient clinic of the university presented with somatoform disorders (Stangier and Gieler 1997). These were especially often body dysmorphic disorders and psychogenic pruritus (see Part I, Prevalence of Somatic and Emotional Disorders).

1.3.1 Somatization Disorders

Somatization disorders include the occurrence of a pattern of recurrent, multiple, clinically significant somatic complaints that usually lead to medical treatment. Often there is a combination of pain, as well as various gastrointestinal, sexual, and pseudoneurological symptoms.

In dermatology, environmental physical complaints, the so-called ecosyndrome, is in the foreground of the somatization disorders, whereby multiple fluctuating complaints are attributed to various intolerances.

Environmentally Related Physical Complaints

For many years, an increasing number of patients have sought medical help for nonspecific hypersensitivities to environmental toxins. Totally different complaints are reported, often affecting several organ systems, and they are objectively very difficult to characterize. Many patients have made an odyssey to various specialty physicians and alternative healers without finding lasting help. The problem is popular in the media ("Allergic to everything?"). The patients are classified under various terms and diagnoses (see below).

Definition. In environment-related physical complaints (ICD-10: F45.0), the patients report specific and nonspecific multiple physical complaints, of which the presumed cause is exposure to environmental toxins, with no proof of a direct causal relationship between exposure and extent of complaints. Numerous doctors are often consulted.

Environment-related physical complaints can be seen as a subgroup of somatoform disorders in which there is hypersensitivity to environmental substances.

Categorization. The following is an overview of the patterns of complaints.

Categorization of Environment-Related Physical Complaints and Related Terms

- General:
  - Ecosyndrome
  - "Ecological illness"

  - Multiple chemical sensitivity syndrome (MCS)
  - Chemical hypersensitivity syndrome
  - "Total allergy syndrome" or 20th-century syndrome
  - Allergic toxemia
  - "Cerebral allergy"
  - Idiopathic environmental intolerance
  - Multiorgan dysesthesia
- Special forms:
  - Sick-building syndrome
  - Gulf War syndrome
- Special forms:
  - Electrical hypersensitivity
  - Light allergy
  - Amalgam-related complaint syndrome
  - Detergent allergy
  - Food intolerances
- Differential diagnosis:
  - Chronic fatigue syndrome
  - Fibromyalgia syndrome
  - Hypochondriasis: infection phobia (mycophobia, AIDS phobia)

Pathogenesis. The concepts of environment-related physical complaints, including multiple chemical intolerances (MCS syndrome) have not been generally proven in a generally acceptable way and are controversial. Biological/physiological explanatory models, stress models with trigger factors, conditioning models, and purely emotional/psychiatric phenomena, even including sociocultural illness behavior, have been discussed. Scientific acceptance and consensus of the concept of illness does not exist at the present time.

In general, this is a heterogeneous patient group with heterogeneous pathogenesis. Thus, in some patients, objectifiable somatic hypersensitivities or even clear IgE-mediated allergies may be found in addition to psychosomatic factors.

Somatic models assume a possibly conditioned loss of tolerance to chemical exposure with gradually increasing sensitivity and generalization to the entire organism. Procedures of laboratory chemical diagnostics and the contested setting of limits cause particular difficulties here.

Moreover, sociocultural factors play a decisive role in this biopsychosocial phenomenon. The discussion of "environmental toxins," which is often reported broadly in the media, always leads to an increase in individual syndromes, such as the amalgam-related complaint syndrome, a presumed "detergent allergy," or atypical systemic *Candida* infection.

The role of environmental toxins remains unclear, but it must be emphasized that the diagnostic possibilities are still very limited in this area. Some authors assume an elevated sensitivity to odors, and others propose neurophysiologic changes in the transmission of stimuli. In many cases it is possible, by means of proper allergological diagnostics, to prove real hypersensitivity reactions that improve after appropriate stimulus withdrawal.

Extensive studies on larger groups of patients have shown that this is not a uniform presentation of disease. Numerous different causes appear to exist. In many patients, psychosomatic factors (often in the depressive category) play a role; in others, however, objectively recordable hypersensitivity or other diseases that had not been diagnosed earlier (such as chronic infections) can be demonstrated.

Clinical findings. Environment-related physical complaints are characterized clinically by recurrent and nonspecific complaints in various organ systems, which may occur as a reaction to environmental exposure to many different chemical substances unrelated to one another or to exposure to nonmaterials (such as radiation).

The complaints may be monosymptomatic or occur in combination and may be coupled with an endless variability of other symptoms.

The patients report various physical complaints, as seen in the following overview.

Guiding Symptoms of Environment-Related Physical Complaints

- Headache, burning eyes, rhynorrhea
- Fatigue, listlessness
- Concentration impairment, forgetfulness
- Pain in the movement apparatus
- Unspecific dizziness/tachycardia
- Dyspnea

Somatic and psychiatric differential diagnostics are of central importance in causality and in the prognosis and treatment.

Ecosyndrome, "Ecological Illness," "Total Allergy Syndrome"

Different terms and diagnoses are sometimes used in this group of disorders and are synonymous with envi-

Table 1.6 Overview of somatoform disorders in dermatology

ICD nr.	Somatoform disorder	Dermatoses	
F 45.0	Somatization disorder	Environment syndrome	Ecosyndrome, multiple chemical sensitivity syndrome, sick-building syndrome
		Special forms	Food allergies, sperm allergy, detergent allergy, light allergy electrosmog, amalgam-related complaint syndrome
F 45.2	Hypochondriacal disorder	Hypochondriacal disorder in the actual sense	Infections (bacteria, fungi, viruses, parasites)
			Neoplasia
			Other nosophobias (environment syndrome; see above)
		Body dysmorphic disorder	Whole body: Dorian Gray syndrome
			Regional: head, breast, genitals
		Special form	Botulinophilia
F 45.3	Somatoform autonomic function disorder	Erythrophobia	
		Goose bumps	
		Hyperhidrosis	
		Special form	Undifferentiated somatoform idiopathic anaphylaxia
F 45.4	Persistent somatoform pain disorder	Cutaneous dysesthesias	Glossodynia – orofacial pain syndrome
			Trichodynia
			Vulvodynia, phallodynia, anodynia
F 45.8	Other somatoform disorders	Sensory complaints	Itching
			A. Localized somatoform itching
			B. Generalized somatoform itching (pruritus sine materia)
			Paresthesias
			Burning
			Stabbing

ronment-related physical complaints, depending on the clinical description.

In the ecosyndrome, patients have different subjective presentations of disease in various organ systems, coupled with the conviction of being sick because of environmental toxins.

In the "total allergy syndrome," numerous "allergies" are held responsible for the complaints ("allergic to everything").

Multiple Chemical Sensitivity Syndrome

In the multiple chemical sensitivity (MCS) syndrome (ICD-10: F45.0), the patient complains of various physical complaints after slight exposure to chemical environmental substances, although no objective proof of increased exposure or a causal relationship between exposure and extent of the complaints can be shown. The patient reports improvement after avoiding exposure.

In the German-speaking area, particular complaints are reported following exposure to wood preservatives, solvents, insecticides, heavy metals, disinfectants or aromas (perfume), and other locally specific environmental substances.

Diagnostic Criteria for Multiple Chemical Sensitivity Syndrome

- Elicitation of symptoms by a variety of factors following slight exposure
- Various symptoms, which manifest in more than one area/organ system and which improve on avoiding exposure
- Complaints that cannot be explained by diagnostic procedures
- Tendency to chronification
- Considerable suffering
- Exclusion of other known diseases

From this it is seen that an unequivocal diagnosis can often not be made. With today's knowledge, it is unclear whether hypersensitivity to various chemicals is really present, which is why the terms "presumed multiple chemical sensitivity" or "idiopathic environment-related intolerance" have been suggested several times.

The syndrome is also defined as a somatization disorder under ICD-10 (ICD-10: F45.0; DSM-IV-TR: 300.81) and is treated with corresponding psychotherapy.

Sick-Building Syndrome

In sick-building syndrome, vapors from buildings and inside rooms are held responsible for the complaints.

Gulf War Syndrome

In Gulf War syndrome, radioactive substances or chemical war materials used in combat situations are held responsible as elicitors of listlessness and other unspecific syndromes. This disorder has been primarily described for soldiers (United States, Great Britain) after their deployment in the first Gulf War.

To be remembered in this connection are also the so-called "war tremblers" (shell shock) after bombardments in World War I.

Special Forms

Electrical Hypersensitivity

In electrical hypersensitivity, the patient holds emanations from things such as high tension wires as responsible for his or her existing complaints.

An increasing number of people are worried about possible dangers to health from electromagnetic fields ("electrosmog"). This worry is seen in increasing questions about this in medical practice and also in reports in the media. People living near the so-called base transmitter stations report impairment to well-being and symptoms that they relate to the installation and operation of these transmitters.

Worries in the population can be attributed to no small degree to the fact that the people living near the planned stations (transmission towers) were not informed promptly or in detail and were not given a say in the planning. This leads to great anxiety and uncertainty, conditions that in themselves may make people sick.

According to today's knowledge, when the guidelines of the World Health Organization (WHO) and other international organizations, including the International Commission on Non-Ionizing Radiation Protection (ICNIRP) and the European Union (EU) recommendation of 1999 (European Commission) are complied with, no effects on the health of the population need be anticipated, but it must be admitted that such effects cannot be ruled out and that there is considerable need for research. For this reason, WHO and the EU are presently carrying out various broad research programs.

Microwave radiation generated from the use of mobile telephones has been suspected of numerous ailments ranging from brain tumors to increased general allergies (Kimata 2002).

"Light Allergy"

There are a number of other comorbidities in "light allergy," so this special form is described in Chap. 9.

Amalgam-Related Complaint Syndrome

In the amalgam-related complaint syndrome, multiple ailments are ascribed to tooth fillings with amalgam due to the putative slow release of metal ions. This has led individuals to replace their mercury-containing fillings with composite or ionomeric ones.

"Detergent Allergy"

A number of skin changes, usually eczema or skin complaints such as pruritus, have recently been attributed by patients to a presumed detergent allergy. Skin contact with bedding washed with a new detergent, or unknown detergents when sleeping in a different bed away from home, is blamed.

Food Intolerances

Food intolerances may also show transitions to the environmental syndrome complex (see Chap. 4).

Psychiatric symptoms of environment-related physical complaints. A national multicenter study showed that a heterogeneous multiplicity of sometimes allergological, sometimes psychosomatic, and rarely toxic reactions is behind this diagnosis. The patients (n=234) very often showed psychosomatic similarity to patients with somatization disorders.

It is also particularly characteristic that the exposure is coupled to a varying degree with fears, so that the patients develop a pronounced avoidance behavior. The avoidance behavior – often even anxious behavior in the expectation of the feared situations – limits the patients considerably in their normal living, professional performance, and social activities and relationships. Moreover, close contact persons or partners may be drawn into the syndrome.

In summary, it can be said that general diagnostics are made according to the guidelines for somatoform disorders, and differentiation from a phobic disorder up to even paranoid psychoses must be drawn.

Differential diagnosis. A more intensive differential diagnosis within the group of environment-related physical complaints is made according to the provocation factors reported by the patient. These define categorization in the specific subgroups: multiple chemical sensitivity syndrome or ecosyndrome, sick-building syndrome, or Gulf War syndrome, including specific phenomena and special forms such as amalgam-related complaint syndrome and electrical hypersensitivity.

Differential diagnostics separate out pure hypochondriasis, such as infection phobia (*Candida*, AIDS), which in some cases may occur as comorbidity or show overlapping boundaries.

Other somatization disorders can be clearly differentiated with the frequently associated terms chronic fatigue syndrome and fibromyalgia syndrome, in which the patients do not descriptively report in the history any exposure to toxins as the presumed cause.

Chronic Fatigue Syndrome

In chronic fatigue syndrome, the complaints of listlessness and fatigue are in the foreground. Among these are persistent complaints of increased tiredness after intellectual efforts or weakness and exhaustion after minimal physical activity. In addition, the patient has muscle pain, tension headache, insomnia, inability to relax, and irritability.

Exhaustion is the guiding symptom, which lasts at least 3 months and cannot be attributed to any physical disease. Depression, anxiety disorders, somatoform disorders, and organically caused diseases must be ruled out in the differential diagnosis.

Fibromyalgia Syndrome

In fibromyalgia syndrome, the patient reports widespread soft tissue pain in addition to the complaints of lethargy and fatigue.

Usually the complaints are of extensive, broad-area muscle pains of changing localization, mainly in the spine and extremities, which are accompanied by subjectively perceived swelling of the extremities in addition to ligament and tendon pain.

Sometimes typical pressure points can be proven, and the sensation of pain can be elicited by moderate finger pressure on certain points. Characteristic are points on the back of the head and lower neck area, midshoulder, the sternum, prominent points on the elbow joints, the buttocks musculature, the hip bones, and around the cleft of the knee joint. The American College of Rheumatology has established general classification guidelines for fibromyalgia that include a minimum of 11 defined tender pressure points.

In addition, there are heterogeneous general complaints including fatigue and insomnia, headache, irritated bowels, cold extremities, dry mouth, palpitations, tremors, irritated bladder, and circulatory problems. Psychiatric disorders include depressive mood, anxiety, and emotional lability.

Overall, the diagnoses and differential diagnoses of the environment-related physical complaints can therefore be made and differentiated based on the history. The differential diagnosis may, however, often be difficult because of great similarities.

Psychotherapy. Environment-related physical complaints are not included in the ICD-10 and DSM-4 classifications and must therefore be categorized with respect to diagnostics and corresponding therapy concepts with the somatoform disorders or somatization disorders.

Therapy of these unclear complaints is oriented totally to the results of intensive examinations. In the foreground is avoidance of recognized relevant eliciting factors, except in the treatment of the underlying disease; avoidance of allergens (rarely); special diets, for example with respect to nutrient additives; renovation of living accommodations (rarely); and almost always psychosomatic primary care, psychoeducation, or psychotherapy or psychiatric therapy.

There remains a considerable need for research in this area. The affected patients must be taken seriously. This can succeed only in a trusting relationship between the doctor and the patient and in an interdisciplinary approach, since several organ systems are usually affected.

Psychotherapy must be adapted individually to the patient. According to the available literature, cognitive behavioral therapeutic measures may possibly be effective.

The often made sole recommendation to completely avoid or remove the agent considered damaging, including acts such as apartment renovation, total avoidance of possible toxins, and removal of all amalgam fillings, is contraindicated according to current experience in the treatment of environment-related physical complaints.

Moreover, iatrogenic phobias or hypochondrias may be present in detoxification cures (including pulling of all teeth) or corresponding recommendations from the treating doctor and must be avoided from the start.

Interdisciplinary cooperation among environmental medical experts, psychosomatic physicians, allergologists, and dermatologists points the way to successful treatment.

Psychopharmacotherapy. There are presently no confirmed studies on pharmacotherapy. SSRIs and anxiolytics may, however, have a positive influence, especially on phobic disorders or an underlying depressive disorder and may clearly relieve the intensity of symptoms.

Reference

Kimata H (2002) Enhancement of allergic skin wheal responses by microwave radiation from mobile phones in patients with atopic eczema/dermatitis syndrome. Int Arch Allergy Immunol 129(4):348–350

Further Reading

Bullinger M (1989) Psychological effects of air pollution on healthy residents. J Environ Psych 9: 103–118

Cotterill JA (1996) Body dysmorphic disorder. Dermatol Clin 14(3): 457–463

Cullen MR (1987) The worker with multiple chemical hypersensitivities: an overview. Occup Med 2: 655–661

Eberlein-König B, Behrendt H, Ring J (2002) Idiopathische Umweltintoleranz (MCS, Öko-Syndrom) – neue Entwicklungen. Allergo J 11: 434–441

Eis D, Mühlinghaus T, Birkner N, Bullinger M, Ebel H, Eikmann T, Gieler U, Herr C, Hornberg C, Hüppe M, Lecke C, Lacour M, Mach J, Nowak D, Podoll K, Quinzio B, Renner B, Rupp T, Scharrer E, Schwarz E, Tönnies R, Traenckner-Probst I, Rose M, Wiesmüller GA, Worm M, Zunder T (2003) Multizentrische Studie zur Multiplen Chemikalien-Sensitivität (MCS) – Beschreibung und erste Ergebnisse der "RKI-Studie". Umweltmed Forsch Prax 8:133–145

Gieler U, Bullinger M, Behrendt H, Eikmann T, Herr C, Ring J, Schwarz E, Suchenwirth R, Tretter F (1998) Therapeutische Aspekte des Multiple Chemical Sensitivity Syndroms. Umweltmed Forsch Prax 3: 3–10

Nasterlack M, Kraus T, Wrbitzky R (2002) Multiple Chemical Sensitivity. Dtsch Ärzteblatt 99: A2474–2483

Ring J, Eberlein-König B, Behrendt H (1999) "Eco-syndrome" ("multiple chemical sensitivity" – MCS). Zentralbl Hyg Umweltmed 202: 207–218

Röttgers HR (2000) Psychisch Kranke in der Umweltmedizin. Dtsch Ärzteblatt 97: A835–840

Stangier U, Gieler U (1997) Somatoforme Störungen in der Dermatologie. Psychotherapie 2: 91–101

Staudenmayer H, Selner JC, Buhr MP (1993) Double-blind provocation chamber challenges in 20 patients presenting with "multiple chemical sensitivity." Regul Toxicol Pharmacol 18: 44–53

Tretter F (1996) Umweltbezogene funktionelle Syndrome. Int Praxis 37: 669–686

Voack C, Borelli S, Ring J (1997) Der umweltmedizinische Vier-Stufen-Plan. MMW 139: 41–44

1.3.2 Hypochondriacal Disorders

The ICD-10 distinguishes between two large illness groups of hypochondriacal disorders:

- Hypochondriacal disorders in the actual sense (infections, neoplasias)
- Dysmorphophobia (body dysmorphic disorders)

Both groups are coded in the DSM-IV-TR: 300.7.

The traditional assignment and classification of dysmorphophobia (body dysmorphic disorder) here will certainly be removed in the future based on today's understanding of causality and will form a group of its own instead.

Cutaneous Hypochondrias

Definition. Hypochondrias (ICD-10: F45.2; DSM-IV-TR: 300.7) comprise persistent, excessive preoccupation with the fear or conviction of suffering from one or more serious, progressive physical diseases. In preoccupation with a normal physical event, the sensation is often interpreted by the afflicted person as abnormal and stressful, but it relies on misinterpretation (Fig. 1.28b).

In cutaneous hypochondrias, this preoccupation is focused on the skin and sexually transmitted diseases.

Diagnostic Criteria of Hypochondrias

- There is persistent preoccupation with the fear or conviction of suffering from a serious physical illness, without sufficient physical findings.
- This conviction of and preoccupation with fear of illness persists despite negative medical diagnostic tests and assurance from the physician about the absence of somatic illness.
- The symptoms cannot be better explained by primary anxiety, panic, compulsive, or depressive disorder.

Clinical findings. In dermatology there are different heterogeneous patterns of complaints, which, however, are focused especially on the skin and mucous membranes (Fig. 1.28c).

Categorization of Dermatovenereological Hypochondrias

- Infections
  - *Candida* phobia (usually generalized)
  - AIDS phobia
  - Venereophobia (unspecific form)
  - Syphilis phobia
  - Borrelia phobia
  - Parasitophobia
- Neoplasia
  - Carcinophobia (unspecific)
  - Melanoma phobia (specific), often in dysplastic nevus syndrome
- Other nosophobias and differential-diagnostic special forms
  - Ecosyndrome
  - Electrosmog
  - Light allergy
  - Amalgam phobia
  - Food allergy

In addition, in individual cases the classification of environmental syndromes in patients with presumed food allergies, sperm allergy (Chap. 4), and amalgam phobia must be discussed as an overlapping transition or hard-to-delimit differential-diagnostic special form of hypochondrias.

In hypochondriacal disorders of the outward appearance, there is also overlapping with body dysmorphic disorders.

Psychiatric symptoms. In the hypochondriacal disorders, the patient is excessively preoccupied with the fear of a serious illness or the conviction of having one. Depressive and anxiety disorders may be included as central criteria and dispositional factors.

Traumatizing life events may often be cited by the patients as elicitors (Rief et al. 1994; Musalek 1996). Especially among these are deaths or serious illnesses in persons close to the patient. Characteristically, the intensity of the symptoms varies between the individual consultations and also depending on the patient's current life situation.

Differential diagnosis. In the first place, anxiety and somatization disorders as well as body dysmorphic disorders must be differentiated. If an anxiety or panic disorder is primarily in the foreground, the cutaneous hypochondria must be considered as secondary. In somatization disorders, the accent is more on the multiple, shifting complaints.

With respect to purely depressive disorders, the question arises of primary or secondary genesis. If primarily depressive symptoms are in the foreground, the cutaneous hypochondria may occur as a comorbidity or epiphenomenon. Uncorrectable transitions to hypochondriacal delusion (ICD-10: F22; DSM-IV-TR 297.1 somatic type) must be differentiated.

Therapy. Treatment as part of psychosomatic primary care is initially in the foreground, whereby the doctor must first consider the patient's overall situation in light of his or her history.

The frequently existing isolation is often made worse by the assurance that the patient is healthy and does not have to worry.

Access to the patient can usually be achieved by thematizing the social situation, coping with the disease, earlier experience with illness, and possible serious eliciting situations.

Cutaneous hypochondrias belong to the somatoform disorders and should be treated accordingly (they need to be diagnosed by taking into account the type of psychiatric symptoms exhibited to determine whether psychotic vs. mood is the prominent disturbance). Often there are pronounced depressive disorders or anxiety disorders, which necessitate additional supportive behavior therapy with cognitive restructuring, psychodynamic therapies, or pharmacological treatment measures.

If there is no motivation for psychotherapy or insight into the psychosocial aspects of the disease, motivation can sometimes be created by setting up concrete follow-up appointments (2–4-week intervals) and long-term, regular consultations. Psychoeducation is meaningful within this framework of medical care.

Psychopharmacotherapy. Drug therapy is oriented to the comorbidity, so SSRIs, tricyclic antidepressants, or neuroleptics may often be indicated.

References

Musalek M (1996) Wahnsyndrome in der Dermatologie. In: Gieler U, Bosse KA (Hrsg) Seelische Faktoren bei Hautkrankheiten. Huber, Bern

Rief W, Hiller W, Geissner E, Fichter M (1994) Hypochondrie: Erfassung und erste klinische Ergebnisse. Z Klin Psychol 23: 34–42

Further Reading

Avia MD, Ruiz MA, Olivares ME, Crespo M, Guisado AB, Sanchez A, Varela A (1996) The meaning of psychological symptoms: effectiveness of a group intervention with hypochondriacal patients. Behav Res Ther 34: 23–31

Barsky AJ (1996) Hypochondriasis. Medical management and psychiatric treatment. Psychosomatics 37: 48–56

Lupke U, Rohr W, Nutzinger D (1996) Stationäre Verhaltenstherapie bei Hypochondrie. Psychotherapeut 6: 373–384

Warwick HM, Clark DM, Cobb AM, Salkovskis PM (1996) A controlled trial of cognitive-behavioral treatment of hypochondriasis. Br J Psychiatry 169: 189–195

Body Dysmorphic Disorders (Dysmorphophobia)

Body dysmorphic disorders have as a central criterion the excessive preoccupation with a deficiency or disfiguration of physical appearance. This deficiency either does not exist at all or is only very minor. This exaggerated preoccupation may lead to marked limitations in social, professional, and functional areas.

In dermatology and psychosomatic medicine, the term disfiguration syndrome was used. The ICD-10 categorizes the illness in the group of somatoform disorders under hypochondria (F45.2). Other common terms are dermatological nondisease (Cotterill 1996), ugliness syndrome, and Thersites complex (Thersites was the ugliest warrior in Odysseus's army, according to Homer's saga). In the United States and United Kingdom, it is termed body dysmorphic disorder (Altamura 2001; Philipps 2000).

For dermatologists and in all of psychosomatic dermatology, patients with body dysmorphic disorders make up the most important group of problem patients, both quantitatively and qualitatively, in addition to somatoform itching (see Part I, Prevalence of Somatic and Emotional Disorders).

The British dermatologist Cotterill postulated the following for the patient group with body dysmorphic disorders:

"I know of no more difficult patients to treat than those with body dysmorphic disorder."

In the case of objectifiable, clearly visible skin diseases, this experience of disfigurement may be appropriate; in the case of minimal or not objectifiable skin manifestations, a body dysmorphic disorder can be assumed. The smallest normal variations or morphological changes in the skin may be experienced subjectively as disfiguring.

Definition. For clinical and practical reasons, the diagnostic criteria of body dysmorphic disorders in the DSM-IV is preferred to the ICD-10 and the concept of dysmorphophobia.

Diagnostic Criteria of Body Dysmorphic Disorders, DSM-IV-TR 300.7

- Excessive preoccupation with an imagined deficiency or disfigurement of the outward appearance. If a slight physical anomaly is present, the concern of the person affected is greatly exaggerated.
- Excessive preoccupation causes intense suffering or detriment to social, professional, or other important functional areas.
- The excessive preoccupation cannot be better explained by another psychiatric disorder.

Occurrence. The prevalence of body dysmorphic disorders is cited as approximately 1% of the total American population. Among American students, up to 4% meet the criteria of body dysmorphic disorder according to DSM-IV (Philipps 2000; Bohne et al. 2002). The relative number of comparable German students corresponds to this figure (Oosthuizen et al. 1998; Otto et al. 2001).

In dermatology clinics and in dermatological practice, body dysmorphic disorder has an incidence of 11.9–15.6% and 23% in various cosmetic dermatological consults. Women between ages 35 and 50 and men younger than 35 are affected (Phillips 2000).

Pathogenesis. Various theories attempt to explain the onset of a body dysmorphic disorder.

The self-discrepancy theory is an approach described by Veale et al. (2003), in which patients with body dysmorphic disorder present with significant discrepancies between their self-actual and both their self-ideal and self-should.

The high comorbidity of depression and social phobias, usually occurring in more than 70% (see information below on psychiatric symptoms), is conspicuous in nearly all studies. This approach is based on a neurobiological understanding that a serotonin imbalance exists. The responsiveness of the disorder to SSRIs is understandable in this context.

In addition to these descriptive-psychiatric approaches, some reports assume an inflammatory process in the frontotemporal area of the brain (Gabbay et al. 2003).

The most frequent explanatory approach in recent years is a cognitive-behavioral approach, which essentially assumes that a faulty development occurs due to erroneous perception and assessment processes with respect to one's own appearance (Veale et al. 2001, 2003). In addition, media-induced factors predispose individuals to this disorder by ingraining certain ideals of beauty (Phillips et al. 2000).

The psychodynamic explanatory approach assumes a possible conflict model underlying the symptom, whereby separation and dependency conflicts in early childhood may be possible causes of a hypochondriacal development, disintegrative anxiety states, and autistic and self-denigrating feelings of disgust.

The bonding theory is another approach. This could demonstrate that insecure or anxiety-bound children have the highest rate of hypochondriacal thoughts and functional disorders.

There is often an eliciting event (often mortification) in an emotional conflict that the patient seeks as a central focus on the basis of an insecure bonding pattern and doubts in self-esteem. The underlying conflicts are displaced, the hypochondriacal assessment stabilizes as disfiguring, and this in turn leads to increased feelings of disgust and shame, which potentiate the process (see Fig. 1.29c).

Clinical findings. Clinical examination reveals no pathological findings or only minimum variations from normal. In body dysmorphic disorder, differentiation can be made from a clinical point of view between whole-body disorders and regional complaints. The presumed regional deficiencies in outward appearance are localized especially in the face, breast, and genitalia (Table 1.7).

The spectrum of presumed deficiencies in outward appearance is endlessly variable. This includes quality and quantity of skin and skin appendages, as well as asymmetries or disproportionality of the nose, eyelids, eyebrows, lips, teeth, breasts, or genitals. Hair loss or hypertrichosis, dispigmentations, pore size, visible blood vessels, pallor, reddening of the skin, or sweating may also be reported as anomalies.

Whole-Body Disorders

Dorian Gray syndrome

The term Dorian Gray syndrome was selected (Brosig et al. 2001) to explain the patient's underlying wish to remain forever young. The name of the syndrome is taken from the title of a novel by Oscar Wilde, in which the protagonist, Dorian Gray, sells his soul to the devil so that he will not have to experience growing old. The love of self, artificiality, and egocentrism of the narcissist are apparent.

Definition. Dorian Gray syndrome is a body dysmorphic disorder associated with narcissistic regression, sociophobia, and a great wish to remain young. In some cases, lifestyle medications are sought to retard the natural aging process.

> **Dorian Gray Syndrome**
>
> - Denial of the aging process
> - Imagined or minimal defects with shame and social withdrawal (narcissistic regression)
> - Body dysmorphic disorder

Clinical findings and psychiatric symptoms. The clinical presentation of the syndrome is characterized diagnostically by symptoms of body dysmorphic disorder, the social withdrawal attendant on narcissistic regression, and denial of personality-structuring maturation. Lifestyle medications and interventions are often taken to achieve this goal.

Psychotherapy. After clarifying the patient's motivation, treatment requires courageous application of intensive psychotherapy, which may be done in combination with antidepressants and neuroleptics.

Psychopharmaceuticals. If a depressive mood predominates, SSRIs or a combination with neuroleptics to increase the effect of SSRIs to treat the psychiatric disorder are indicated in conjunction with the desirable psychotherapeutic treatment (with reference to Phillips 2000).

Hypertrichosis

Excessive preoccupation with hair may lead to the perception of having too much or too little. In many cases, men as well as women consult for epilation; removal of the hair is seen as a solution without which self-esteem (apparently) cannot be stabilized.

Hyperhidrosis

If physiological sweating is deemed abnormal, a body dysmorphic disorder may predominate. Differentiation is made between whole-body disorder ("I sweat so much") and the more frequent regional disorders of the hands, feet, or axillae.

> **Focus on Sweating**
>
> - Body dysmorphic disorder
> - Multifactorial dermatosis
> - Somatoform autonomic function disorder
> - Delusional disorder

Table 1.7 Clinical classification of body dysmorphic disorders in dermatology

Clinical classification	Characteristic pattern of complaints	
Whole-body disorders	Anti-aging	Dorian Gray syndrome
	symptoms	Hypertrichosis
		Seborrhea
		Hyperhidrosis
		Muscle mass
	Special form	Eating disorders
Region-related disorders	Head	Hypertrichosis, flushing, ectopic sebaceous glands, seborrhea, hypertrichosis, exfoliatio linguae areata)
	Breast	Proportion, areola
	Genitals	Proportion, hair growth
	Special form	Botulinophilia

Differential-diagnostically, emotional excitement is a frequent trigger factor in sweating, so multifactorial dermatological or somatoform autonomic symptoms must be ruled out. These are presented in detail in the sections on somatoform autonomic function disorder and multifactorial dermatoses (see Sect. 1.3.3 and Chap. 2, respectively).

Muscle Mass

Pathological worry about the extent of muscle mass is one form of whole-body disorder (Pope et al. 1997; Fig. 1.29 a,b).

Studies of this form of body dysmorphic disorders have been performed recently, especially among bodybuilders. It appears that Western media and culture have an important influence on the genesis of this biopsychosocial phenomenon. Excessive preoccupation results in detriment to social, professional, and other important functional areas. Often there is abuse of anabolic steroids, growth hormones (hGH), or other substances.

Special Form: Eating Disorders

Eating disorders are by definition not body dysmorphic disorders but are considered a separate entity. Eating disorders are, however, often accompanied by impaired body schemes and, according to the latest studies, show a blurred transition to body dysmorphic disorders in a subgroup, so they should be mentioned here.

Definition. Two main syndromes are described under the heading of eating disorders (ICD-10: F50; DSM-IV-TR: 307.1): anorexia nervosa (ICD-10: F50.0) and bulimia nervosa (ICD-10: F50.2; DSM-IV-TR: 307.51).

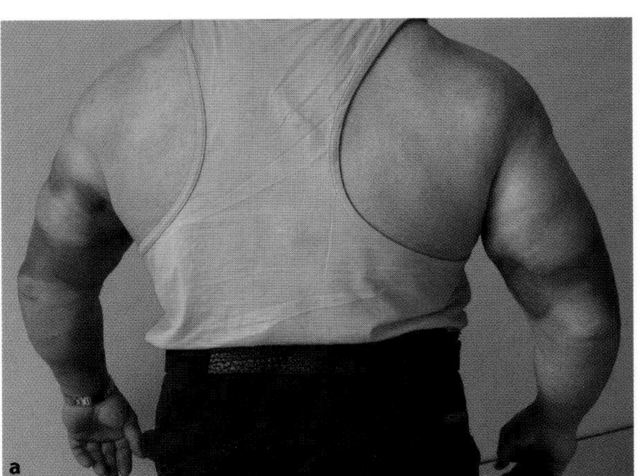

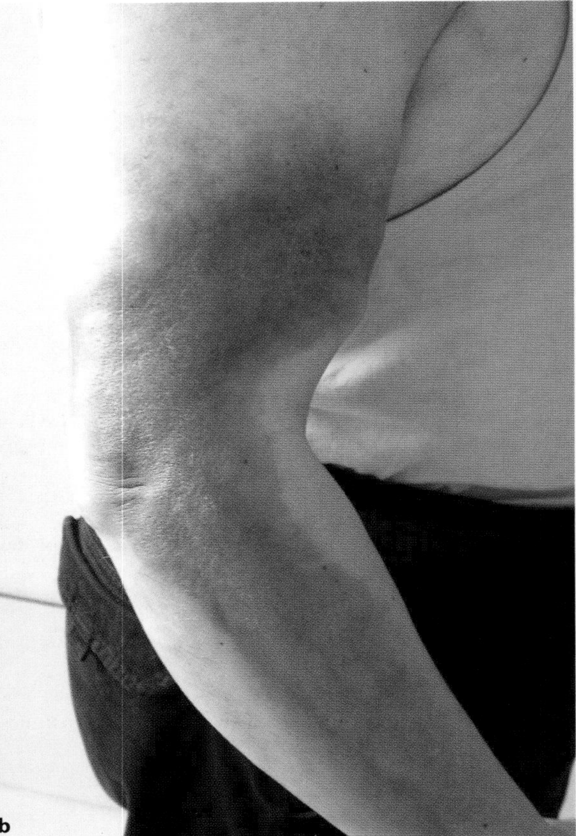

Fig. 1.29a–c Body dysmorphic disorder. **a** Injection of sesamoid oil into muscles. **b** Granulomatous reaction. **c** Formation of disfiguration problematics *(see next page)*

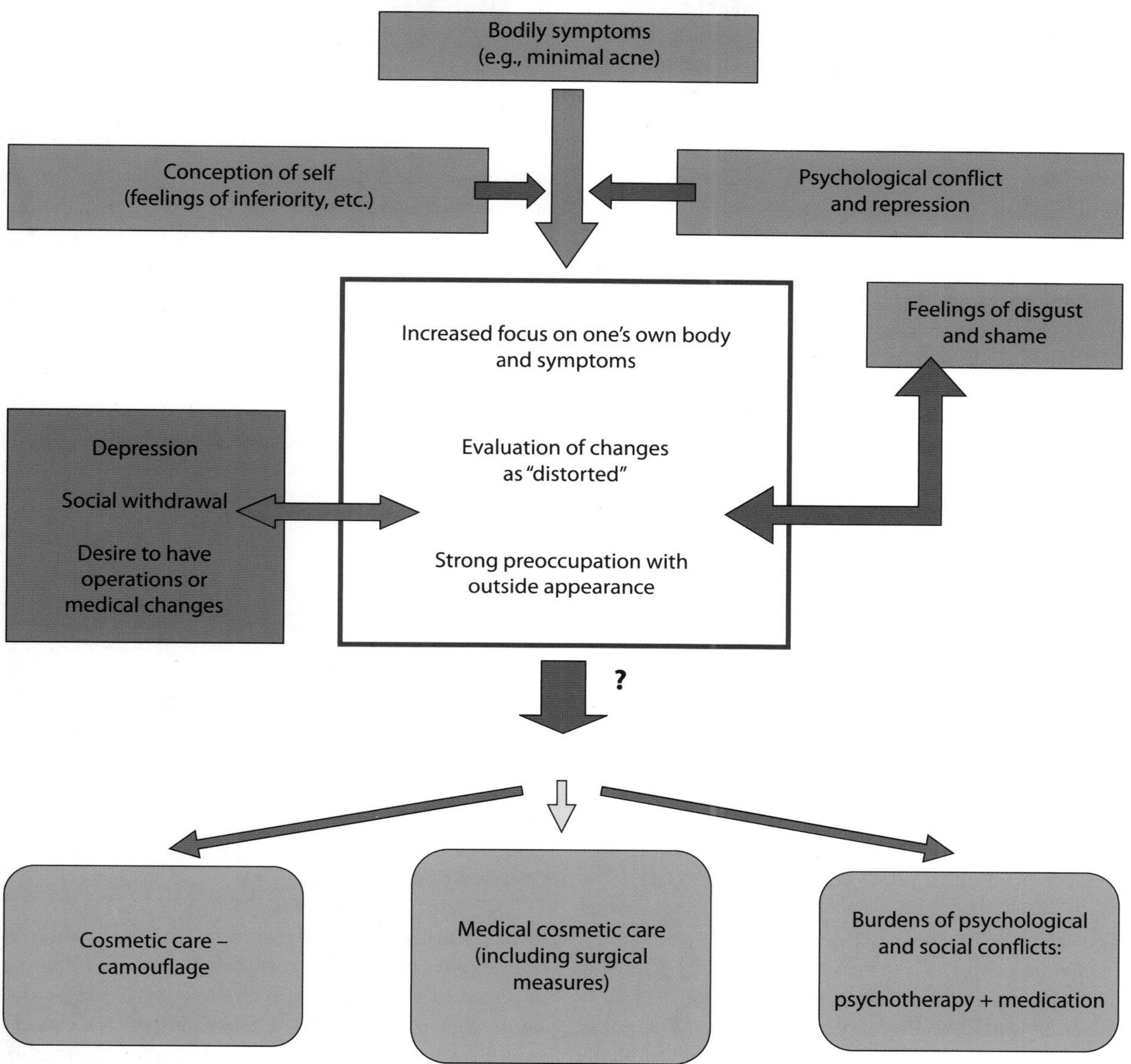

Fig. 1.29 *(continued)* **c** Formation of disfiguration problematics

1

Anorexia Nervosa

Anorexia nervosa is characterized by intentional, self-willed weight loss, mostly in young girls and adolescents. Sometimes the weight loss is caused by self-induced vomiting, excessive physical exercise, and, additionally, self-induced purging.

A deep-seated body scheme disorder is present in the form of a specific psychiatric disorder.

Bulimia Nervosa

Bulimia nervosa (bulimia) is characterized by repeated episodes of voracious hunger and excessive preoccupation with control of body weight. In bulimia, great quantities of food are consumed within a short time, followed by self-induced vomiting. In the transient hunger periods, laxatives, thyroid medications, and appetite inhibitors are taken. There is a close psychopathological relationship to anorexia nervosa.

Clinical presentation. For dermatologists, two biopsychosocial aspects of eating disorders are relevant:

> **! Patients with eating disorders show skin changes and increased body dysmorphic disorders because of the psychiatric disorder.**

Overall, 81% of patients with eating disorders also report dissatisfaction with their skin (Gupta and Gupta 2001). Predominantly there are verifiable symptoms such as xerosis and roughness as well as wrinkles or hyperpigmentation in connection with the disorder, xerosis (58.3%), telogen effluvium (50%), changes in nails (45.8%), cheilitis (41.6%), acne (41.6%), gingivitis (33.3%), acrocyanosis (29%), diffuse hypertrichosis (25%), carotenoderma (20.8%), generalized pruritus (16.6%), hyperpigmentations (12.5%), striae distensae (12.5%), facial dermatoses, and seborrheic dermatitis (8.3%), as well as impaired wound healing and melasma (4.1%; Strumia et al. 2001). Women younger than 30 years are especially affected (Fig. 1.30).

In addition to skin changes due to the eating disorder, these patients also show increased signs of a body dysmorphic disorder of the skin, hair, teeth, chin, nose, ears, or eyes (Gupta and Johnson 2000). An ego deficit and self-esteem problems related to the eating disorder may possibly prepare the way in this context for an additional body dysmorphic disorder as a comorbidity (Ravaldi et al. 2003).

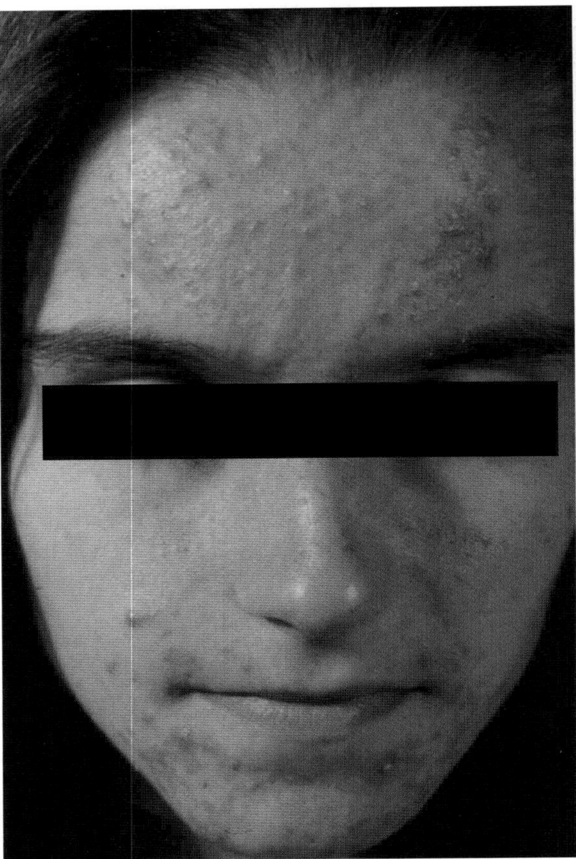

Fig. 1.30 Woman with extensive acne, the first manifestation since developing anorexia nervosa

Partial Body Disorders

Unlike whole-body disorders, a special localization is characteristically often reported with special symptoms in disorders in certain parts of the body. Whether the assumed symptoms, such as hyperhidrosis, are considered disturbing may differ from patient to patient only for the hands or axillae. Frequently reported symptoms of regional body dysmorphic disorders refer to the hair, sweat, or blood vessels.

Psychogenic Effluvium, Telogen Effluvium, Androgenic Alopecia

Clinical findings. Patients with objectively normal hair often report subjectively disfiguring hair loss and subjectively suffer very much from their presumed illness (Fig. 1.31).

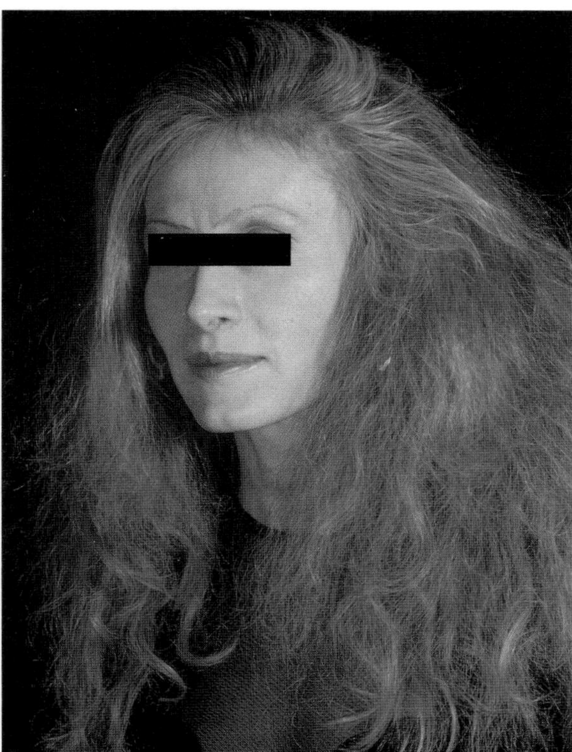

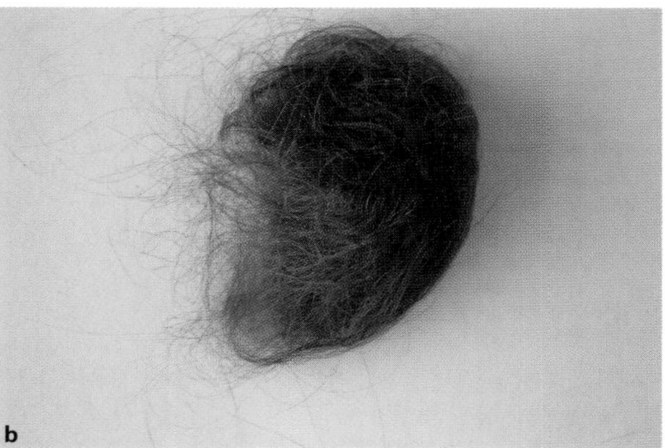

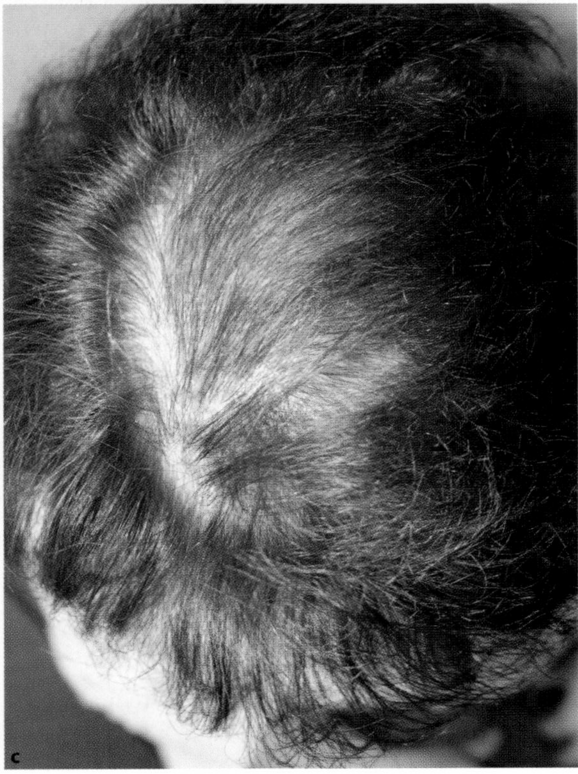

Fig. 1.31 **a** Body dysmorphic disorder in a 40-year-old woman with presumed hair loss. **b** Loose hair presented to the dermatologist by another female patient as proof of severe hair loss and hair disease. Diagnostics evaluated a telogen effluvium, normal hair status in this patient with somatoform disorder. **c** Androgenic alopecia in a woman

In excessive preoccupation with an imagined deficit (with objectively normal trichogram) in telogenic effluvium or alopecia diffusa (ICD-10: F45.9, L65.0) or age-appropriate androgenic alopecia (ICD-10: F45.9, L64.9), there is a psychogenic effluvium in the sense of a body dysmorphic disorder. If there is slight hair loss, the patient's worry is greatly exaggerated.

Patients with presumed hair loss are a common special problematic group in the dermatological practice. Usually those afflicted by this body dysmorphic disorder are women, but recently there has been an increase in the number of young, usually single, men.

Men with hair loss have lower self-esteem, higher depression values, higher introversion, higher neuroticism, and a feeling of unattractiveness. They feel less attractive when the hair loss begins early, and it is more intensively perceived by young and single men appearing in public (Cash 1992).

Neuroticism includes a tendency to excessive emotional lability with nervousness, hypersensitivity, anxiety, and excitability.

Telogen effluvium and androgenic alopecia in women are especially problematic. In androgenic alopecia in women, the hair becomes thin on the midscalp, frequently accompanied by thinning of all hair. Often a strip of thicker hair remains in the front (Fig. 1.31c).

Patients with skin or hair diseases that are objectively harmless, such as diffuse alopecia, suffer greatly subjectively from their illness and experience marked helpless-

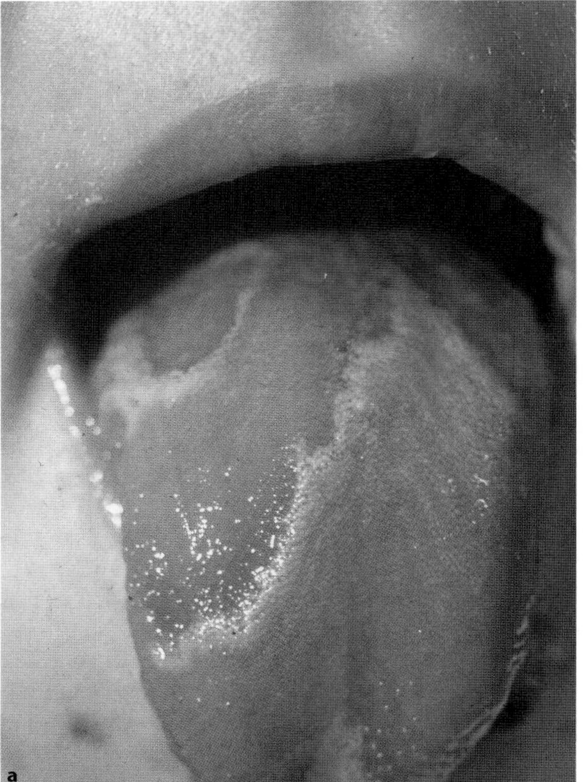

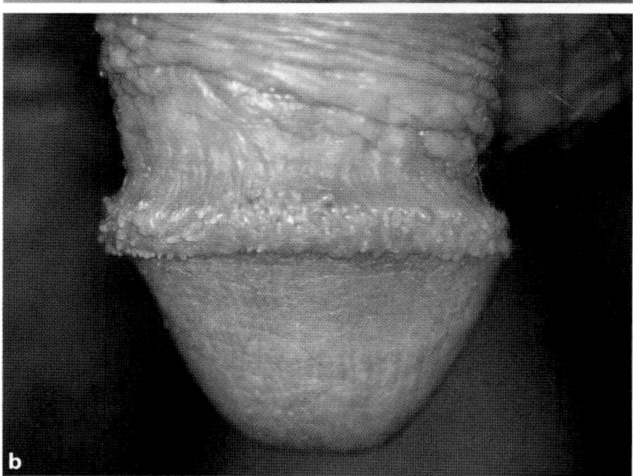

Fig. 1.32 **a** Geographic tongue in patient with depression and serious carcinophobia. Previously, seven different specialists had been consulted, sometimes with invasive diagnostics with negative findings. **b** Pearly penile papules (papillae coronae glandis) in a 23-year-old male patient suspected to have a malignant neoplasia

ness. An adjustment disorder should be included in the differential diagnosis of these patients (Niemeier et al. 2002). Based on the findings presented, alopecia patients often require additional psychotherapeutic intervention.

Geographic Tongue

Geographic tongue, also called lingua geographica, is a symptom that is often a source of concern for the person affected and which is not infrequently accompanied by carcinophobia.

Characteristically, there are variously large, often maplike, red depapillated areas on the normal surface of the tongue. The plaques change their form, size, and location from day to day. A single consultation about the harmlessness of the normal variations is often not sufficient, and even unremarkable findings in more detailed diagnostics cannot calm the patient (Fig. 1.32). This finding is often associated with or part of psoriasis vulgaris.

Differential diagnosis. The differential diagnosis of this somatoform disorder covers a broad spectrum. Some patients complain of impaired sensitivity after eating hot or cold foods, or a continuously burning tongue, so cutaneous dysesthesia must be ruled out. Differential-diagnostic categorization among the cutaneous hypochondrias should be checked in the individual case if the patient thinks he or she has some disease (carcinophobia) because of the changes observed.

Differential Diagnoses in Normal Variants in the Mouth

- Body dysmorphic disorder
- Cutaneous dysesthesia (burning tongue)
- Cutaneous hypochondrias (fear of disease)

Buccal Sebaceous Gland Hypertrophy

Ectopic sebaceous glands as a normal variant are frequent in the buccal mucosae and the lips (Fordyce glands). There are numerous papules 1–3 mm in diameter, with no sign of inflammation.

If no emotional stabilization occurs after an explanatory discussion of the harmlessness of this sebaceous gland variation, consideration must be given to a body dysmorphic disorder.

The differential diagnosis must also rule out cutaneous hypochondria, in which persistent preoccupation with the fear or conviction of suffering from a serious physical disease predominates.

Breast

Body dysmorphic disorders of the breast usually concern their size and shape (Fig. 1.33). In recent times, the complaints of large breasts have increased, and surgical reductions are occasionally performed. Other individual cases refer to presumed ugly scars or pigmentations, as well as to visible blood vessels.

Genitals

Proportion

Worry about the size of the penis predominates in men. The concern is usually that the penis is too small. Indication for medical operation is given only in the case of micropenis (erection length less than 7.5 cm; Wessels 1996).

Although according to estimates there is no somatic indication for penis augmentation (penis enlargement) in more than 90% of the patients (Porst 2001), 10,000 operations costing $3,500–9,500, with sometimes high complication rates, were performed worldwide in 1997. Among healthy men, there is often a feeling of inferiority that is to be corrected with the scalpel. But penile augmentation in subjects with normal findings cannot correct a psychiatric disorder.

Women complain of too-large labia pudenda that they want reduced surgically in an increasing number of cases. Reduction of the labia could be a desire for regression to the prepubescent stage. Often the procedure is performed to please a partner, who pays for the operation.

Sebaceous Gland Hypertrophy

Ectopic sebaceous glands are found as a normal variant in the genital area. The shaft of the penis and the inner prepuce fold are especially affected and present clinically with multiple, yellowish papules up to 3 mm in diameter. Free sebaceous glands in the area of the labia minora and on the inner aspect of the labia majora are often visible only on stretching the mucosae.

Ectopic sebaceous glands in the genital area are often considered bothersome, especially by young men, leading to limitation in seeking a partner and sexual contacts. Many men believe the variant to be a disease.

If no emotional stabilization occurs after an explanatory discussion of the harmlessness of this sebaceous gland variation, consideration must be given to a body dysmorphic disorder. The differential diagnosis must also rule out cutaneous hypochondria, in which persistent preoccupation with the fear or conviction of suffering from a serious physical disease predominates.

Papillae Coronae Glandis

Papillae coronae glandis (synonyms pearly penile papules) are a rare normal finding that must be differentiated from ectopic sebaceous glands. A border consisting of a single row or multiple rows of whitish-red small papules is found on the proximal glans, with spread to the sulcus coronaries (Fig. 1.32b).

Hair Growth

Genital hair growth is another focus. Patients often consider too much hair (hypertrichosis ICD-10: F54, L68) to be a defect. Increasingly, however, even normal genital hair is being removed by a large majority of young women and, more recently, also by men. Cosmetic trends as well as traditional ethnic and religious aspects predominate, particularly in Middle Eastern countries.

In part, however, psychodynamic aspects of regression with a desire to reinstate a prepubescent body status and rejection of the role of an adult woman are present. Men shave genital hair for pseudoaugmentation of the penis.

Too-little hair is, however, also considered a deficit and is altered by complicated hair transplantation from the head to the mons pubis (Fig. 1.34).

Cellulite

Cellulite (status protrusis cutis), also called "peau d'orange skin," occurs in various areas of the body and does not represent a true subcutaneous inflammatory process. In peau d'orange skin, especially in the gluteal area and external thighs, the subcutaneous fat tissue protudes

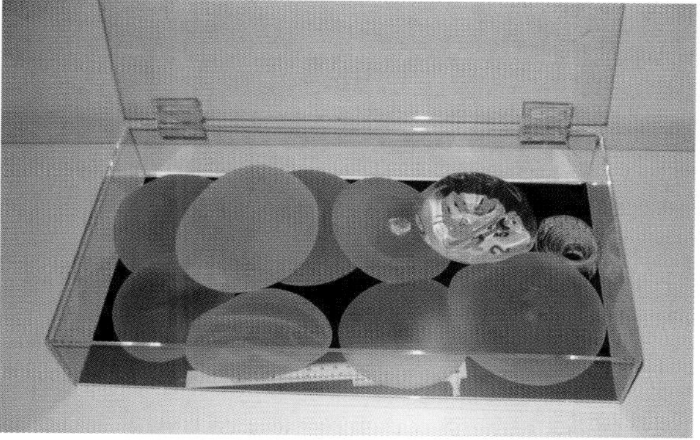

Fig. 1.33 Sample material for breast implantations

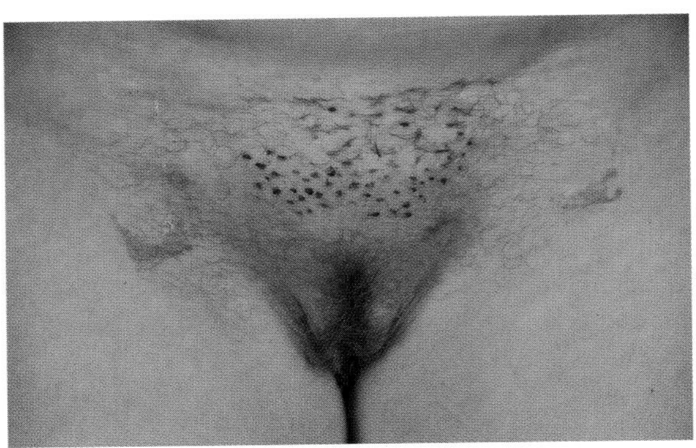

Fig. 1.34 Hair transplantation from the head to the mons pubis, in assumed too-little hair (contrary to the fashion trend)

through the connective tissue and forms small bumps of fat. Women are especially affected because there is parallel networking of the connective tissue.

Due to the diagonal and cross-structuring of their connective tissue, men are mostly spared these changes. The disorder may be genetically determined. To prevent the quiltlike, flat fat pad or so-called orange peel skin, women should pay special attention to their normal weight. Vacuum pressure massages, electrodes in the subcutaneous fatty tissue, liposuction, and cure packs are often used as treatment.

Feet, Hands, Axillae

Feet, hands, and axillae can be the focus for a body dysmorphic disorder, especially with respect to hyperhidrosis.

Special Form: Botulinophilia in Dermatology

No other lifestyle phenomenon has occupied dermatologists in recent times as much as the attention paid to sweating. It is conspicuous that a broad segment of the population has made a normal bodily function like sweating into a disease and a medical problem. If excessive preoccupation with imagined hyperhidrosis is present, there is a psychosocial disorder in the sense of a body dysmorphic disorder.

A quasi-side effect of the introduction and broad use of botulinus toxin in serious hyperhidrosis is that this form of therapy has been discovered by healthy people who demand it as a lifestyle therapy. Although there is otherwise a rather exaggerated fear of potent toxins in the environment, food, air, or water, individuals appear to set aside such reservations with respect to botulinus toxin for the treatment of presumed hyperhidrosis, and this procedure is in demand, even as an out-of-pocket treatment.

The new diagnosis "botulinophilia" was introduced in 2001 (Harth 2001) to denote the new lifestyle venenophilia, especially in body dysmorphic disorders with normal physiological sweating and additional persistent demand for botulinus toxin therapy by the patient despite negative findings. The current corrected diagnosis criteria for botulinophilia are as follows.

Diagnosis of Botulinophilia

Psychosocial diagnostic criteria for a body dysmorphic disorder DSM IV (300.7), ICD-10 (F45.2):

1. The affected individual is excessively preoccupied with imagined hyperhidrosis. If a slight physical anomaly is present, the person's worry is greatly exaggerated.
2. The excessive preoccupation causes suffering in a clinically significant way or is detrimental to social, professional, or other important functional areas.
3. The excessive preoccupation cannot be better explained by another psychiatric disorder.
   Somatic diagnostic criterion in hyperhidrosis:
4. Gravimetric measurement up to 50 mg sweat excreted per minute.

If all four criteria are met, and the patient demands therapy despite negative results and detailed explanation that the indication does not exist, the diagnosis is botulinophilia (Figs. 1.35, 1.36).

Even extensive measurements such as gravimetry cannot dissuade the affected person from the misinterpretation as disease. This misinterpretation often cannot be corrected in medical consultations, and sweating continues to be perceived as a physical anomaly. A typical patient statement is then, "But I sweat."

If there is no medical indication but great pressure for the desired treatment, a psychosocial disorder must be considered and clarified.

Summary of Body Dysmorphic Disorders

Psychiatric symptoms. In body dysmorphic disorder, comorbidities are often present, predominantly affective disorders, followed by anxiety disorders and, especially, social phobias. Suicidal tendencies must be watched for in a subgroup of patients with body dysmorphic diseases,

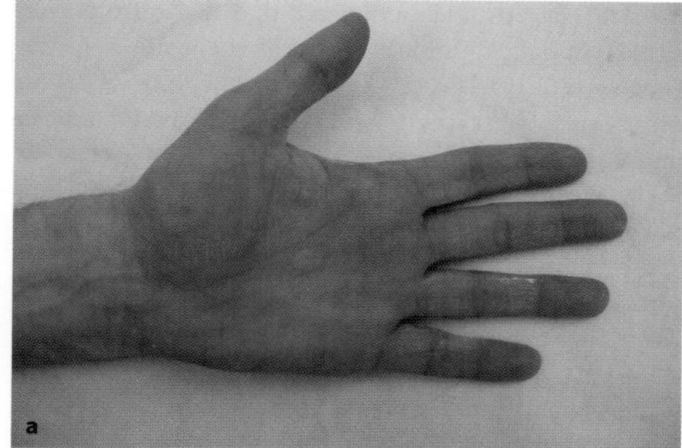

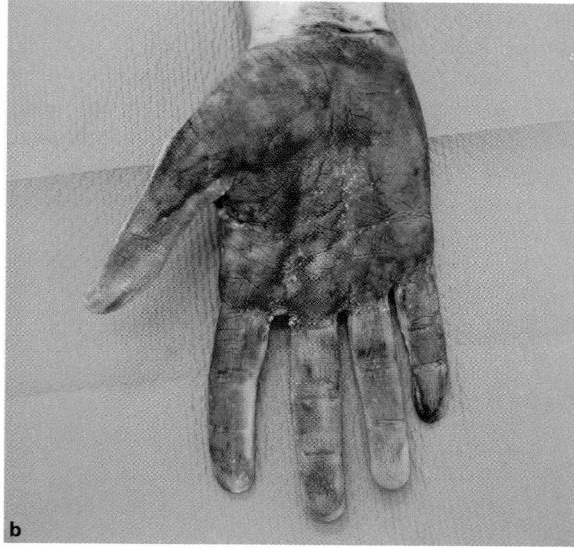

Fig. 1.35 **a** Botulinophilia: Patient with negative sweating test, presumed hyperhidrosis of the hands and pronounced sociophobia. **b** Comparison findings. Positive sweating test in hyperhidrosis of the hands with sociophobia as reactive adjustment disorder

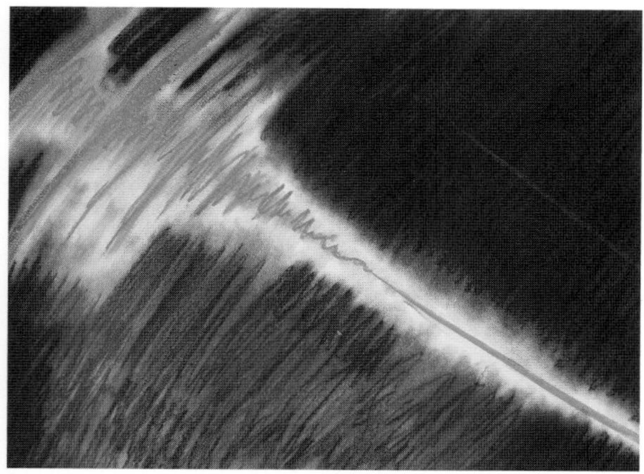

Fig. 1.36 Body dysmorphic disorder anxiety in art therapy

as well as narcissistic personality disorders up to and including body-related delusions (Philipps et al. 2000).

Moreover, a great overlapping with the compulsive disorders can be observed (Hollander et al. 1999). Patients have compulsive thoughts with great worry about their appearance as well as compulsive acts. Some patients spend several hours daily in compulsive acts such as continuous control of their appearance in front of the mirror, or touching and performing time-consuming grooming measures.

Areas with visual exposure are especially a focus for observing physical symptoms and area-related complaints. The complaints may also be an expression of a specific symbolic meaning that should be examined. Thus, questions of stigmatization and interpersonal communication in public may play a role if the head is involved, or of partnership or sexual disorders if the genitals are involved. In whole-body disorders, more complex biopsychosocial phenomena are often present.

Because the body dysmorphic disorder primarily affects the face, as it is the site of shame expression (as well as the breasts and genitals), shame becomes the main affect.

Shame assumes the interpersonal look of another and may lead to avoidance of the public with sociophobia due to the fear of visual exposure. An increased tendency to suicide is also assumed by most authors (Garcia-Parajua et al. 2003; Philipps et al. 2000). This was confirmed by a Swedish study that demonstrated that women have a higher suicide rate following cosmetic breast implantations (Koo et al. 2003).

Diagnostically, the body dysmorphic disorder is characterized primarily by the great discrepancy between the disfigurement as rated by the examiner and the disfigurement as experienced by the patient. The visual analog scale (VAS) has been found helpful as a simple scheme to determine this discrepancy to control the course. The person affected is given a VAS from 1 to 10 and indicates on this how much he or she feels disfigured. At the same time, the examiner also makes an independent rating of the quasi-objective disfigurement. If a discrepancy of more than 5 units on the VAS is found, there is a high grade of suspicion of a body dysmorphic disorder, which should then be more closely investigated and confirmed (see Chap. 14).

More precise diagnosis is now possible by the validated international questionnaires on problems of disfigurement that have been developed in the United States by Dufresne et al. (2001) and Jorgensen et al. (2001) and in Germany by Stangier et al. (2000).

In these patients there is a marked discrepancy between the desired ideal image and the actual or self-rated real image. A typical patient quote is "I can't stand myself." A self-esteem problem is nearly always found in body dysmorphic disorders and is often the focus in psychotherapy.

Differential diagnosis. The discussion around the classification of body dysmorphic disorders is still open and inconclusive. In the ICD-10, dysmorphophobia (F45.2) (synonyms include ugliness delusion and disfiguration anxiety) is classified as a subgroup of hypochondria.

The dominance and presence of compulsive disorders, social anxieties, depression, and narcissistic personality disorders must be differentiated. These may also be present in body dysmorphic disorder as comorbidities.

If the preoccupation with a presumed defect in appearance takes on delusional dimensions, persistent delusional disorders (Sect. 1.2) with skin-related or body-related delusions, body odor delusion, or delusional hypochondrias must be ruled out.

Patient's wish for therapy. In patients with body dysmorphic disorders, the desired treatment can really only achieve an apparent solution to the psychiatric disorder. The spectrum ranges from apparently harmless conservative measures such as lifestyle medications to major invasive procedures, including operations such as face lifts, liposuction, and breast modifications that require several hours of narcosis.

Severity of the Desired Treatment

- Mild: conservative therapy (lifestyle medications)
- Moderate: chemical peeling, botulinus toxin, laser therapy
- Serious: invasive operations under narcosis, augmentation, lifting

Operative procedures (Crisp 1981; Tvrdek et al. 1998) or long periods of medication use may, however, potentiate the psychiatric disorder and lead to further unsuccessful treatment. Moreover, the expert-killer syndrome phenomenon must be taken into account (see Chap. 17).

Corresponding patients with body dysmorphic disorders may then have corrected new noses, ears, breasts, or hips with which they are still dissatisfied (Strian 1984). Invasive operative procedures or conservative therapies are contraindicated in body dysmorphic disorder. Therapy of the psychosocial disorder takes first place (psychotherapy, psychopharmaceuticals).

Medical therapy. It is important that the suspected diagnosis of body dysmorphic disorder be made early. The prognosis for psychosomatic/psychiatric illnesses, as for other organic diseases, is better the earlier that diagnosis and therapy are begun.

A warning is also in order against repeated, but unnecessary, organic diagnostics. These run the risk that the patient will become fixated on a purely somatic/physical understanding of illness and may contribute to the strengthening and chronification of the psychiatric disorder.

The therapeutic consequences must be determined individually and may include psychodynamic psychotherapy, psychoanalysis, or behavior therapy as well as psychopharmaceutical therapy strategies. In practice, the first goal is to take the patient's complaints seriously and understand them. Thematization of the frequently underlying conflict situation is often possible through taking an extended history of the patient's psychosocial situation. Confrontation with the psychiatric disorder too early is not appropriate.

The discussion often veers away from the symptom toward psychosocial aspects. Psychoeducation has been found especially beneficial here (see Chap. 18).

Stepwise Plan for Body Dysmorphic Disorders

1. Psychosomatic primary care
2. Psychoeducation (taking the environment into account)
3. Motivation for psychotherapy
4. Behavior therapy (cognitive restructuring)
5. Integrative psychodynamic psychotherapy
6. Psychopharmaceuticals (SSRIs)

The motivation of the patient with body dysmorphic disorders for the expanded psychosocial treatment concept is usually low and presents a great challenge to the dermatologist. Initially, this may be attempted as part of psychosomatic primary care.

Basically, the principles of patient management as described by Rief and Hiller (1992) for medical and psychosomatic care can be applied to somatoform disorders/body dysmorphic disorders in skin diseases.

Initial Patient Management in Somatoform/Body Dysmorphic Disorders

- Establishment of a doctor–patient relationship characterized by acceptance and understanding

- Presentation of an adequate (multifactorial) explanatory model
- Working out of the relationships between the skin problem and eliciting emotional and cognitive as well as unconscious reaction patterns
- Preparation for more intensive psychotherapy, taking the patient's motivation into account

The efficacy of behavior therapy with cognitive restructuring has been demonstrated, and the success of behavioral programs has been presented in some studies with 2-year follow-up (McKay 1999; Wilhelm et al. 1999).

The approach designated integrative psychodynamic psychotherapy was described, for example, by Kholmogorova and Garanjan (2001) as a combination of cognitive and psychodynamic components especially for somatoform disorders. The possible group psychotherapeutic psychodynamic therapy approach also offers approaches for inpatient treatment of somatoform disorders.

The therapy approach that we prefer has the advantage that there is not only a learned behavior pattern but also observation of a conflict model underlying the symptom, which can be worked out with the patient. Working out the unconscious elements by reflecting the transferences enables the patient to find a way to explain his or her disorder instead of simply working on the learned symptom reactions.

To stabilize the explanatory model found through psychodynamic therapy, cognitive procedures such as exercises with the VAS are performed, since the aim is to identify not only an explanatory model for the case in question but also a means to apply this to everyday living. The new patterns of relationships must be experienced and stabilized.

Psychopharmaceuticals. In somatoform disorders, there may be a heterogeneous pattern of different psychiatric disorders that even reaches a transition to psychotic disorders, such as the delusional form of body dysmorphic disorder. The target symptoms of the psychopharmaceuticals must be selected accordingly. A singular, uniform group of medications is not indicated. A large study of tricyclic antidepressants has shown a significantly better efficacy of clomipramine over desipramine in body dysmorphic disorder, but the two medications are rarely used in dermatology these days because of the less favorable side effect spectrum compared with SSRIs (Hollander et al. 1999).

Predominant in the treatment strategy of the delusional form is drug treatment with neuroleptics (see Chap. 15), and in the nondelusional type, adequate psychotherapy or drug combination therapy, usually with SSRIs.

Fluoxetine, sertraline, paroxetine, and citalopram generally show good efficacy in the therapy of somatoform disorders and have been used with promising results. Body dysmorphic disorders are currently treated with fluoxetine or fluvoxamine, with attention to side effects (Phillips et al. 2002; Hollander et al. 1999).

! SSRIs are the drug therapy of first choice in the treatment of nondelusional body dysmorphic disorders.

In light of comorbidities, a combination therapy or monotherapy with anxiolytics may also be indicated (Fig. 1.36).

References

Altamura C, Paluello MM, Mundo E, Medda S, Mannu P (2001) Clinical and subclinical body dysmorphic disorder. Eur Arch Psychiatry Clin Neurosci 251: 105–108

Bohne A, Keuthen NJ, Wilhelm S, Deckersbach T, Jenike MA (2002) Prevalence of symptoms of body dysmorphic disorder and its correlates: a cross-cultural comparison. Psychosomatics 43: 486–490

Brosig B, Kupfer J, Niemeier V, Gieler U (2001) The "Dorian Gray Syndrome": psychodynamic need for hair growth restorers and other "fountains of youth." Int J Clin Pharmacol Ther 39(7): 279–283

Cash TF (1992) The psychological effects of androgenetic alopecia in men. J Am Acad Dermatol 26(6): 926–931

Cotterill JA (1996) Body dysmorphic disorder. Dermatol Clin 14(3): 457–463

Crisp AH (1981) Dysmorphophobia and the search for cosmetic surgery. Br Med J (Clin Res Ed) 282(6270): 1099–1100

Dufresne RG, Phillips KA, Vittorio CC, Wilkel CS (2001) A screening questionnaire for body dysmorphic disorder in a cosmetic dermatologic surgery practice. Dermatol Surg 27: 457–462

Gabbay V, Asnis GM, Bello JA, Alonso CM, Serras SJ, O'Dowd MA (2003) New onset of body dysmorphic disorder following frontotemporal lesion. Neurology 61(1): 123–125

Garcia-Parajua P, Martinez Vio M, Ovejero Garcia S, Caballero Martinez L (2003) Severity in dysmorphophobia: description of two cases. Actas Esp Psiquiatr 31(3): 168–170

Gupta MA, Gupta AK (2001) Dissatisfaction with skin appearance among patients with eating disorders and non-clinical controls. Br J Dermatol 145(1): 110–113

Gupta MA, Johnson AM (2000) Nonweight-related body image concerns among female eating-disordered patients and nonclinical controls: some preliminary observations. Int J Eat Disord 27(3): 304–309

Harth W, Linse R (2001) Botulinophilia: contraindication for therapy with botulinum toxin. Int J Clin Pharmacol Ther 39(10): 460–463

Hollander E, Allen A, Kwon J, Aronowitz B, Schmeidler J, Wong C, Simeon D (1999) Clomipramine vs. desipramine crossover trial in body dysmorphic disorder: selective efficacy of a serotonin reuptake inhibitor in imagined ugliness. Arch Gen Psychiatry 56(11): 1033–1039

Jorgensen L, Castle D, Roberts C, Groth-Marnat G (2001) A clinical validation of the Dysmorphic Concern Questionnaire. Aust N Z J Psychiatry 35: 124–128

Kholmogorova A, Garanjan N (2001) A combination of cognitive and psychodynamic components in the psychotherapy of somatoform disorders. Psychother Psychosom Med Psychol 51: 212–218

Koot VCM, Peeters PHM, Granath F, Grobbee DE, Nyren O (2003) Total and cause specific mortality among Swedish women with cosmetic breast implants: prospective study. BMJ 326: 527–528

McKay D (1999) Two-year follow-up of behavioral treatment and maintenance for body dysmorphic disorder. Behav Modif 23: 620–629

Niemeier V, Harth W, Kupfer J, Mayer K, Linse R, Schill WB, Gieler U (2002) Prävalenz psychosomatische Charakteristika in der Dermatologie. Hautarzt 53: 471–477

Oosthuizen P, Lambert T, Castle DJ (1998) Dysmorphic concern: prevalence and associations with clinical variables. Aust N Z J Psychiatry 32: 129–132

Otto MW, Wilhelm S, Cohen LS, Harlow BL (2001) Prevalence of body dysmorphic disorder in a community sample of women. Am J Psychiatry 158: 2061–2063

Phillips KA, Dufresne RG, Wilkel CS, Vittorio CC (2000) Rate of body dysmorphic disorder in dermatology patients. J Am Acad Dermatol 42: 436–441

Phillips KA, Albertini RS, Rasmussen SA (2002) A randomized placebo-controlled trial of fluoxetine in body dysmorphic disorder. Arch Gen Psychiatry 59: 381–388

Pope HG Jr, Gruber AJ, Choi P, Olivardia R, Phillips KA (1997) Muscle dysmorphia. An underrecognized form of body dysmorphic disorder. Psychosomatics 38(6): 548–557

Porst H (2001) Manual der Impotenz. Uni-Med Science, Hamburg

Ravaldi C, Vannacci A, Zucchi T, Mannucci E, Cabras PL, Boldrini M, Murciano L, Rotella CM, Ricca V (2003) Eating disorders and body image disturbances among ballet dancers, gymnasium users and body builders. Psychopathology 36(5): 247–254

Rief W, Hiller W (1992) Somatoforme Störungen – Körperliche Symptome ohne organische Ursachen. Huber, Bern

Stangier U, Hungerbühler R, Meyer A, Wolter M (2000) Diagnostische Erfassung der körperdysmorphen Störung. Eine Pilotstudie. Nervenarzt 71(11): 876–884

Strian F (1984) Die Dysmorphophobie als Kontraindikation kosmetischer Störungen. Handchir Mikrochir Plast Chir 16: 243–245

Strumia R, Varotti E, Manzato E, Gualandi M (2001) Skin signs in anorexia nervosa. Dermatology 203(4): 314–317

Tvrdek M, Duskova M, Vrtiskova J (1998) Is there a borderline between reconstructive and aesthetic surgery? Acta Chir Plast 40(4): 91–95

Veale D, Kinderman P, Riley S, Lambrou C (2003) Self-discrepancy in body dysmorphic disorder. Br J Clin Psychol 42: 157–169

Veale D, Riley S (2001) Mirror, mirror on the wall, who is the ugliest of them all? The psychopathology of mirror gazing in body dysmorphic disorder. Behav Res Ther 39: 1381–1393

Wessells H, Lue TF, McAninch JW (1996) Complications of penile lengthening and augmentation seen at 1 referral center. J Urol 155(5): 1617–1620

Wilhelm S, Otto MW, Lohr B, Deckersbach T (1999) Cognitive behavior group therapy for body dysmorphic disorder: a case series. Behav Res Ther 37: 71–75

Further Reading

Busso C, Mordoh A, Llopis C, Haas R, Bello M, Woscoff A (2000) Prevalence of cutaneous manifestations in 200 patients with eating disorders. Int J Dermatol 39(5): 348–353

Choi PY, Pope HG Jr, Olivardia R (2002) Muscle dysmorphia: a new syndrome in weightlifters. Br J Sports Med 36(5): 375–376

Chung B (2001) Muscle dysmorphia: a critical review of the proposed criteria. Perspect Biol Med 44(4): 565–574

Harth W, Linse R (2002) Penisaugmentation, die dritte Ebene der körperdysmorphen Störung. Abstraktband 10. Jahrestagung, Gießen, Arbeitskreis psychosomatische Dermatologien (Sektion der DDG), S 33

Heckmann M, Ceballos-Baumann AO, Plewig G (2001) Botulinum toxin A for axillary hyperhidrosis (excessive sweating). N Engl J Med 344(7): 488–493

Hollander E, Aronowitz BR (1999) Comorbid social anxiety and body dysmorphic disorder: managing the complicated patient. J Clin Psychiatry 60(Suppl 9): 27–31

Kapfhammer H-P, Gündel H (Hrsg) (1997) Psychotherapie der Somatisierungsstörungen. Thieme, Stuttgart, S 104–116

Koblenzer CS (1985) The dysmorphic syndrome. Arch Dermatol 121(6): 780–784

Mayerhausen W, Vogt HJ, Fichter MM, Stahl S (1990) Dermatologic aspects of anorexia and bulimia nervosa. Hautarzt 41(9): 476–484

Neziroglu F, Stevens KP, McKay D, Yaryura-Tobias JA (2001) Predictive validity of the overvalued ideas scale: outcome in obsessive-compulsive and body dysmorphic disorders. Behav Res Ther 39: 745–756

Nierenberg AA, Phillips KA, Petersen TJ, Kelly KE, Alpert JE, Worthington JJ, Tedlow JR, Rosenbaum JF, Fava M (2002) Body dysmorphic disorder in outpatients with major depression. J Affect Disord 69: 141–148

Nissen B (2000) Hypochondria: a tentative approach. Int J Psychoanal 81: 651–666

Sass H, Wittchen H-U, Zaudig M (2001) Diagnostisches und Statistisches Manual Psychischer Störungen DSM-IV. Hogrefe, Göttingen

Schulze UM, Pettke-Rank CV, Kreienkamp M, Hamm H, Brocker EB, Wewetzer C, Trott GE, Warnke A (1999) Dermatologic findings in anorexia and bulimia nervosa of childhood and adolescence. Pediatr Dermatol 16(2): 90–94

Stangier U (2002) Hautkrankheiten und körperdysmorphe Störung. Hogrefe, Göttingen

Stangier U, Hungerbühler R, Meyer A, Wolter M, Deusinger I (1997) Depression, social anxiety and body image disturbance in body dysmorphic disorders. In: Dermatology and Psychiatry, 7th International Congress on Dermatology and Psychiatry. Abstract Book, Halle, p 13

1.3.3 Somatoform Autonomic Disorders (Functional Disorders)

Erythrophobia, goose bumps, and certain subgroups of hyperhidrosis in particular are among the somatoform autonomic functional disorders (ICD-10: F45.3).

A person's feelings are often apparent in skin changes. If these emotionally triggered skin presentations are experienced as subjectively bothersome and if at the same time they have psychosomatic relevance, the person afflicted sometimes consults a dermatologist to obtain relief. The characteristic of somatoform autonomic disorders is a repeated presentation of physical symptoms coupled with a stubborn demand for medical examinations, despite repeated negative results and assurance by the doctor that the symptoms are not pathological.

Facial Erythema (Blushing)

Blushing is a common phenomenon in our society, with erythema usually located in the cheeks and neck. The physiological and predisposed reactivity of this form of erythema is, however, usually well compensated emotionally and thus differs from erythrophobia.

Erythrophobia

If there is pronounced anxiety with respect to blushing or in some cases only an anxiety disorder without clinical blushing, the diagnosis is erythrophobia. Erythrophobia may cause detriment in important ways to social, professional, or other important functional areas and may lead to pronounced avoidance behavior in certain situations and in dealing with other people and to social withdrawal in the person's private or professional life.

Psychodynamically, there are characteristically two types of reaction: blushing (or fear of blushing) in rage and blushing associated to embarrassment.

The feeling of being "caught" can occur in a situation of familiar attention with concurrent fear of disdain or criticism. Usually, the capacity for self-assertion and self-perception is damaged, and anxiety coupled with inhibited aggression arises.

The diagnostics and differential diagnosis between this somatoform autonomic functional disorder and a body dysmorphic disorder are often difficult because the boundary is blurred. In some cases, a single case decision or double diagnosis is then necessary (Fig. 1.37).

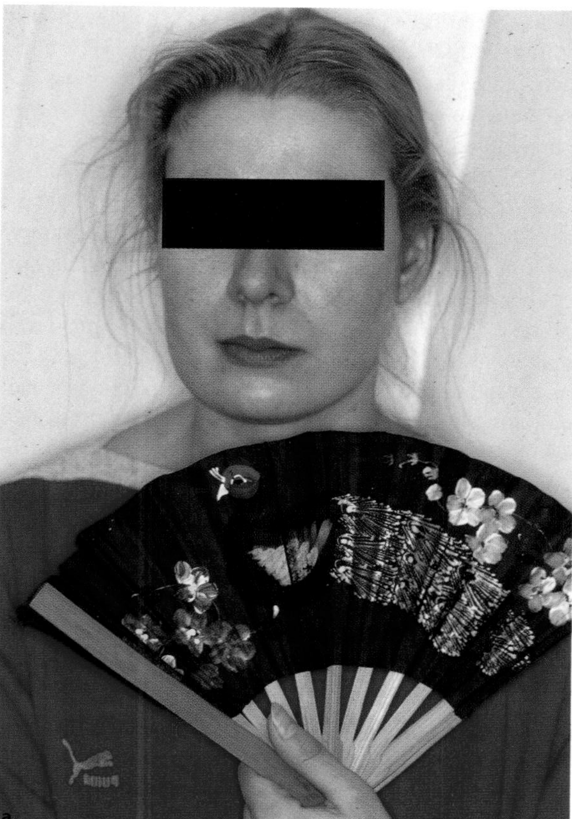

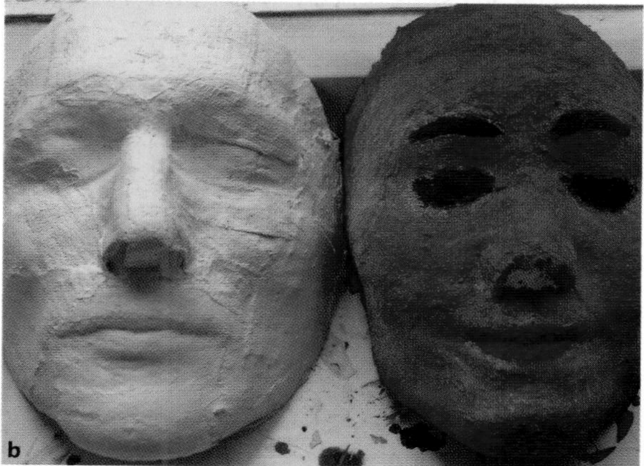

Fig. 1.37 **a** Woman with fan and erythrophobia without physical findings in the sense of a body dysmorphic disorder. **b** Erythrophobia in art therapy

Goose Bumps (Cutis Anserina)

Goose bumps consist of follicular papules secondary to contraction of the piloerector muscles

The nervous excitation of this muscle proceeds via nerve fibers that are excited by nerve messenger substances (neuropeptides). The neurons in turn are connected directly to the brain via the spinal cord and the central nervous system so that stimulations are transported to the skin. Goose bumps cannot be voluntarily elicited. The presentation appears to be unconscious or only vegetatively controlled, but it can also be elicited by physical stimuli including cold and electrical current. How emotions and affects activate these nerve pathways has not yet been investigated, although it is a very well-known phenomenon. Goose bumps may also be elicited by a gentle breath of air, which sets in motion the vellus hairs. Genetic factors also play a role here, since not all people tend to such reactions. It is, however, a good example for the close connection between the central nervous system and the skin via a blastodermic layer, the ectodermis, which was determined in the embryonic development of the human being. Blushing occurs similarly to goose bumps, but instead of the contraction of hair bulb muscles, the small skin vessels dilate and thus cause erythema. Both phenomena can, however, be directly influenced by emotional reactions.

Hyperhidrosis

Hyperhidrosis affecting primarily the hands, feet, or axillae often occurs in the framework of certain individually different situations with vegetative liability. This usually occurs in stressful situations such as examinations, public speaking, or particularly anxiety-laden situations. Even Hippocrates (about 460–377 BC) reported that fear may cause sweating.

Hyperhidrosis is a problem area that, although broad, has received little attention thus far in dermatology. There are blurred boundaries with a number of psychiatric disorders, and the differential diagnosis must distinguish between a secondary hyperhidrosis as a consequence of organ diseases (Chap. 2), body dysmorphic disorder (Sect. 1.3.2, botulinophilia), or delusional disorders (Sect. 1.2, body odor delusion).

A detailed discussion is found in Chap. 2 on multifactorial dermatoses.

1.3.4 Persistent Somatoform Pain Disorders (Cutaneous Dysesthesias)

In persistent somatoform pain disorders (ICD-10: F45.4; DSM-IV-TR: 307.80 associated with psychological factors):

- Pain is predominant in the presentation and reported by the patient as clinically significant.
- The pain causes suffering and/or professional and social detriment.
- However, it is not explained by a somatic cause or other psychiatric disorder.

Categorization. In dermatology, somatoform pain disorders usually express as regional cutaneous dysesthesias and mucosal dysesthesias. Predominant among them are glossodynia (orofacial pain syndrome), vulvodynia, phallodynia, trichodynia, and anodynia (Table 1.8).

It should be noted here that the classic classification of somatoform pain disorders (ICD-10: F45.4) must be reconsidered because other sensory complaints, such as burning and tingling, are often present and thus may represent a transition to an "other somatoform disorder" (ICD-10: F45.8).

The following clinical entities are among the clinically important pain syndromes in dermatology.

Dermatodynia

Dermatodynia is very rare, and hardly any publications on this condition are available. The painfulness of the entire skin (dermatodynia) usually occurs only in organic nerve disorders or as a result of viscerocutaneous reflexes.

Glossodynia

Definition. Glossodynia (ICD-10: K14.6, F45.4 and F22.0 DSM-IV-TR: 307.80 pain disorder with psychological factors) involves dysesthesias with burning pain or tingling in the tongue and other parts of the oral mucosa.

Clinical findings. The complaints in the mouth show no organically confirmable pathology. If somatic disorders are present, they do not explain the type or extent of the patient's symptoms, suffering, and internal involvement.

Psychiatric symptoms. About 50% of the patients with glossodynia present with deviating personality disorders. In 33–82%, life events, especially loss of a partner, can be proven (Huang et al. 1996). There is frequent association with depressive moods and anxiety disorders. In addition, there is evidence that glossodynia patients present with symptoms of alexithymia (Miyaoka et al. 1996). Thus, these patients are characteristically unable to express their feelings (Pasquini et al. 1997).

In a study of 335 psychosomatic skin patients (Niemeier et al. 2002), glossodynia patients were more likely

Table 1.8 Classification of dysesthesias

Generalized cutaneous dysesthesias		
		Dermatodynia
		Hemialgia (pain on one side of the body)
Regional cutaneous dysesthesias	Head	Glossodynia
		Scalp dysesthesia
		Trichodynia
	Urogenital pain syndromes	Vulvodynia
		Orchiodynia
		Urodynia
		Urethral syndrome
		Phallodynia (phallalgia, penile pain syndrome)
		Prostatodynia
		Coccygodynia
		Perineal pain syndrome
		Anodynia
		Proctodynia
	Special forms	Erythromelalgia
		Trigeminal neuralgia
		Postzosteric neuralgia
		Proctalgia fugax

to present unremarkably in all psychological test inventories of self-rating than patients in other disease groups. Medically, however, the importance of emotional factors for the course of the disorder in glossodynia is rated the highest (Gieler et al. 2001).

The contradiction in rating between patient and doctor can be explained psychodynamically by a pronounced defense mechanism (denial, suppression) on the patient's part. Practical experience shows that hypochondriacal disorders may additionally be important.

Psychotherapy. Strong denial and great resistance to a psychosomatic explanatory model are accompanied by the patient's expectation of a purely somatic treatment and rejection of the causally important psychiatric disorder. Frequently these are "difficult" patients, and the doctor and the patient are bound from a psychodynamic point of view by a transference/countertransference dynamic that is hard to resolve. This often causes a problem in the practice. The psychiatric disorder cannot be treated without appropriate motivation on the patient's part.

Foremost in the therapy is the patient's motivation as part of psychosomatic primary care, whereby more detailed thematization of central conflicts beyond psychoeducation as the minimum basis is not possible. In part, psychosomatic access succeeds via thematization of the current psychosocial life situation. Keeping a pain diary

1

that includes emotional factors is decisive, as is scheduling follow-up appointments.

Once the patient is successfully motivated, psychotherapy is aimed at the dominating underlying disorder. A causally important somatized depression is usually predominant (Fig. 1.38).

Psychopharmaceuticals. The use of antidepressants is often given preference over psychodynamic therapy, also due to the patient's age and lack of motivation. According to most reports and experience discussed in the literature, tricyclic antidepressants such as doxepin or even neuroleptics are preferred. Attention must be particularly paid to the anticholinergic side effects including dry mouth, which may worsen complaints related to the oral mucosa. Newer antidepressants such as mirtazapine should perhaps be preferred, but there are no corresponding studies yet.

Case reports with gabapentin have been published frequently of late and report good therapeutic success. This is an off-label use in dermatology and often requires relatively high doses.

References

Gieler U, Niemeier V, Kupfer J, Brosig B, Schill WB (2001) Psychosomatische Dermatologie in Deutschland. Eine Umfrage an 69 Hautkliniken. Hautarzt 52: 104–110

Huang W, Rothe MJ, Grant-Kels JM (1996) The burning mouth syndrome. J Am Acad Dermatol 34(1): 91–98

Miyaoka H, Kamijima K, Katayama Y, Ebihara T, Nagai T (1996) A psychiatric appraisal of "glossodynia." Psychosomatics 37: 346–348

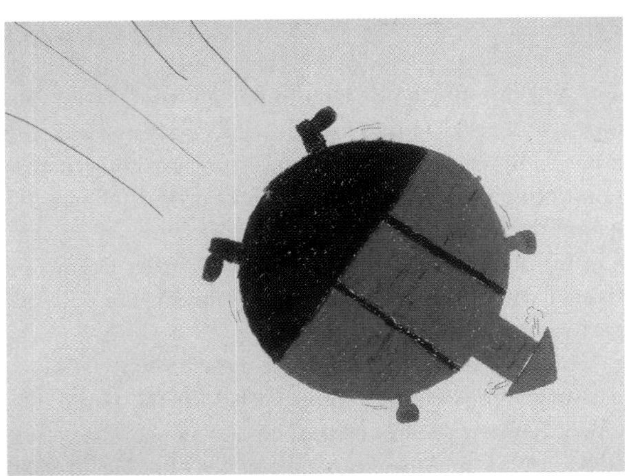

Fig. 1.38 Painting therapy: woman with pronounced glossodynia and rage

Niemeier V, Kupfer J, Harth W, Brosig B, Schill WB, Gieler U (2002) Sind Patienten mit Glossodynie psychisch unauffällig? Eine psychodiagnostisch schwer fassbare Erkrankung. Psychother Psychosom Med Psychol 52: 425–432

Pasquini M, Bitetti D, Decaminada F, Pasquini P (1997) Insecure attachment and psychosomatic skin disease. Ann Ist Super Sanita 33: 605–608

Further Reading

Meiss F, Fiedler E, Taube KM, Marsch WC, Fischer M (2004) Gabapentin in the treatment of glossodynia. Dermatol Psychosom 5: 17–21

Niemeier V, Kupfer J, Brosig B, Gieler U (2001) Glossodynia as an expression of a somatoform disorder – a hard-to-grasp psychodiagnostic disease? With presentation of a single case from a psychodynamic point of view. Dermatol Psychosom 2: 134–141

Ploeg HM van der, Wal N van der, Eijkman MA, Waal I van der (1987) Psychological aspects of patients with burning mouth syndrome. Oral Surg Oral Med Oral Pathol 63(6): 664–668

Scala A, Checchi L, Montevecchi M, Marini I, Giamberardino MA (2003) Update on burning mouth syndrome: overview and patient management. Crit Rev Oral Biol Med 14(4): 275–291

Trichodynia/Scalp Dysesthesia

Occurrence. Thirty-four percent of patients with hair loss, including chronic telogen effluvium as well as androgenetic alopecia and particularly follicular degeneration syndrome, suffer painful sensations in the scalp with no pathological somatic finding (Rebora et al. 1996). Due to the discrepancy with clinical findings, the authors postulate a somatoform disorder and scientifically corroborate the term trichodynia, which is reported by a large number of patients with hair loss.

Pathogenesis. The neuropeptide substance P is may be identified as a possible cause of the unpleasant sensations.

Definition. In trichodynia, there are painful dysesthesias, especially in the hair and even more so when the hair is touched. In scalp dysesthesia, there are painful dysesthesias of the scalp.

Differential diagnosis. The term trichodynia, which is often used in the literature, does not always appear to be entirely precise because the scalp usually hurts (scalp dysesthesia; Hoss and Segal 1998), and the pain is projected to the hair (Trueb 1997). The transition to scalp dysesthesia is then blurred, and a sharp differential-diagnostic separation from trichodynia is often hardly possible and of little practical use.

Clinical findings. No pathological clinical finding can be identified in trichodynia. In some patients, a paraartefact in the sense of a localized skin-picking syndrome in the hair of the head may occur due to the trichodynia (Fig. 1.39).

Psychiatric symptoms. Based on the incongruity between objectifiable clinical findings and the subjectively described symptoms, trichodynia is a somatoform disorder and thus a psychiatric disorder without clinical correlate. Trichodynia is therefore comparable to other somatoform pain disorders (cutaneous dysesthesias) such as glossodynia and vulvodynia. Seventy-six percent of patients with trichodynia present with psychiatric signs, especially depression, compulsive disorders, and anxiety disorders (Kivanc-Altunay et al. 2003).

Trichodynia may occasionally occur in connection with fear of hair loss. Hair loss or even the fear of hair loss may cause or promote painful sensations or other sensitivity disorders. A depressive episode may potentiate painful dysesthesias.

Differential diagnosis. The patients complain of pain around the roots of the hair. Differential diagnosis must rule out a body dysmorphic disorder if the presumably disfiguring hair loss predominates in the complaint symptoms. Moreover, there may be monosymptomatic hypochondriacal disorders, conversion disorders, or a somatized depression.

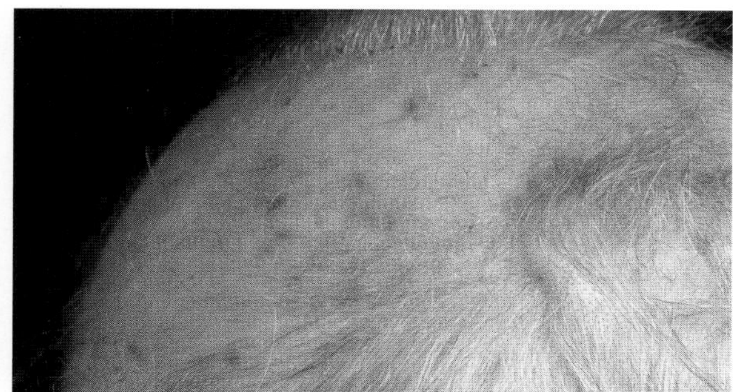

Fig. 1.39 A 67-year-old man with trichodynia in depression. Due to the trichodynia, there is dermatitis paraartefacta syndrome self-manipulation (skin-picking syndrome), which is conspicuous in the area of alopecia

Differential Diagnosis for Trichodynia

- Cutaneous dysesthesia
- Cutaneous hypochondrias (fear of disease)
- Somatized depression
- Dysesthesia as part of an ecosyndrome (environment-related physical complaints)
- Body dysmorphic disorder
- Monosymptomatic hypochondriacal psychosis
- Body dysmorphic delusion

Psychotherapy and psychopharmaceuticals. No studies of large groups of patients have been performed regarding therapy of trichodynia or scalp dysesthesia. Psychotherapy should be determined according to the somatoform disorder and carried out as for other cutaneous pain syndromes (refer to stepwise plan).

Single case reports show depressive and anxiety disorder as comorbidities, for which antidepressants, doxepin, and alprazolam are favored as therapeutic options (Hoss and Segal 1998).

References

Hoss D, Segal S (1998) Scalp dysesthesia. Arch Dermatol 134: 327–330

Kivanc-Altunay I, Savas C, Gokdemir G, Koslu A, Ayaydin EB (2003) The presence of trichodynia in patients with telogen effluvium and androgenetic alopecia. Int J Dermatol 42(9): 691–693

Rebora A, Semino MT, Guarrera M (1996) Trichodynia. Dermatology 192: 292–293

Trueb RM (1997) Trichodynie. Hautarzt 48(12): 877–880

Urogenital and Rectal Pain Syndromes

Pain syndromes in the urogenital and rectal areas, perineum, and anus have been well described but not well studied and are usually very resistant to therapy. Chronic pelvic complaints in men are a frequent psychosomatic syndrome. These patients often present with depressive disorders, compulsive disorders, or hypochondriacal disorders, comparable to glossodynia.

Therapy is successful only when it takes biopsychosocial aspects into account; invasive therapeutic procedures should be avoided (Krege et al. 2003; Wesselmann et al. 1997).

Vulvodynia, phallodynia (phallalgia, penile pain syndrome), orchiodynia, urethral syndrome, prostatodynia, urodynia, perineal pain syndrome, coccygodynia, anodynia, proctodynia, and proctalgia fugax also belong to this symptom complex. The majority of publications on this disorder complex concern vulvodynia.

Phallodynia/Orchiodynia/Prostatodynia

Genital pain in men usually affects the testicles and perineum. Isolated pain in the penis occurs less frequently. Persistent, pulling pain of varying intensity is usually reported.

Clinical findings. The patients report qualitatively different complaints, such as a feeling of pressure in the perineum, pulling in the groin that sometimes radiates to the testicles, an increased urge to urinate, burning in the distal urethra, a feeling of pressure or burning behind the pubis, or a feeling of tension in the lower back. In addition, somatization disorders including increased sweating, inner restlessness, tachycardia, sleep disorders, and heartburn may also occur.

Psychiatric symptoms. After organic diseases have been ruled out, etiological components such as impaired sexuality, physical false posture, neuroticism, and exhaustion symptoms may be assumed, behind which, in turn, there may be a compulsive personality structure, sexual problems, or spousal conflicts (Brähler et al. 2002).

Psychodynamically, conflicts with ambition, a striving for delineation and autonomy, and devotional desires are related to genital pain syndromes. In patients with chronic pains, depressive moods, the feeling of increasing powerlessness, fatigue and exhaustion, and fear of further limitations also play a decisive role in general.

Differential diagnosis. Prostate inflammation must first be ruled out. If one-sided testicular pain is reported as the only symptom, the doctor must rule out neoplasia and affections of nerve roots L1 and L2. A chronic inflammatory process may be the cause of persistent penile pain, such as penile erysipelas, balanoposthitis, cavernitis, urethritis, or, in rare cases, Peyronie's disease.

Anodynia/Proctalgia Fugax

Isolated anodynia is rare and usually occurs with phallodynia or vulvodynia in the sense of a so-called anogenital pain syndrome or as part of anal or perianal eczema (Chap. 2). The first evidence of the origin of pain is often found in the description of the pain character. The predominant complaint symptom is a persistent, severe, and tormenting pain that cannot be explained by a physical disorder. A psychogenically caused rectal pain can persist even during diagnostic spinal or peridural anesthesia.

Differential-diagnostically, there may be chronic pain in the perineum, especially in chronic prostate inflammation.

Some patients additionally develop proctalgia fugax, which is characterized by acute intense rectal pain (anorectal neuralgia), often nocturnal and usually affecting males.

Psychiatric symptoms. The anogenital area is a preferred part of the body for symbolic pain (conversion neurosis). It occurs in connection with emotional conflicts or psychosocial problems. The result is usually considerable medical care and attention.

If somatoform pain disorders persist, compulsive disorders and depressive disorders must be considered.

Vulvodynia

The term vulvodynia denotes chronic states of pain in the exterior female genitals. Chronic pain syndromes such as chronic pelvic pain syndrome and chronic vulvodynia account for about 15–20% of all consultations in outpatient gynecological care (Scialli 1999).

Psychiatric symptoms. In tests and psychological questionnaires of self-rating, patients with vulvodynia showed clearly greater psychosocial signs and tendency to somatization than a control group (Stewart et al. 1994). Characteristically, these patients show more anxiety disorders, hypochondriacal disorders, and sexual disorders. Ten percent report sexual abuse in their history, and attention must be paid to this. Moreover, there are significant connections between the occurrence of chronic lower abdominal pain and psychosocial stress, including marital/spousal conflicts.

Differential diagnosis. Differential diagnosis must rule out a localized pruritus in the genitals (pruritus genitalis) and urticaria factitia, which, however, may also be triggered by emotional factors.

Other somatic differential diagnoses of vulvodynia include the following:

- Essential vulvodynia
- Vulvodynia due to dermatoses
- Vulvodynia due to vulvovestibulitis; in this type of vulvodynia, pain is especially severe during coitus
- Vulvodynia due to vulvovaginitis

Special Forms

Erythromelalgia

Erythromelalgia is a specific pain syndrome limited to the skin, which is characterized by, intense painful hyperemia localized in the feet and sometimes including the hands, possibly by a defect in prostaglandin metabolism. The mutation of a sodium channel has been found to mediate familial erythromelalgia. One must rule out the presence of lupus, polycythemia vera, and multiple sclerosis. Therapies include calcium channel inhibitors and SSRIs.

Differential-diagnostically, acrodynia may also cause painful and itching or burning erythema by mercury intoxication in childhood, and painful skin reddening can also develop during phototherapy treatment.

Erythromelalgia may be triggered in some patients by emotional stress. Emotional elicitability has also been demonstrated by some reports of successful therapy of erythromelalgia with relaxation procedures, including hypnosis (Chakravarty et al. 1992).

Posthepetic Neuralgias

Following viral infections, especially with the varicella zoster virus, persistent, chronic pain symptoms that are hard to treat may occur. Disorders in coping with disease, depressive disorders, and also adjustment disorders are foremost as additional emotional triggers.

Trigeminal Neuralgia

Trigeminal neuralgia is a facial pain limited to the area of the trigeminal branch. There may be acute, sudden pain or a chronic recurrent course.

Notalgia Paresthetica

Localized notalgia paresthetica (Goulden et al. 1998) is a neuroradicular disease in which emotionally triggerable burning pain, paresthesias, or pruritus occurs in a discrete area on the upper back, usually over the scapula.

Local treatment includes topical local anesthetics, corticosteroids, and capsaicin.

Dissociative Sensitivity and Sensory Disorders (F44.6)

The phenomenon of assumed anesthetic skin areas is ascribed differential-diagnostically to the dissociative disorders and should be mentioned here. Various losses of different sensory modalities may be reported without corresponding to a neurological lesion or disease. The anesthetic skin areas more likely correspond to the patient's idea of body functions than to medical knowledge (see Chap. 3, Fig. 3.7). Neurological investigation is warranted, as well as consideration of the possibility of infectious diseases such as leprosy.

Therapy Summary

Psychotherapy. The basis of every therapy in almost all cases is initially to keep a complaint diary and determine the VAS score (Chap. 13).

> **Stepwise Plan for Pain Syndromes**
>
> 1. Psychosomatic primary care
> 2. Visual analog scale (VAS)
> 3. Pain dairy (complaint diary)
> 4. Psychoeducation
> 5. Relaxation therapy
> 6. Psychodynamic therapy (analysis of past conflicts)
> 7. Psychopharmaceuticals (depending on dominating comorbidity)

When and in what situations the complaints occur can be entered in the complaint diary. At the next appointment, the entries can be discussed with the patient and structured. The VAS helps in recording the extent of pains or complaints from the patient's point of view. The score also provides a course control of the therapeutic program.

Relaxation techniques can be a helpful support (Krege et al. 2003). The motivation for an expanded treatment concept is often low, so psychoeducation and psychosomatic primary care take precedence.

The question of when psychotherapy is indicated in pain syndromes depends on comorbidities, present conflicts and patient's motivation. Depending on the underlying psychosomatic disorder or comorbidity, a focal therapy may offer an effective therapeutic option.

Psychopharmaceuticals. Trials with local anesthetics have been described in individual cases, but they have no significant relevance. Treatment with classic pain relievers often has no effect in urogenital and rectal pain syndromes. According to empirical reports, antidepressants and relaxation procedures can be considered the therapy of first choice (Wesselmann et al. 1997).

Most literature reports and experiences recommend the use of tricyclic antidepressants or SSRIs in cutaneous pain syndromes. The treatment of first choice in urogenital and rectal pain syndromes is the SSRIs (fluoxetine, sertraline, paroxetine, citalopram).

Therapy of cutaneous pain syndromes is done today by taking the comorbidities into account (depressive disorders, anxiety disorders) and primarily using SSRIs, doxepin, or amitriptyline.

Gabapentin (Neurontin) appears to be successful in individual cases and thus offers an alternative to the use of antidepressants in pain symptoms, although this is an off-label use. Individual reports show good efficacy of gabapentin for the treatment of glossodynia; it is supposed to show better efficacy than antidepressants because, for example, SSRIs may potentiate the complaint symptoms of glossodynia due to anticholinergic side effects such as dry mouth. There are also positive single case reports on other cutaneous pain syndromes in other localizations (Sasaki et al. 2001). The mean daily dose is 900–1,200 mg and may be increased long term to 2,400 mg/day.

Amitriptyline (Elavil), a tricyclic antidepressant, is the drug of first choice in severe states of pain, including postherpetic neuralgias; 25–75 mg may be taken in the evening.

Doxepin (Sinequan) and carbamazepine (Tegretol) are also effective. If these do not show an effect, treatment with atypical antipsychotics can be attempted.

Treatment with botulinus toxin is reported to produce good therapeutic benefits in proctalgia fugax (Katsinelos et al. 2001; Table 1.9).

References

Brähler E, Berberich H, Kupfer J (2002) Sexualität und Psychosomatik der chronischen Beckenbeschwerden des Mannes. In: Seikowski K, Starke K (Hrsg) Sexualität des Mannes. Pabst, Lengerich, S 81–90

Chakravarty K, Pharoah PD, Scott DG, Baker S (1992) Erythromelalgia – the role of hypnotherapy. Postgrad Med J 68: 44–46

Table 1.9 Pharmacologic therapy of persistent somatoform pain disorders (*SSRIs* selective serotonin reuptake inhibitors)

Psychiatric disorder		Therapy
Head	Glossodynia	SSRIs, paroxetine, sertraline, citalopram, fluoxetine
		2nd choice: doxepin, amitriptyline mirtazapine, gabapentin, low dose antipsychotics
	Trichodynia, scalp dysesthesia	SSRIs, doxepin or alprazolam
Urogenital pain syndromes	Phallodynia, Orchiodynia, Prostatodynia, Anodynia, Proctodynia, Vulvodynia	SSRIs; note that erectile dysfunction possible
		2nd choice: tricyclic antidepressants, doxepin
Special form	Postherpetic neuralgia	Amitriptyline
		2nd choice: doxepin, carbamazepine, gabapentin, low dose antipsychotics
	Erythromelalgia	Calcium channel blockers, SSRIs
	Proctalgia fugax	SSRIs, individual cases botulinum toxin?

Goulden V, Toomey PJ, Highet AS (1998) Successful treatment of notalgia paresthetica with a paravertebral local anesthetic block. J Am Acad Dermatol 38(1): 114–116

Katsinelos P, Kalomenopoulou M, Christodoulou K, Katsiba D, Tsolkas P, Pilpilidis I, Papagiannis A, Kapitsinis I, Vasiliadis I, Souparis T (2001) Treatment of proctalgia fugax with Botulinum A toxin. Eur J Gastroenterol Hepatol 13(11): 1371–1373

Krege S, Ludwig M, Kloke M, Rubben H (2003) Chronic pain syndrome in urology. Urologe A 42(5): 669–674

Sasaki K, Smith CP, Chuang YC, Lee JY, Kim JC, Chancellor MB (2001) Oral gabapentin (Neurontin) treatment of refractory genitourinary tract pain. Tech Urol 7(1): 47–49

Scialli AR (1999) Evaluating chronic pelvic pain. A consensus recommendation. Pelvic Pain Expert Working Group. J Reprod Med 44(11): 945–952

Stewart DE, Reicher AE, Gerulath AH, Boydell KM (1994) Vulvodynia and psychological distress. Obstet Gynecol 84: 587–590

Wesselmann U, Burnett AL, Heinberg LJ (1997) The urogenital and rectal pain syndromes. Pain 73(3): 269–294

Further Reading

Bodden-Heidrich R, Kuppers V, Beckmann MW, Ozornek MH, Rechenberger I, Bender HG (1999) Psychosomatic aspects of vulvodynia. Comparison with the chronic pelvic pain syndrome. J Reprod Med 44(5): 411–416

Edwards L (2003) New concepts in vulvodynia. Am J Obstet Gynecol 189(Suppl 3): 24–30

Luzzi GA (2002) Chronic prostatitis and chronic pelvic pain in men: aetiology, diagnosis and management. J Eur Acad Dermatol Venereol 16(3): 253–256

Pukall CF, Payne KA, Binik YM, Khalife S (2003) Pain measurement in vulvodynia. J Sex Marital Ther 29(Suppl 1): 111–120

Zermann DH, Ishigooka M, Doggweiler R, Schmidt RA (1999) Neurourological insights into the etiology of genitourinary pain in men. J Urol 161(3): 903–908

1.3.5 Other Undifferentiated Somatoform Disorders (Cutaneous Sensory Disorders)

Cutaneous sensory disorders are also differentiated from somatoform pain disorders (cutaneous dysesthesias) and are classified with the other undifferentiated somatoform disorders (ICD-10: F45.8).

In particular, the following sensory disorders may occur in dermatology:

- Itching
- Burning
- Tingling
- Stabbing pain

! There are often qualitative variations and descriptions of the symptoms, with mixed presentations of itching and stabbing, tingling and stabbing, or burning and pain.

Unpleasant sensations of burning often overlap with the pain syndromes such as glossodynia, which must be differential-diagnostically clarified.

Tingling, stabbing, and biting pains are most often found in patients with delusion of parasitosis with presumed parasites in the skin. Primary among the group of cutaneous sensory disorders is somatoform itching, which is discussed in detail below.

Somatoform Itching

Pruritus is one of the most important and most frequent complaints cited as a symptom in dermatology.

Pathogenesis. Initially, an attempt was made to interpret pruritus as a subliminal pain stimulus. There are, of course, known analogies to pain; however, researchers in this field have shown that puritus is transmitted via specialized C-fibers and is mediated only in part by the pain fibers (Magerl 1991; Handwerker 1993, 1998; Schmelz et al. 1997). Itching is elicited by direct mechanical stimulation or physical or chemical stimuli (release of histamine) of sensitive nerve endings. The perception of the feeling of pruritus is coupled with the motor response of scratching as a spinal reflex and can be inhibited by cortical and subcortical centers. In addition, synaptic connections of nerve fibers to immunocompetent cells in the skin are known, which make not only efferent but also afferent itching plausible (Williams et al. 1995; Bienenstock et al. 1991; Naukkarinen et al. 1991). Neuropeptides and neurokinins in the skin are presently in the focus of pruritus research (Luger and Lotti 1998).

The intensity of pruritus depends on the part of the body, the time of day, and the subjective stress. Itching can be provoked not only by mechanical, electrical, or chemical stimuli but also emotionally (Rechenberger 1981). Itching occurs conspicuously often in emotional excitation (rage, annoyance, excitement, and, less often, joy). It is assumed that substances that elicit pruritus and transmitters in the vegetative nervous system can potentiate or decrease the sensitivity to itching.

Definition. The characteristic of somatoform pruritus is repeated presentation of physical symptoms coupled with a stubborn demand for medical examination despite the repeated absence of primary dermatological lesions.

The diagnosis of somatoform itching is basically possible in practice according to the following additional criteria:
- The presence of psychological factors that play an important role with respect to the onset, severity, elicitation, or maintenance of itching
- Great suffering or great detriment to social or professional life
- Preoccupation (both in thoughts and acts) with the pruritus or the state of the skin
- A search for medical assurance (for example, allergy tests)

Clinical findings. Two groups can be differentiated in somatoform itching:
- Generalized somatoform itching (e.g., pruritus sine materia)
- Localized somatoform itching

Generalized Somatoform Pruritus (Pruritus Sine Materia)

Pruritus sine materia (ICD-10: F45.8) is the chronic occurrence of usually subliminal psychogenic itching after diseases that would causally explain the pruritus have been ruled out (e.g., diabetes, lymphoma, hepatogenic itching). The clinical presentation is usually unremarkable or shows excoriations. Women older than 50 are typically affected (Fig. 1.40).

Localized Somatoform Pruritus

Characteristically, tormenting itching of unclear genesis is in the foreground of localized pruritus, with the genital or anal region being especially affected in dermatology.

Psychiatric symptoms. Itching, including the generalized form, can also be elicited mentally (Arnetz and Fjellner 1985). The emotional and cognitive perception of pruritus is seen in the following aspects:
- The intensity of itching is dependent on seeking attention and on subjective controllability (Scholz and Hermanns 1994).
- A close connection has been determined between depression and itching, both in laboratory studies (Arnetz and Fjellner 1985) and in clinical trials with dermatological patients (Gupta et al. 1989; Gupta et al. 1994; Sheehan-Dare et al. 1990).
- Animal experimental studies confirm that the secretion of histamine, one of the most important itch-eliciting mediator substances, can be conditioned in a Pavlovian model (Russell et al. 1984).

These findings indicate the possibility that itching reactions are subject to central nervous control and may be transferred by learning and memory processes to nonorganic stimuli.

> **!** **Itching can be elicited or potentiated mentally and through stress. Attention must be paid to the vicious cycle of itching and depression.**

Depression and anxiety are often found as comorbidities with pruritus sine materia. Moreover, there are impairments in coping with disease, and coping with the disease itself may also lead to depression and psychosocial conflicts. In skin diseases associated with the symptom of pruritus, it is recommended that the patient be questioned about elicitors of the itching (stress, burdens, changes in life). Particular attention must be paid to the itching and scratching cycle in patients with atopic eczema (Chap. 2).

According to Schultz-Amling and Köhler-Weisker (1996), localized genital or anal itching can often be interpreted as an expression of a (not necessarily unconscious) sexual conflict and is thus frequently a conversion disorder. This could apply, for example, in a patient with localized pruritus in the vaginal area after she has separated from her partner. The localized pruritus can be understood as a conversion symptom in such an individual case, even knowing that not every case of pruritus genitalis may be so interpreted when no clear recordable psychosocial aspects of this sort are found (Fig. 1.40b).

Differential diagnosis. The diagnosis of a somatoform pruritus (sine materia) should not be made until after a thorough ruling-out of internal diseases. Unclear itching in young patients is especially atypical and can be seen as an early symptom of lymphoma or polycythemia vera (paraneoplastic pruritus; Fig. 1.40d).

The cause of unclear itching may, however, also be dermatoses, which in part have a psychosomatic component, such as aquagenic pruritus, which occurs after contact with water (Shelley and Shelley 1998). On the other hand, the adrenergic forms of urticaria (Shelley and Shelley 1985) can be identified by determining the adrenaline or noradrenaline content in the serum.

Itching can, however, also arise from the intravenous administration of hydroxylethyl starch infusions (for example, in tinnitus therapy) and frequently persist for months (Metze et al. 1997). Likewise to be explained somatically are forms of itching that follow skin infections, especially scabies (postscabetic eczema), which is coupled with intense itching despite successful treatment.

Somatoform pruritus may also occur in an atopic skin diathesis. The differential-diagnostic delineation from a minimal form of atopic dermatitis may cause difficulties if the boundaries are blurred (see Chap. 2). Psychoses and drug abuse should be ruled out in the differential diagnosis.

Psychotherapy. Elicitation of pruritus may often occur as a consequence of emotional conflict situations. If the physician can recognize connections between emotional stress and itching, the patient should be made aware of this. This alone often contributes to considerably better coping with the symptoms. Pruritus patients are often open to a biopsychosocial understanding of the disease. Psychodynamic psychotherapy and cognitive behavior therapy have proven beneficial. Relaxation techniques are also effective.

Psychopharmaceuticals. The use of antihistamines is the first line of therapy, although the nonsedating ones often do not show adequate efficacy (Chap. 15). In persistent forms, sedating antihistamines, neuroleptics with antihistaminic action, and antidepressants or benzodiazepines may successfully break through the vicious itching–depression or itching–scratching cycle.

Somatoform Burning, Stabbing, Biting, Tingling

Burning, tingling, stabbing, and the like are counted among the other undifferentiated somatoform disorders (ICD-10: F45.8). These are rare but typical sensory complaints that have been only unsatisfactorily defined in the classification of pain syndrome and which should be counted among the other somatoform disorders.

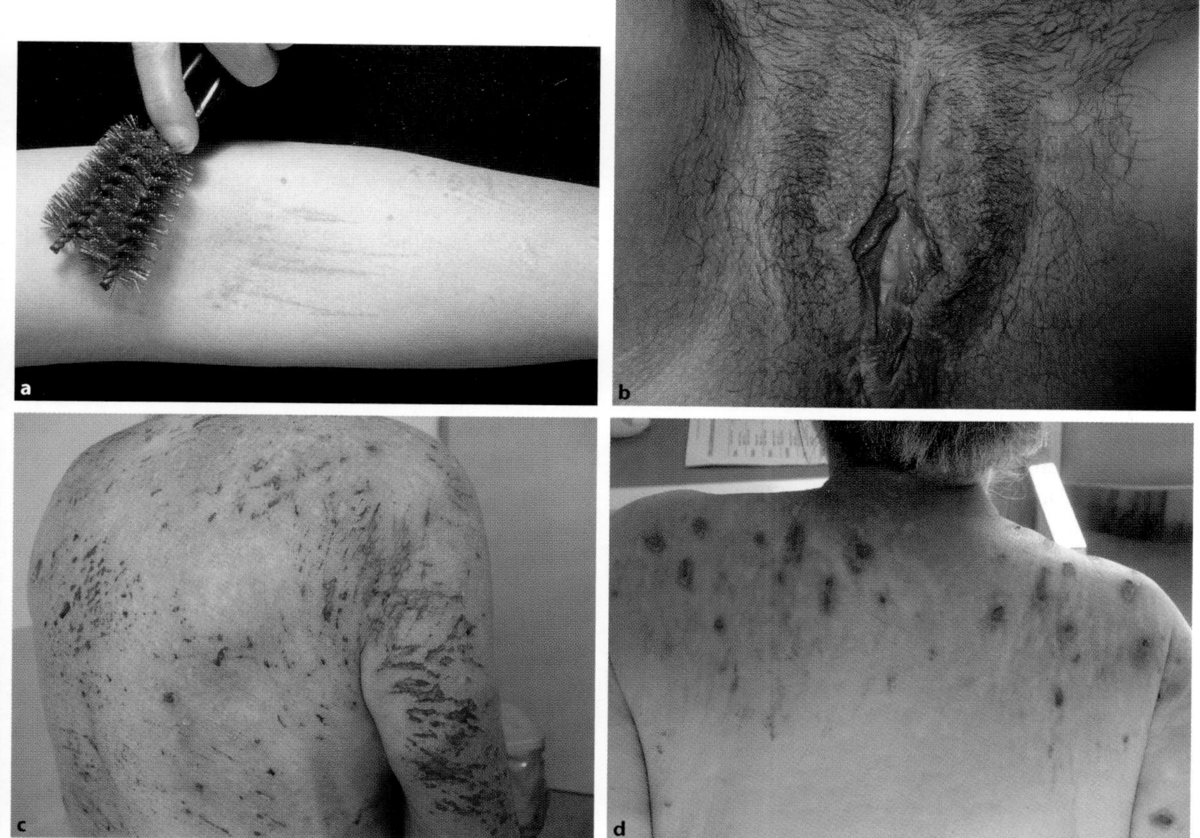

Fig. 1.40 **a** Mentally triggered pruritus with wire brush as aid to scratching. **b** Vulvar eczema in 27-year-old patient with depression. **c** Severe scratching in a patient with xerosis and kidney disease. **d** Pruritus as sign of paraneoplasia in patient with carcinoma

The patients usually complain of burning and other sensory complaints, with blurred transitions and usually vague descriptions (quote: "As though a needle were stuck into my skin"). These can be localized or generalized and are often a symptom that greatly reduces the quality of life. Sometimes the burning is accompanied by thermically perceived changes.

Clinical findings. No pathological skin findings can be diagnosed. Facial burning in part is often described, which is not taken very seriously. The so-called pantomime syndrome is characteristic.

> **The following belong to the pantomime syndrome:**
> - **Symptomatic, usually facial, burning**
> - **Typical pantomimic presentation of a fantasized elicitor of the complaint (needle, fire)**
> - **Introverted presentation**
> - **Silence and great concentration**

In the pantomime syndrome, there is regional burning in the face or only the cheeks. Characteristically, the patient emphasizes the description of the symptoms with an even movement of the palms toward both cheeks and finally places the hands on the cheeks or parts of the face.

In describing stabbing, the patient often imitates stabbing with a needle. The stabbing is sometimes demonstrated in the arms by poking the first and second fingers of the right hand suddenly to the skin, as though holding a needle. Some patients perform the demonstration introvertedly in absolute silence and show a high level of concentration.

In rare cases, the patients manipulate their own skin autoaggressively with tools and instruments when there is tingling or stabbing. Secondarily, there are then artificial lesions or irritative eczemas due to the self-manipulation. Transitions to tactile hallucinoses should be watched for and delusional disorders differential-diagnostically ruled out in these cases.

Psychiatric symptoms. As elicitors and potentiators of the complaints, some patients thematize stress, burdens, changes in life, and current conflicts as well as repressed rage. Frequently there are comorbidities with affective disorders or depressive or anxiety disorders.

Differential diagnosis. Not infrequently, the burning of the skin correlates with delusions, whereby the patient is thoroughly and undeviatingly convinced that there are particles or substances in the skin that are causing the suffering. This in turn must be differentiated from the so-called acarophobia or infestation delusion, which is in a group of its own but which may also be associated with burning in the skin (Musalek 1991).

On the one hand, differentiation must be made from localized notalgia paresthetica; on the other, from the burning caused by an erythropoietic protoporphyria – which as a congenital dermatosis, however, usually appears in childhood (Keller and Hornstein 1983). If corresponding differential diagnoses have been dermatologically ruled out, the diagnosis of a somatoform burning of the skin should be made. Moreover, specific stress-related dermatoses such as seborrheic eczema may be accompanied by tingling and burning, especially under stress.

Psychotherapy. Only individual case reports are available on psychotherapy. Focal therapy of the depression or anxiety disorder is often necessary. The procedure should be carried out according to the somatoform disorder. The use of a complaint diary and the VAS has proven beneficial.

Patients can often recognize the relationships between emotional stress and itching in the framework of psychosomatic primary care. Talking things through, in the sense of psychoeducation, may lead to clear improvement in coping with the symptoms. However, overpsychologizing of the symptoms is contraindicated.

Psychopharmaceuticals. The currently available literature recommends the use of tricyclic antidepressants in sensory complaints such as burning, stabbing, biting, and tingling. Broader studies are unavailable because of the rare, isolated occurrence of the disorder. Therapy of the accompanying depression predominates. The greatest number of studies have been performed with amitriptyline (Elavil). Moreover, the use of doxepin or a therapy attempt with SSRIs may be made.

> **These days, sensory complaints are primarily treated with doxepin, SSRIs, or amitriptyline.**

In the United States the use of capsaicin or topical anesthetic creams is recommended as local therapy. Our experience has shown that good results can be attained with UVA1 therapy, as well as photobalneotherapy or the addition of SAD light therapy in the winter months.

References

Arnetz B, Fjellner BB (1985) Psychological predictors of pruritus during mental stress. Acta Derm Venereol 65: 504–508

Bienenstock J, MacQueen G, Sestini P, Marshall JS, Stead RH, Perdue MH (1991) Mast cell/nerve interactions in vitro and in vivo. Am Rev Respir Dis 143: 55–58

Gupta MA, Gupta MK, Kirkby S, Weiner HK, Mace TM, Schorck NJ, Johnson EH, Ellis CN, Vorhees JJ (1989) Pruritus in psoriasis: a prospective study of some psychiatric and dermatologic correlates. Arch Dermatol 124: 1052–1057

Gupta MA, Gupta AK, Schork NJ, Ellis CN (1994) Depression modulates pruritus perception: a study of pruritus in psoriasis, atopic dermatitis, and chronic idiopathic urticaria. Psychosom Med 56: 36–40

Handwerker H (1993) Neurophysiologische Mechanismen des Juckens. Z Hautkr 68: 730–735

Handwerker H (1998) Pathophysiologie des Juckreizes. In: Garbe C, Rassner G (Hrsg) Dermatologie – Leitlinien und Qualitätssicherung für Diagnostik und Therapie. Springer, Berlin, S 43–45

Luger TA, Lotti T (1998) Neuropeptides: role in inflammatory skin diseases. J Eur Acad Dermatol Venerol 10: 207–212

Magerl W (1991) Neurophysiologie des Juckens. Allergologie 14: 395–405

Metze D, Reimann S, Szepfalusi Z, Bohle B, Kraft D, Luger TA (1997) Persistent pruritus after hydroxyethyl starch infusion therapy: a result of long-term storage in cutaneous nerves. Br J Dermatol 136: 553–559

Musalek M (1991) Der Dermatozoenwahn. Thieme, Stuttgart

Naukkarinen A, Harvima IT, Aalto MI, Harvima RJ, Horshmanheimo M (1991) Quantitative analysis of contact sites between mast cells and sensory nerves in cutaneous psoriasis and lichen planus based on a histochemical double staining technique. Arch Dermatol Res 283: 433–437

Niemeier V, Kupfer J, Gieler U (2000) Observations during an itch-inducing lecture. Dermatol Psychosom 1: 15–18

Rechenberger I (1981) Pruritus as a psychic phenomenon. MMW Munch Med Wochenschr 123(24): 1005–1006

Russell M, Dark KA, Cummins RW, Ellman G, Callaway E, Peeke HVS (1984) Learned histamine release. Science 225: 733–734

Schmelz M, Schmidt R, Bickel A, Handwerker HO, Torebjörk HE (1997) Specific C-receptors for itch in human skin. J Neurosci 17: 8003–8008

Scholz OB, Hermanns N (1994) Krankheitsverhalten und Kognitionen beeinflussen die Juckreiz-Wahrnehmung von Patienten mit atopischer Dermatitis! Z Klin Psychol 23: 127–135

Schultz-Amling W, Köhler-Weisker A (1996) Pruritus ani. In: Gieler U, Bosse KA (Hrsg) Seelische Faktoren bei Hautkrankheiten, 2. Aufl. Huber, Bern, S 105–112

Sheehan-Dare RA, Henderson MJ, Cotterill JA (1990) Anxiety and depression in patients with chronic urticaria and generalized pruritus. Br J Dermatol 123: 769–774

Shelley WB, Shelley ED (1985) Adrenergic urticaria: a new form of stress-induced hives. Lancet 9;2(8463): 1031–1033

Shelley WB, Shelley ED (1998) Aquadynia: noradrenergic pain induced by bathing and responsive to clonidine. J Am Acad Dermatol 38: 357–358

Williams RM, Bienenstock J, Stead RH (1995) Mast cells: the neuroimmune connection. Chem Immunol 61: 208–235

Further Reading

Goulden V, Toomey PJ, Highet AS (1998) Successful treatment of notalgia paresthetica with a paravertebral local anesthetic block. J Am Acad Dermatol 38: 114–116

Rief W, Hiller W (1992) Somatoforme Störungen. Huber, Bern

1.4 Dermatoses as a Result of Compulsive Disorders

The psychiatric disorder is primarily in the foreground of dermatoses as a result of compulsive disorders (ICD-10: F42); a skin disease occurs secondarily. The compulsive disorder is causally responsible for the occurrence of the dermatosis.

Definition. Compulsive disorders predominately comprise compulsive thoughts (ICD-10: F42.0) or compulsive acts (ICD-10: F42.1) as well as mixed (ICD-10: F42.2) symptomatics.

Compulsive thoughts are recurrent and persistent thoughts, impulses, or ideations that are experienced as obtrusive and inappropriate and which elicit pronounced anxiety and great malaise.

Compulsive acts are repeated behavior patterns, such as washing the hands, controlling for tidiness, or imagined acts.

Compulsive disorders may also be present as a comorbidity with certain dermatoses (Sect. 3.3.3).

Clinical symptomatics. A model example for dermatoses as a result of compulsive disorders is washing eczema, in which initially compulsive thoughts of contamination, possibly in connection with cutaneous hypochondrias such as bacteriophobias, lead to compulsive acts with constant washing of the hands and thus irritation and subsequent dermatitis. Additionally, sensitizations may arise, and contact-allergic superimposition by ingredients in the soap (aromas) may become important.

Categorization of Compulsive Disorders

Certain compulsive disorders
- Washing eczema
- Primary lichen simplex chronicus

Frequent compulsive disorders
- Trichotillomania
- Body dysmorphic disorder
- Cutaneous hypochondrias
- Special multifactorial dermatoses (anal eczema, seborrheic eczema)

Psychiatric symptoms. Compulsive disorders are usually not found as isolated symptomatics but are associated with other comorbidities. Depression (38.9%), panic disorder (15.5%), and social phobias (10.1%) are among the frequent comorbidities of these disorders (Hollander et al. 1997).

Differential diagnosis. The differential diagnosis comprises in first place the group of dermatitis paraartefacta syndrome (DPS) – that is, disorders of impulse control – and body dysmorphic disorders. Some authors classify DPS principally as compulsive disorders, especially when there are stereotype acts, as with skin-picking syndrome with self-injury. Trichotillomania, onychotillomania, onychophagia, neurotic excoriations, and acne excoriée also belong to this group.

Moreover, compulsive disorders occur in body dysmorphic disorders. Often there are compulsive thoughts with preoccupation with external appearance and compulsive acts, whereby the patient spends hours in front of the mirror to control his or her outward appearance or to positively alter the appearance. Some authors thus also favor the concept of body dysmorphic disorders as compulsive disorders (Phillips 1996). Further research and discussion will lead to a final classification in the future (Table 1.10).

Compulsive Washing

Definition and clinical findings. Compulsive washing is characterized by excessive and exaggerated washing, especially of the hands but sometimes of other body areas as well. The symptomatics appear due to the attendant drying of the skin and correspond to the presentation of a contact dermatitis. The hands are usually erythematous, scaly, and, in extreme forms, afflicted with fissures. The frequency of washing by far exceeds that of normally expected behavior; washings from 50 to 200 times per day may be reported. The patients definitely report the correct figures because they usually suffer significantly from the disease and have attempted to get it under control (Figs. 1.41, 1.42).

Psychiatric symptoms. The psychiatric symptoms are characterized by the compulsive impulse and the compulsive acts, which are sometimes considered disruptive by the patients, who have already tried to combat the disorder by changing their behavior. However, they are not successful because the compulsions are too strong. In the background is almost always a feeling of disgust or an unfounded fear of infection, but the patient should be questioned about this. The patient feels disgust at touching foreign objects (such as door handles) and then has an irresistible urge to wash off the presumed offending or dangerous disease pathogen. Patients experience compulsive washing both as reducing negative affectivity and as intensifying a positive affectivity in the sense of reduction of fear. Sometimes – in corresponding emotional conflicts – rejection of one's own person and one's own skin are predominant. In such cases, compulsive washing is an artefact.

Differential diagnosis. Other forms of cumulative toxic eczema must, of course, be addressed in the differential diagnosis and must be appropriately clarified allergologically. Irritant and chronic contact dermatitis must also be ruled out.

Psychotherapy. Behavior therapy programs have proven beneficial in the psychotherapy of compulsive washing. The program begins with keeping a diary in order to record the frequency and the situations in which the compulsive washing primarily occurs. Cognitive behavior therapy is effective in these disorders. If the compulsive washing occurs as part of a more complex situation and biographic conflicts clearly play an apparent role, a psychodynamic or psychoanalytical psychotherapy should also be considered. In psychotherapy one first assumes that the compulsive washing, like anxiety reactions, simply conceals another more conflict-laden topic, and stabilization must be instituted before it is possible to abandon the compulsive washing. In the dermatological practice, however, the initiation of the symptom diary can be successful, and a reduction of washing behavior may be achieved in milder cases.

Psychopharmaceuticals. Antidepressants have proven beneficial in the therapy of compulsive washing, especially those that also have a positive effect on the compulsive behavior and compulsive impulses. Clomipramine, a tricyclic antidepressant, can especially be recommended and may be used in increasing doses. Desipramine, fluoxetine, and fluvoxamine have been reported in studies.

References

Hollander E, Greenwald S, Neville D, Johnson J, Hornig CD, Weissman MM (1997) Uncomplicated and comorbid obsessive-compulsive disorder in an epidemiologic sample. Depress Anxiety 4(3): 111–119

Phillips KA (1996) Body dysmorphic disorder. Diagnosis and treatment of imagined ugliness. J Clin Psychiatry 57(8): 61–64

Further Reading

McElroy SL, Phillips KA, Keck PE (1994) Obsessive compulsive spectrum disorder. J Clin Psychiatry 55(suppl 10): 33–51

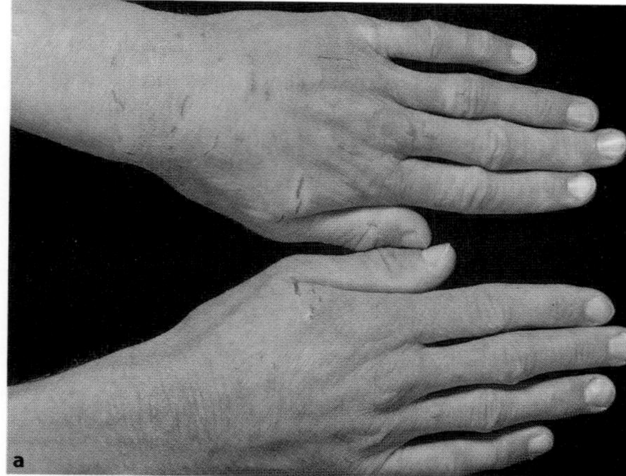

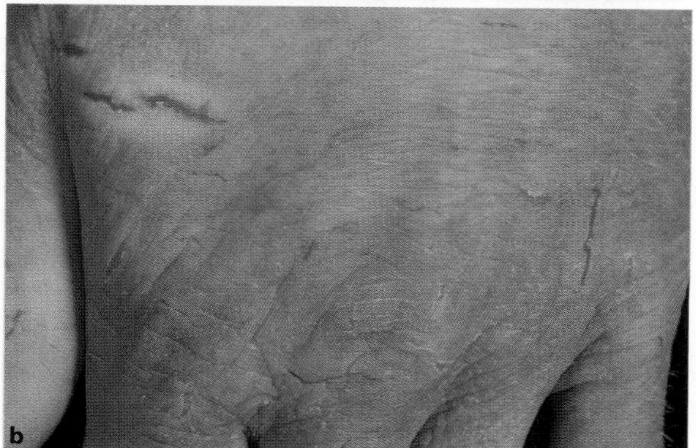

Fig. 1.41a,b Washing eczema of the hand; cumulative-toxic dermatitis resulting from handwashing 30 times per day. **a** Overview. **b** Close-up

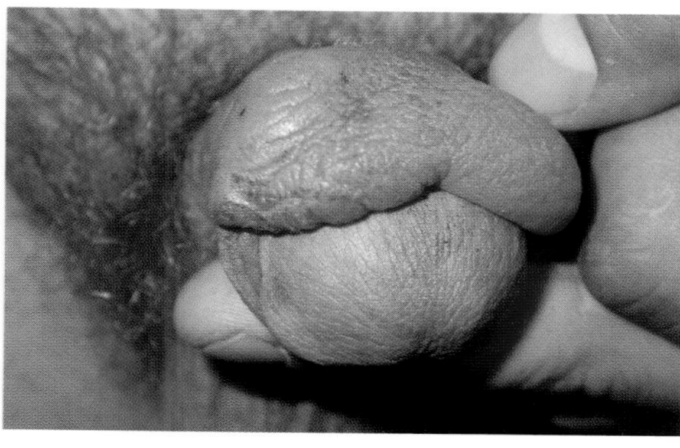

Fig. 1.42 Genital washing compulsion. Eczematous skin lesions in a man with compulsive disorder and sexual conflict

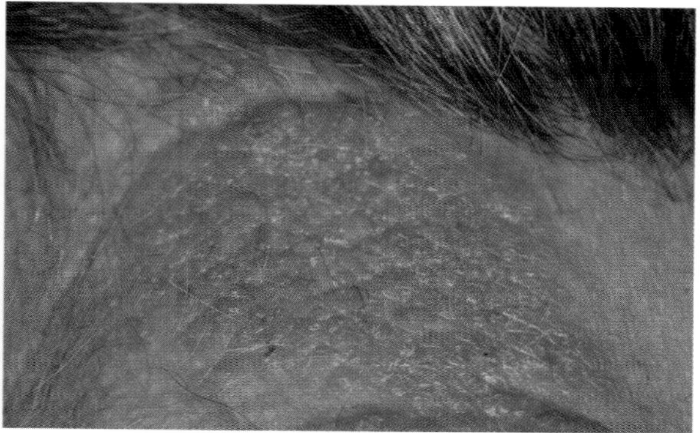

Fig. 1.43 Lichen simplex chronicus on the forehead: continuous rubbing with the hand when thinking and concentrating

Riddle M (1998) Obsessive compulsive disorder in children and adolescents. Br J Psychiatry 173(suppl 35): 91–96

Sieg J, Scholz OB (2001) Subjektives Gefühls- und Körpererleben bei Wasch- und Kontrollzwangshandlungen. Verhaltenstherapie 11: 288–296

Steketee GS, Grayson JB, Foa EB (1985) Obsessive-compulsive disorder: differences between washers and checkers. Behav Res Ther 23: 197–201

Primary Lichen Simplex Chronicus

Definition and clinical findings. Lichen simplex chronicus (LSC; ICD-10: F68.1, L28.0; DSM-IV-TR 312.30) is a chronic pruritic lichenoid plaque with thickening of the skin areas, which is provoked and maintained by rubbing or scratching (Fig. 1.43).

In LSC, there is primarily an emotional disorder with skin manifestations. A relationship to atopic eczema is possible. The predilection sites are the posterior neck, extensor aspect of the extremities, axillae, and genital area.

Psychiatric symptoms. A compulsive disorder is predominant in the psychiatric symptoms of LSC.

Differential diagnosis. The group of prurigo diseases (prurigo simplex acuta, prurigo simplex subacuta, and prurigo simplex chronica) must also be ruled out differential-diagnostically. Characteristic of the prurigo group, papules are found as primary lesions, and inflammatory cellular infiltrate in the later chronic forms is found histologically.

Prurigo diseases are characteristically multifactorial dermatoses in which – besides emotional factors (primarily depressive disorders) – metabolic disorders, diseases of internal organs, hormonal disorders, or atopic skin diathesis play an etiopathogenetic role.

Differential diagnosis must rule out paraartefacts, whereby emotionally there is predominantly an impairment of impulse control and the manipulation urge cannot be controlled.

Psychotherapy. Treatment of the psychiatric symptoms of LSC corresponds mainly to concepts of behavior therapy (Chap. 14). Favorable results can also be attained with the habit-reversal technique for treating itching by controlling the scratching.

Occlusive bandages have been found beneficial as a local therapeutic measure (Unna boot), sometimes in combination with topical preparations containing glucocorticoids, coal tar, and zinc oxide.

Psychopharmaceuticals. Antihistamines alone are usually inadequate. Antihistamines with sedative effect (hydroxyzine) and tricyclic antidepressants (doxepin) can be used in a stepwise regimen (see Chap. 15 on antihistamines). A psychopharmacological attempt at therapy with SSRIs may be successful in individual cases.

Further Reading

Phillips KA (1996) Body dysmorphic disorder. Diagnosis and treatment of imagined ugliness. J Clin Psychiatry 57(8): 61–64

Rosenbaum MS, Ayllon T (1981) The behavioral treatment of neurodermatitis through habit-reversal. Behav Res Ther 19: 313–318

Simeon D, Hollander E, Stein DJ, Cohen L, Aronowitz B (1995) Body dysmorphic disorder in the DSM-IV field trial for obsessive-compulsive disorder. Am J Psychiatry 152(8): 1207–1209

Stein DJ, Hollander E (1992) Dermatology and conditions related to obsessive-compulsive disorder. J Am Acad Dermatol 26: 237–242

Table 1.10 DSM-IV-TR and ICD-10 Classification of Psychiatric Disorders

Mood Disorders		
DSM-IV-TR	**ICD-1**	
296.00	F30.9	Bipolar I Disorder, Single Manic Episode, Unspecified
296.01	F30.1	Bipolar I Disorder, Single Manic Episode, Mild
296.02	F30.1	Bipolar I Disorder, Single Manic Episode, Moderate
296.03	F30.1	Bipolar I Disorder, Single Manic Episode, Severe Without Psychotic Features
296.04	F30.2	Bipolar I Disorder, Single Manic Episode, Severe With Psychotic Features
296.05	F30.7	Bipolar I Disorder, Single Manic Episode, In Partial Remission
296.06.1.1	F30.7	Bipolar I Disorder, Single Manic Episode, In Full Remission
296.40	F31.0	Bipolar I Disorder, Most Recent Episode Hypomanic
296.40	F31.9	Bipolar I Disorder, Most Recent Episode Manic, Unspecified
296.41	F31.3	Bipolar I Disorder, Most Recent Episode Manic, Mild
296.42	F31.3	Bipolar I Disorder, Most Recent Episode Manic, Moderate
296.43	F31.4	Bipolar I Disorder, Most Recent Episode Manic, Severe Without Psychotic Features
296.44	F31.5	Bipolar I Disorder, Most Recent Episode Manic, Severe With Psychotic Features
296.45	F31.7	Bipolar I Disorder, Most Recent Episode Manic, In Partial Remission
296.50	F31.9	Bipolar I Disorder, Most Recent Episode Depressed, Unspecified
296.51	F31.3	Bipolar I Disorder, Most Recent Episode Depressed, Mild

Mood Disorders		
DSM-IV-TR	**ICD-1**	
296.52	F31.3	Bipolar I Disorder, Most Recent Episode Depressed, Moderate
296.53	F31.4	Bipolar I Disorder, Most Recent Episode Depressed, Severe Without Psychotic Features
296.54	F31.5	Bipolar I Disorder, Most Recent Episode Depressed, Severe With Psychotic Features
296.55	F31.7	Bipolar I Disorder, Most Recent Episode Depressed, In Partial Remission
296.56	F31.7	Bipolar I Disorder, Most Recent Episode Depressed, In Full Remission
296.60	F31.9	Bipolar I Disorder, Most Recent Episode Mixed, Unspecified
296.61	F31.6	Bipolar I Disorder, Most Recent Episode Mixed, Mild
296.62	F31.6	Bipolar I Disorder, Most Recent Episode Mixed, Moderate
296.63	F31.6	Bipolar I Disorder, Most Recent Episode Mixed, Severe Without Psychotic Features
296.46	F31.7	Bipolar I Disorder, Most Recent Episode Manic, In Full Remission
296.7	F31.9	Bipolar I Disorder, Most Recent Episode Unspecified
296.80	F31.9	Bipolar Disorder NOS
296.89	F31.8	Bipolar II Disorder, No Manic Episodes But Hypomanic
296.20	F32.9	Major Depressive Disorder, Single Episode, Unspecified
296.21	F32.0	Major Depressive Disorder, Single Episode, Mild
296.22	F32.1	Major Depressive Disorder, Single Episode, Moderate
296.23	F32.2	Major Depressive Disorder, Single Episode, Severe Without Psychotic Features
296.24	F32.3	Major Depressive Disorder, Single Episode, Severe With Psychotic Features
296.25	F32.3	Major Depressive Disorder, Single Episode, In Partial Remission
296.26	F32.3	Major Depressive Disorder, Single Episode, In Full Remission
296.30	F33.9	Major Depressive Disorder, Recurrent, Unspecified
296.31	F33.0	Major Depressive Disorder, Recurrent, Mild
296.32	F33.1	Major Depressive Disorder, Recurrent, Moderate
296.33	F33.2	Major Depressive Disorder, Recurrent, Severe Without Psychotic Features
296.34	F33.3	Major Depressive Disorder, Recurrent, Severe With Psychotic Features
296.35	F33.4	Major Depressive Disorder, Recurrent, In Partial Remission
296.36	F33.4	Major Depressive Disorder, Recurrent, In Full Remission
296.90	F39	Mood Disorder NOS

Mood Disorders		
DSM-IV-TR	**ICD-1**	
301.13.1.1	F34.0	Cyclothymic Disorder
300.4.1.1	F34.1	Dysthymic Disorder
Anxiety and Somatoform and Dissociative Disorders		
DSM-IV-TR	**ICD-10**	
300.00	F41.9	Anxiety Disorder NOS
300.02	F41.1	Generalized Anxiety Disorder
300.11	F44.x	Conversion Disorder
300.12	F44.0	Dissociative Amnesia
300.13	F44.1	Dissociative Fugue
300.14	F44.x	Dissociative Identity Disorder
300.15	F44.9	Dissociative Disorder NOS
300.16	F68.1	Factitious Disorder With Predominantly Psychological Signs and Symptoms
300.19	F68.1	Factitious Disorder NOS
300.19	F68.0	Factitious Disorder With Combined Psychological and Physical Signs and Symptoms
300.21	F40.01	Panic Disorder With Agoraphobia
300.22	F40.00	Agoraphobia Without History of Panic Disorder
300.23	F40.1	Social Phobia
300.29	F40.2	Specific Phobia
300.3	F42.9	Obsessive-Compulsive Disorder, Unspecified
300.4	F34.1	Dysthymic Disorder
300.6	F48.1	Depersonalization Disorder
300.7	F45.2, F22.0	Body Dysmorphic Disorder
300.7	F45.2	Hypochondriasis
300.81	F45.0	Somatization Disorder
300.82.1.1	F45.9	Somatoform Disorder, Unspecified

Miscellaneous		
(ICD-10: F21;	DSM-IV-TR: 301.22)	Schizotypal Personality Disorder
(ICD-10: 60.31;	DSM-IV-TR: 301.83)	Borderline Personality Disorder
(ICD-10: F22.0;	DSM-IV-TR: 297.1)	Delusional Disorder
(ICD-10:F63.9;	DSM-IV-TR: 312.30)	Impulse-Control Disorder NOS
(ICD-10: F45.4;	DSM-IV-TR: 307.xx	Pain Disorder
(ICD-10: F45.4;	DSM-IV-TR: 307.80	Pain Disorder Associated With Psychological Factors
(ICD-10: F45.4;	DSM-IV-TR: 307.89	Pain Disorder Associated With Both Psychological Factors and a General Medical Condition
(ICD-10: F50.0;	DSM-IV-TR: 307.1)	Anorexia Nervosa
(ICD-10: F50.2;	DSM-IV-TR: 307.51)	Bulimia Nervosa
(ICD-10: F98.4;	DSM-IV-TR: 307.3)	Stereotypic Movement Disorder
(ICD-10: Z76.5;	DSM-IV-TR: V65.2)	Malingering

Multifactorial Cutaneous Diseases

2

Multifactorial dermatoses may be frequently triggered by psychosocial factors. These diseases often have a polygenetic susceptibility; however, despite this genetic predisposition, their course is subject to emotional influences. These are considered psychosomatic diseases in the classical sense.

The course of disease, which is usually chronic and recurrent, is characterized by a series of dysregulations, usually of the immune system (psychoneuroimmunology). The exogenous and endogenous trigger factors are numerous, and their importance differs from person to person.

In order to initiate qualitatively adequate diagnostics and therapy for multifactorial dermatoses, attention should be paid early to not only the subgroup (cluster) of psychosomatic disorders but also to parainfectious, paraneoplastic, and allergic factors.

Historically, seven diseases make up the classic psychosomatic disorders in the narrower sense: duodenal ulcers, ulcerative colitis, essential hypertension, rheumatoid arthritis, hyperthyreosis, asthma, and atopic dermatitis.

The multifactorial diseases have greatly expanded the list of psychosomatic diseases in the current concept. Among the most frequent and important multifactorial dermatoses are atopic eczema, acne vulgaris, and psoriasis vulgaris. Many controlled biopsychosocial studies are now available that clearly confirm the influence of psychosocial factors, so these three diseases head the group of multifactorial psychodermatoses in the following text. The amount of data is understandable because these disorders occur very frequently in the general population, and thus recruitment for studies is easily done. The other multifactorial dermatoses whose course is subject to emotional influence are listed in alphabetical order.

Multifactorial Dermatoses

Frequent multifactorial dermatoses:
- Atopic dermatitis
- Acne vulgaris
- Psoriasis vulgaris

Other multifactorial dermatoses:
- Alopecia areata
- Anal pruritus/dermatitis
- Dyshidrosiform hand dermatitis
- Herpes simplex
- Hyperhidrosis
- Hypertrichosis
- Lichen planus
- Lupus erythematodes
- Malignant melanoma
- Perioral dermatitis
- Progressive systemic scleroderma
- Prurigo
- Rosacea
- Seborrheic dermatitis
- Ulcers of the leg
- Urticaria
- Vitiligo

Atopic Dermatitis

Atopic dermatitis (ICD-10: L20, F54) is the model disease for the multifactorial causality of a dermatosis to the biopsychosocial model. Experienced by 3–4 million patients, it occupies a high place in prevalence in medicine and especially in dermatology.

Definition. Atopic dermatitis (AD) is a chronic recurrent skin disease with severe pruritus, which is diverse in its morphological aspects and overall course. It is one of the so-called atopic diseases, whereby the term "atopy" denotes the polygenic inherited susceptibility to develop allergic asthma, allergic rhinitis, or AD. The criteria defined by Hanifin and Rajka (1980) are usually used to diagnose the disease. These include the cardinal symptoms (typical eczema, itching, positive family history, chronic course) and facultative symptoms (e.g., white dermographism, itching upon sweating, intolerance of animal wool, food intolerances).

Pathogenesis. It is generally accepted that AD is based on an unalterable genetic disposition (Schultz-Larsen et al. 1986) and that an episode may be triggered by numerous factors (Scheich et al. 1993; Hermanns and Scholz 1993), including stressful life events (Seikowski and Gollek 1999) and stress influences, which vary from person to person with regard to individual susceptibility. The genetic disposition of this immunological disease is inherited in a multifactorial transmission and is the result of overlapping gene constellations.

Thus far, functional impairments of humoral and cellular immunity (Buske-Kirschbaum et al. 1997) are cardinal findings in AD. These include a high total IgE level (Ishizaka et al. 1967), defect of the T suppressor cells (Böhm and Bauer 1997), shifted Th1/Th2 balance in favor of the Th2 constellation (Abeshira-Amar et al. 1992), impairment of the vegetative nervous system with blockade of the beta-adrenergic system, and impaired sweat excretion and sebum production (Szentivanyi 1968).

Causes of Atopic Dermatitis

- Genetic disposition of overlapping gene constellations
- Functional impairment of humoral and cellular immunity with:
  - Elevated total IgE level
  - Defect of T suppressor cells
  - Shifted Th1/Th2 balance in favor of Th2
- Impairment of the vegetative nervous system with:
  - Blockade of the beta-adrenergic system
- Impaired sweat excretion
- Impaired sebum production
- Elicitation by stress is possible

The psychosocial triggering and elicitability of AD can be well explained by the classical stress model, the close causality to the vegetative nervous system with blockade of the beta-adrenergic system, and excretion of immunoactive messenger substances under stress.

Buske-Kirschbaum et al. (1997) demonstrated reduced secretion of free cortisol in response to psychosocial stress in atopic children exposed to stressors. There appears to be a hypothalamic impairment compared with nonatopic individuals. Consequently, the reduced endogenous cortisol production under stress would result in the impaired anti-inflammatory protective effect of this hormone.

Szentivanyi (1968) reported a partial blockade of the beta-adrenergic system in atopic patients in studies of persons suffering from asthma. There is both direct stimulation via acetylcholine and noradrenaline via the peripheral nervous system and indirect stimulation via the adrenal medulla with adrenalin and noradrenaline. The catecholamines are then bound by both alpha-adrenergic and beta-adrenergic receptors. When the beta receptors are impaired or blocked in their functions, the consequence is increased vasoconstriction (alpha-adrenergic). This results in inadequate perfusion and damage to the epithelium and the skin, which is expressed as white dermographism. Moreover, this also reduces adenosine 3',5'-cyclic monophosphate (cAMP), which in turn leads to increased secretion of inflammation mediators.

Sympathetic nerve fibers are close to mast cells in the dermis. Stress activation of the sympathetic nervous system may enhance activation of these immunocompetent cells.

Patients with atopy also show proliferation of specific Th2 helper cells. The shift in the Th1/Th2 ratio in favor of Th2 helper cells is considered to be a mechanism of the allergic–inflammatory reaction in AD. The Th2 cells are characterized especially by interleukin types IL-3, IL-4, and IL-5. Increased excretion of IL-3 cytokine activates mast cells, evoking increased liberation of histamine as an immediate reaction. IL-4 also activates the B cells and thus IgE production, and IL-5 activates the eosinophilic granulocytes with corresponding eosinophilia and eosinophil cationic protein (ECP) excretion.

Clinical findings. AD is a chronic-recurrent inflammatory skin disease that often begins in infancy. The early childhood manifestation of the disease may appear during the first months of life. The scalp and cheeks are usually affected. At later ages, the flexures, nape of the neck, hands, and feet become affected. The basic symptoms of atopic dermatitis are chronic-recurrent eczematous lesions associated with severe itching. Pruritus is the main symptom of AD (Fig. 2.1).

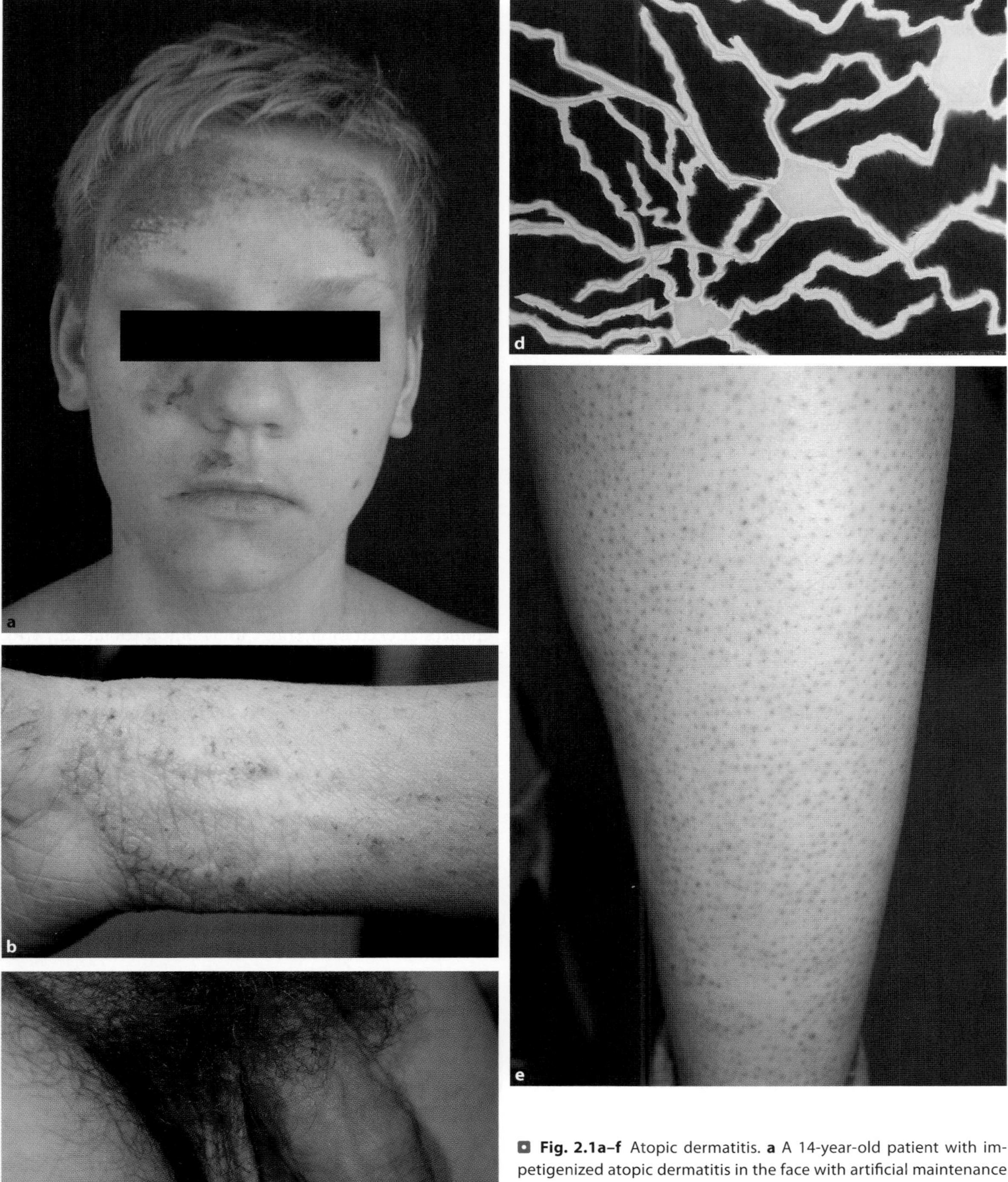

Fig. 2.1a–f Atopic dermatitis. **a** A 14-year-old patient with impetigenized atopic dermatitis in the face with artificial maintenance in stress-triggering. Additionally, he has an adjustment disorder and sociophobia as well as impaired coping. **b** Skin lesions on the arms with pruritus and scratching. **c** A 23-year-old patient with atopic eczema in the genital area and sociophobia. **d** Patient with atopic dermatitis painting broken nerves in art therapy. **e** Atopic dermatitis adjustment disorder in case of keratosis follicularis; differential diagnosis: body dysmorphic disorder. **f** (*see next page*)

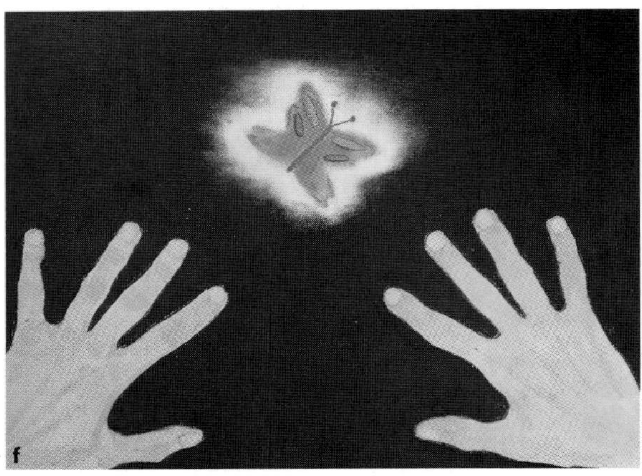

Fig. 2.1 *(continued)* **f** A 26-year-old woman with atopic eczema and hope of wellness in art therapy.

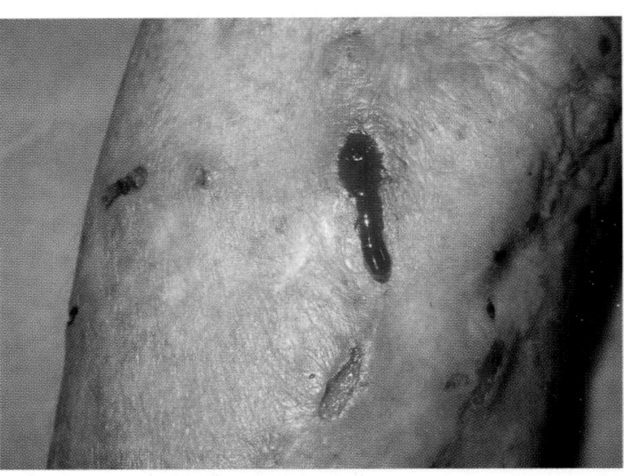

Fig. 2.2 Scratching to the point of bleeding, in which the itching is initially partly masked by pain. Then, however, the inflammation promotes the itching–scratching cycle

Emotional symptomatics. The original term for AD, "neurodermites," was coined by Brocq and Jacquet (1891) and expresses the interpretation that psychosocial and inflammatory factors are decisively involved as cofactors in the onset and maintenance of the disease.

In psychological studies, elevated neuroticism values, elevated excitability, and inadequate coping with stress are repeatedly and reproducibly found. Psychosocial stress is considered a possible elicitor, but it is also a consequence of episodes of AD and is mediated by neuroendocrine, immunological, and vegetative regulatory mechanisms. Neuropeptides have a key function in understanding of the coupling of psyche and soma.

Stress. Approximately 30% of patients with AD notice that exacerbation of the disease appears to be elicited by stressful situations.

Critical life events, such as significant personal losses, low social contacts, dissatisfaction with the occupational situation, difficulties at work, vacation, separation, and, frequently, age-typical crises associated with the transition from the parent's home to kindergarten and school, were found to be eliciting factors of AD (Bosse and Hünecke 1976).

The largest study was performed after the great earthquake in 1995 in the Japanese city of Kobe. There, the disease recurred in 38% of questioned AD patients in the region affected by the earthquake. By contrast, only 7% of the control group participants in areas spared by the quake had new episodes. However, 9% of those affected in the earthquake region also reported improvement, compared with only 1% in the control group (Kodama et al. 1999).

In addition, the intensity of itching depends on subjectively felt stress and is more easily elicited mentally in emotional excitation (rage, annoyance, excitation, and, less often, joy; see Sect. 1.3.5 on somatoform itching).

Itching–scratching cycle. In many clinical studies, connections could be demonstrated between emotional stress and the intensity of the itching sensation. In patients with AD, itching could be elicited by confrontation with personally stressful events of the past. Moreover, it was found that life-altering events can elicit itching or reduce the itching threshold (Roos 2004).

In AD, itching is an important guiding symptom for the doctor. The itching–scratching cycle plays an important role in these patients in maintenance of their skin presentations (Fig. 2.1b).

Bosse and Hünecke (1981) distinguish between at least two different scratching forms with respect to the dynamics of the itching–scratching cycle:

- Smooth rubbing with the palms
- Insatiable, excoriative scratching with the fingernails

The first often has the character of a skipping act, which leads to a reduction of tension. The second form of excoriative scratching is an excessive scratching that leads briefly to a reduction of the itching, which inhibits or overrides the sensation of itching. Due to this initially relieving effect, scratching is conditionally rewarded. Later, however, structural changes arise in the skin as a result of scratching, the itching threshold is lowered, and inflammatory reactions occur in the scratched skin, which in turn leads to itching and to more – usually even more violent – scratching (Fig. 2.2).

This vicious cycle may be initiated by diffuse emotional tensions when scratching – originally used to reduce tension – itself elicits itching. Scratching and itching potentiate each other and can spiral in intensity. Thus, a cycle arises that ends in scratching episodes. Psychodynamically, the itching–scratching cycle is taken to be an unconscious tension-reducing affect that, from a theoretical impulse aspect, may take on the character of lust (Rechenberger 1979; Fig. 2.1c).

Personality structures. Patients with AD often show tension, insecurity, aggressive tendencies, or feelings of inferiority, but no characteristic specific personality structure has been found in continued studies of patients with AD.

It was found that it is senseless to look for individual, specific personality traits that should apply to all AD patients.

Patients with AD are a heterogeneous group with no characteristic specific personality traits that apply to all patients.

Obermayer (1955) showed that early separation of the baby from the breast is a serious trauma in the child's emotional development, which may lead to serious disorders and emotional instability.

Earlier studies demonstrated that a rejecting mother is present in 98% of children with AD. This hypothesis was refuted in later studies.

Studies of personality characteristics in dependence on serum IgE levels in patients with AD show significantly higher excitation levels and inadequate coping with stress, corresponding to negative coping in patients with total IgE levels >100 IU/ml (Scheich et al. 1993).

In particular, patients with depressive-irritable personality type showed significantly higher causative or reactive emotional stress than the other patients with AD.

Ehlers et al. (1994) showed verbal and nonverbal negative communication of patients with AD. Negative communication in AD may possibly prevent the solution of everyday problems and result in elevated excitation levels.

In AD subgroups there is inadequate coping with stress, negative communication, and elevated excitation levels, which impede solution of everyday problems (Fig. 2.1d).

About 20% of patients with AD (neurodermatitis) could be designated as emotionally remarkable based on a questionnaire handed out in a cluster analysis (Gieler et al. 1990).

Deep psychological histories of 25 patients with AD (Heigl-Evers 1976) showed that nearly all patients reported impaired or limited contact behavior. They interpreted their shyness and limitations in contact as an effect of their insecurity in dealing with other people that was caused by the eczema.

Dealing with aggression is an essential stress-related factor due to depressive tension and easy irritability, as is impaired coping with disease in AD, whereby stress increases with the duration of the disease.

Coping with illness. Every episode of AD is accompanied by psychosocial reactions, which in turn affect the disease process. The ever-recurrent episodes convince many of those afflicted that they have no possibility of exerting any influence on the course of the disease, giving them a feeling of helplessness (Fig. 2.1e).

Visible skin changes often elicit negative social interactions (Ehlers et al. 1994). Among these are the patient's usually central proximity–distance conflicts, including impairment of sexuality.

The secondary consequences attendant on itching mainly involve sleep deprivation, trouble concentrating, fatigue, reduced performance, and effects in social and occupational areas. These often lead to resignation, depressive mood, and reactive anxiety, up to and including suicide.

Quality of life. Despite many advances in diagnostics and therapy, no permanent cure can be soon anticipated, so the question of improvement in quality of life is a central topic (Herd et al. 1997).

Of all dermatoses, AD is the one associated with the most limitations in quality of life with respect to physical and emotional well-being and social relationships. The marked reduction in quality of life arises especially because of the chronicity of the disease.

Summary. It can be concluded that possibly elevated excitation levels with greater stress vulnerability are currently central topics in dealing with the disease and quality of life in AD.

Summary: Atopic Dermatitis

- Exacerbations stem from life events, the influence of stress, and psychosocial problems ("daily hassles").
- The course of the disease appears to be influenced by subjective stress factors. Social stress and interaction problems appear to have particular importance as disease elicitors.
- The emotional changes primarily involve fear, depression, and neuroticism (emotional liability with nervousness, hypersensitivity, anxiety, and excitability).
- The ability to cope with the disease is influenced by negative compliance and helplessness.
- Indications for psychotherapy are identified in about 20% of AD patients. Psychotherapeutic treatment procedures are effective in relieving exacerbations.
- Itching and scratching are often detrimental to the person's attention span and ability to concentrate. Coping with the disease and dealing with itching is a central problem for patients (itching–scratching cycle).
- These patients subjectively report the greatest limitations in quality of life among patients with skin diseases.

Diagnostics (clinical): questionnaires. Several questionnaires have been used in studies and found useful in clarifying emotional factors in AD.

1. Marburg skin questionnaire (*Marburger Hautfragebogen*, MHF): The MHF was developed for patients with AD and has been used in numerous studies. In 51 questions it primarily covers coping with the disease in the areas of social fears, helplessness, itching–scratching cycle, depression and anxiety, search for information, and quality of life. It is available in various languages (German, English, French, Dutch, Polish, Japanese). A variant of the MHF, age-appropriately adapted by Kupfer et al. (2003), is given in the form of two questionnaires for children: the CopeKi, for children between 8 and 12 years of age, and the CopeJu, for adolescents between 13 and 18 years of age.
2. Itching cognition questionnaire (*Juckreiz-Kognitions-Fragebogen*): This questionnaire is focused on itching, consisting of 20 questions depicting two scales: coping with itching and catastrophization of itching. It has been used in several studies and was also adapted and standardized for the age groups of 8–12 years and 13–18 years (Kupfer et al. 2003) so that aspects of coping with itching can also be recorded in these age groups.
3. Two questionnaires were developed especially for the parents of children with AD. One is the *Fragebogen für Eltern von neurodermitiskranken Kinder* (FEN, or questionnaire for parents of children with AD), which contains scales regarding aggression in relation to scratching, protective scratching, control of scratching, and negative treatment experience, with a total of 22 questions. It was successfully used during the Neurodermatitis Training Study. The other questionnaire addresses quality of life of parents of children with AD (*Lebensqualität von Eltern mit Neurodermitiskindern*; von Rüden et al. 1999); it contains 26 questions pertaining to this issue.
4. The stigmatization of patients suffering from AD can be recorded with the *Fragebogen zur Erfassung von Hautbeschwerden* (FEH, or questionnaire for recording skin complaints; Schmid-Ott et al. 1999). In 39 questions, it records scales for experienced rejection, external appearance and situation withdrawal, impairment of self-esteem, perceived rejection and devaluation concealment, and composure.

Differential diagnosis. Dermatologically, eczemas resembling AD and similar diseases, including seborrheic dermatitis of childhood, allergic contact dermatitis, scabies, and pyodermas, as well as special forms such as Netherton syndrome or Wiskott–Aldrich syndrome, must, of course, be ruled out. These are probably too rarely diagnosed.

With respect to the psychosomatic aspects, artificial reactions in existing AD are also easily overlooked, but many patients show more scratching behavior than appropriate for AD and eczematous reaction, so artificial aspects should certainly be differentiated here. An excessive limitation of use for fear of allergies may lead to exaggerated avoidance of topical medication, for example. Another aspect would be compulsive coping disorders, which may also be masked by AD and lead to increased use of topical medications or to constant inappropriate preoccupation with the AD.

Dermatological therapy. Topical dermatological therapy brings improvement in quality of life. With respect to the topical and systemic therapeutic alternatives, we refer the reader to the Association of the Scientific Medical Societies in guidelines on AD, which offer a broad spectrum of application possibilities. Psychosomatic measures should always supplement this basic treatment, but not replace it.

Psychotherapy. Psychotherapeutic procedures have proven beneficial as adjuvant therapy in AD (Fig. 2.1f). In a survey concerning the success of various therapies in randomly questioned patients with AD, psychotherapy was reported as effective as topical corticosteroids (Bitzer et al. 1997). Among the symptom-oriented approaches, behavior therapy has been found effective, especially for reducing the itching–scratching cycle, and relaxation procedures are also considerably more effective than normal dermatological treatment alone. In behavior medicine, various techniques have been developed that address coping with the disease, work to offset stigmatization, and also improve quality of life. The training programs that have been established for AD patients have been reported helpful in all published studies; they contain behavior therapy components as an effective therapy module (stress management, role play, relaxation). Both autogenic training and muscle relaxation are suitable. Psychodynamic therapy procedures are also meaningful in conscious or unconscious personal conflicts or for problems in coping with the disease. Williamson (2000) reported that patients who had undergone psychodynamic psychotherapy showed considerably more outbreak-free time than patients without psychotherapy.

Psychodynamically, there are often patterns of conflict related to the proximity–distance conflict, shame affects, or feelings of disgust with one's own skin. Depending on the time of the first manifestation, the severity overall, the frequency of exacerbations, and the positive or negative coping with the disease, emotional symptoms such as depression or anxiety are encountered more frequently. This is understandable when one remembers that infants and small children with AD rarely learn to differentiate between affectionate attention from the mother as the reference person and the itch-eliciting, unpleasant experience of cream application, or they experience these as concurrent stimuli. This sets the stage for the presence of emotional conflicts with the mother, independent of AD, and corresponding reaction patterns that manifest later in adulthood in proximity–distance conflicts.

Psychotherapy is, however, always indicated if stress influences show marked exacerbation of AD as a provocation factor.

Psychopharmaceuticals. Patients with AD are often given antihistamines, which are usually ineffective. These are useful only when their sedative secondary effect is apparent. Thus, medications that have both an antihistaminic and a neuroleptic effect are especially suitable for use in AD, particularly hydroxyzine, doxepin, and chlorpromazine. Sedatives, too, have been found suitable in acute treatment, but their habituation potential should not be underestimated.

References

Abehsira-Amar O, Gibert M, Joliy M, Thèze J, Jankovic DL (1992) IL-4 plays a dominant role in the differential development of Th0 into Th1 and Th2 cells. J Immunol 148: 3820–3829

AWMF: Leitlinie zur Neurodermitis. http://www.AWMF-Leitlinien.de

Bitzer EM, Grobe TG, Dorning H (1997) Die Bewertung therapeutischer Maßnahmen bei atopischer Dermatitis und Psoriasis aus der Perspektive der Patienten unter Berücksichtigung komplementär medizinischer Verfahren. ISEG-Studie Endbericht

Böhm I, Bauer R (1997) TH1 Zellen, TH2 Zellen und atopische Dermatitis. Hautarzt 48: 223–227

Bosse K, Hünecke P (1976) Psychodynamik und Soziodynamik bei Hautkranken. Verlag für Medizinische Psychologie, Vandenhoeck & Ruprecht, Göttingen

Brocq L, Jacquet L (1891) Notes pour servir á l'histoire des neurodermites. Ann Dermatol Syphiligr 97: 193–208

Buske-Kirschbaum A, Jobst S, Wustmans A, Kirschbaum C, Rauh W, Hellhammer D (1997) Attenuated free cortisol response to psychosocial stress in children with atopic dermatitis. Psychosom Med 59: 419–426

Ehlers A, Osen A, Wennigner, Gieler U (1994) Atopic dermatitis and stress: the possible role of negative communication with significant others. Int J Behav Med 2: 107–121

Gieler U, Ehlers A, Höhler T, Burkard G (1990) Die psychosoziale Situation der Patienten mit endogenem Ekzem. Hautarzt 41: 416–423

Hanifin JM, Rajka G (1980) Diagnostic features of atopic dermatitis. Acta Derm Venereol 92: 44–47

Heigl-Evers A, Schneider R, Bosse K (1976) Biographical information from patients with endogenous eczema. Z Psychosom Med Psychoanal 22(1): 75–84

Herd RM, Tidman MH, Ruta DA, Hunter JA (1997) Measurement of quality of life in atopic dermatitis: correlation and validation of two different methods. Br J Dermatol 136: 502–507

Hermanns N, Scholz OB (1993) Psychologische Einflüsse auf die atopische Dermatitis – eine verhaltensmedizinische Sichtweise. In: Gieler U, Stangier U, Brähler E (Hrsg) Hauterkrankungen in psychologischer Sicht. Jahrbuch der Medizinischen Psychologie Bd 9, Hogrefe, Göttingen

Ishizaka K, Ishizaka T, Hornbrook M (1967) Allergen-binding activita of E, G and A antibodies in sera from atopic patients. J Immunol 98: 490–501

Kodama A, Horikawa T, Suzuki T, Ajiki W, Takashima T, Harad S, Ichihashi M (1999) Effect of stress on atopic dermatitis: investigation in patients after the Great Hanshin Earthquake. J Allergy Clin Immunol 104: 173–176

Kupfer J, Keins P, Brosig B, Darsow U, Diepgen DL, Fartasch M, Korsch E, Lob-Corzilius T, Niemeier V, Scheidt R, Schmid-Ott G, Staab D, Szczepanski R, Werfel T, Wittenmeier M, Gieler U (2003) Development of questionnaires on coping with disease and itching cognitions for children and adolescents with atopic eczema. Dermatol Psychosom 4: 79–85

Obermayer M (1955) Psychocutaneous medicine. Thomas, Springfield, IL

Rechenberger I (1979) Prurigo bei Atopie. Materialien zur Psychoanalyse und analytisch orientierten Psychotherapy. Universität Düsseldorf, 5: 67–96

Roos TC (2004) Psychosomatic aspects of skin care and therapy of atopic dermatitis with regard to the patient's dealing with himself and the parents' dealing with their child. Dermatol Psychosom 5: 117–124

Rüden U von , Kehrt R, Staab D, Wahn U (1999) Entwicklung und Validierung eines krankheitsspezifischen Fragebogens zur Erfassung der Lebensqualität von Eltern neurodermitiskranker Kinder. Z f Gesundheitswiss 4: 335–350

Scheich G, Florin I, Rudolph R, Wilhelm S (1993) Personality characteristics and serum IgE level in patients with atopic dermatitis. J Psychosom Res 37: 637–642

Schmid-Ott G, Künsebeck HW, Jäger B, Werfel T, Frahm K, Ruitmann J, Kapp A, Lamprecht F (1999) Validity study for the stigmatization experience in atopic dermatitis and psoriasis patients. Acta Derm Venereol 79: 443–447

Schultz-Larsen F, Holm N, Henningsen K (1986) Atopic dermatitis. A genetic-epidemiologic study in a population-based twin sample. J Am Acad Dermatol 15: 487–494

Seikowski K, Gollek S (1999) Belastende Lebensereignisse bei hautkranken Personen. Z Dermatol 185: 56–61

Szentivanyi MD (1968) The beta adrenergic theory of the atopic abnormality in bronchial asthma. J Allergy 42: 203–205

Further Reading

Augustin M, Zschocke I, Lange S, Seidenglanz K, Amon U (1999) Lebensqualität bei Hauterkrankungen: Vergleich verschiedener Lebensqualitätsfragebögen bei Psoriasis und atopischer Dermatitis. Hautarzt 50: 715–722

Bullinger M (1997) Gesundheitsbezogene Lebensqualität und subjektive Gesundheit. Überblick über den Stand der Forschung zu einem Epulationskriterium in der Medizin. Pychother Psychosom Med Psychol 47: 76–91

Buske-Kirschbaum A, Geiben A, Hollig H, Morschhauser E, Hellhammer D (2002) Altered responsiveness of the hypothalamus-pituitary-adrenal axis and the sympathetic adrenomedullary system to stress in patients with atopic dermatitis. J Clin Endocrinol Metab 87(9): 4245–4251

Consoli S (1996) Skin and stress. Pathol Biol (Paris) 44: 875–881

Ehlers A, Stangier U, Gieler U (1995) Treatment of atopic dermatitis: a comparison of psychological and dermatological approaches to relapse prevention. J Consult Clin Psychol 63: 624–635

Faulstich ME, Williamson DA, Duchmann EG, Conerly SL, Brantley PJ (1985) Psychophysiological analysis of atopic dermatitis. J Psychosom Res 29: 415–417

Fjellner B, Arnetz BB, Eneroth P, Kallner A (1985) Pruritus during standardized mental stress. Acta Derm Venereol 65: 199–205

Gieler U, Niemeier V (2003) Psychophysiological aspects of atopic dermatitis. In: Koo J, Lee C-S (eds) Psychocutaneous Medicine. Dekker, New York, pp 97–118

Gieler U, Hohmann M, Niemeier V, Kupfer J, Stangier U, Ehlers A (1999) Cost evaluation in atopic eczema. J Dermatol Treat 10(suppl 1): 15–20

Hermanns N, Scholz O (1992) Kognitive Einflüsse auf einen histamininduzierten Juckreiz und Quaddelbildung bei der atopischen Dermatitis. Verhaltensmodifikation und Verhaltensmedizin 13(3): 171–194

Mohr W, Bock H (1993) Persönlichkeitstypen und emotionale Belastung bei Patienten mit atopischer Dermatitis. Z Klin Psychol 22: 302–314

Münzel K, Schandry R (1990) Atopisches Ekzem: psychophysiologische Reaktivität unter standardisierter Belastung. Hautarzt 41: 606–611

Rosenbaum MS, Ayllon T (1981) The behavioral treatment of neurodermatitis through habit-reversal. Behav Res Ther 19: 313–318

Stangier U, Ehlers A, Gieler U (2003) Measuring adjustment of chronic skin disorders: validation of a self-report measure. Psychol Assess 15: 532–549

Tobin D, Nabarro G, Baart de la Faille H, Vloten WA van, Putte SCJ van der, Schuurmann HJ (1992) Increased number of immunoreactive nerve fibers in atopic dermatitis. J Allergy Clin Immunol 90: 613–622

Uexküll T von (1995) Psychosomatische Medizin, 5. Aufl. Urban & Schwarzenberg, München

Williamson P (2000) Psychotherapy bei Neurodermitis-Patienten – eine retrospektive Studie an 43 Neurodermitis-Patienten. Dissertation Justus-Liebig-Universität Gießen

Acne Vulgaris

Definition. Acne vulgaris (ICD-10: L70, F54) is a papulopustulous disease of the sebaceous glands, characterized by keratinization impairment of the hair follicles, retention of the follicle contents with formation of comedones, and secondary inflammatory transformation.

Occurrence. Acne occurs in puberty in nearly 90% of adolescents in western countries and must therefore be termed a physiological skin lesion, which, however, is clinically relevant and requires medical treatment in one-third of all adolescents. Persistent acne, termed acne tarda, can persist well into the 4th decade of life. Severe forms of acne may result in significant scarring.

Pathogenesis. Acne has a genetic basis, which may be affected by external influences, including emotional factors. Thus, it is classically a multifactorial dermatosis. Follicular hyperkeratosis and sebaceous gland hyperplasia in particular are among the primary factors, and secondary factors, including microbial hypercolonization, inflammations, and immunoresponses, may play a decisive role in the later course.

Also relevant is the hormonal influence of androgens, including testosterone from testicles and ovaries and dehydroepiandrosterone from the adrenal cortex, which causes growth stimulation of the sebocytes, hyperplasia of the sebaceous glands, hyperseborrhea, and infundibulum keratosis. In consequence, the elevated lipid secretion promotes growth of *Propionibacterium acnes*, the lipase of which cleaves the triglycerides of the sebum in free fatty acids. In addition, chemoattractive substances are released, which attract inflammatory cells.

Clinical findings. The classic primary clinical presentation of acne is characterized by comedones, papulopustules, and papulae. The secondary presentation is characterized by cysts, fistulae, hemorrhagic crusts, and scars that could develop into keloids.

Morphology and Stages of Acne

- Initial acne lesions:
  - Microcomedones
  - Closed comedones
  - Open comedones
- Subsequent lesions:
  - Papulae
  - Pustules
  - Nodules
  - Abscesses
  - Fistulae
- Tertiary, noninflammatory lesions:
  - Scars
  - Cysts
  - Fistulocomedones

Based on the dominant clinical presentation and the severity, acne can be subdivided into acne comedonica, acne papulopustulosa, severe acne papulopustulosa, or acne conglobata, up to acne fulminans with systemic symptoms (Fig. 2.3).

The localization of acne has a typical distribution pattern (face, neck, back, axillae, chest). If the acne mainly manifests in intertriginous areas – that is, perianal, inguinal, or axillary – the term acne inversa is also used, although this mostly refers to hidradenitis suppurativa. Differential diagnosis must rule out other acneiform dermatoses (Fig. 2.3d) that often occur in connection with medications, foods, or endocrine factors (steroid acne). In women, special attention must be paid to the SAHA syndrome, which includes seborrhea, acne, hirsutism, and alopecia.

Classification of Acne

- Severity
  - Acne comedonica
  - Acne papulopustulosa
  - Acne conglobata
- Special form
  - Acne neonatorum
  - Acne fulminans, acne necroticans
  - Acne inversa
  - Acne medicamentosa
  - Acne venenata, acne mechanica
  - Acne aestivalis
- Differential diagnoses
  - Acne excoriée des jeunes filles
  - Steroid acne
  - Adrenogenital syndrome
  - Gram-negative folliculitis
  - Demodex folliculitis
  - Rosacea

Special Form: Acne Inversa – Hidradenitis Suppurativa

The etiopathogenesis of acne inversa (Fig. 2.3c) is characterized by hyperkeratosis of the follicles, formation of comedones, superinfection, and granulomatous inflammatory reactions of the connective tissue with pronounced subcutaneous nodes, fistulae, and consecutive fibrosis. In the beginning there is often a giant comedo, which can be felt coarsely subcutaneously and results in the later course in bulging abscesses. A possible degeneration of acne inversa, especially after a longer course, and the onset of squamous epithelial carcinomas has been reported several times. In the perianal region, deep fistulae may form into the rectum. An association with Crohn's disease has been described. The therapy of choice is surgery.

Emotional symptomatics. Often, the subjective experience of disease in acne patients in no way agrees with the objective medical findings. Acne patients often present with depressive and sociophobic tendencies and have the highest known suicide rates among skin patients (Cotterill and Cunliffe 1997; Niemeier et al. 1998). Self-esteem and disease coping are often impaired.

In psychological questionnaire surveys, acne patients rate themselves as particularly helpless and therefore should perhaps be given more attention in routine therapy. Conspicuous emotional signs are often found in pa-

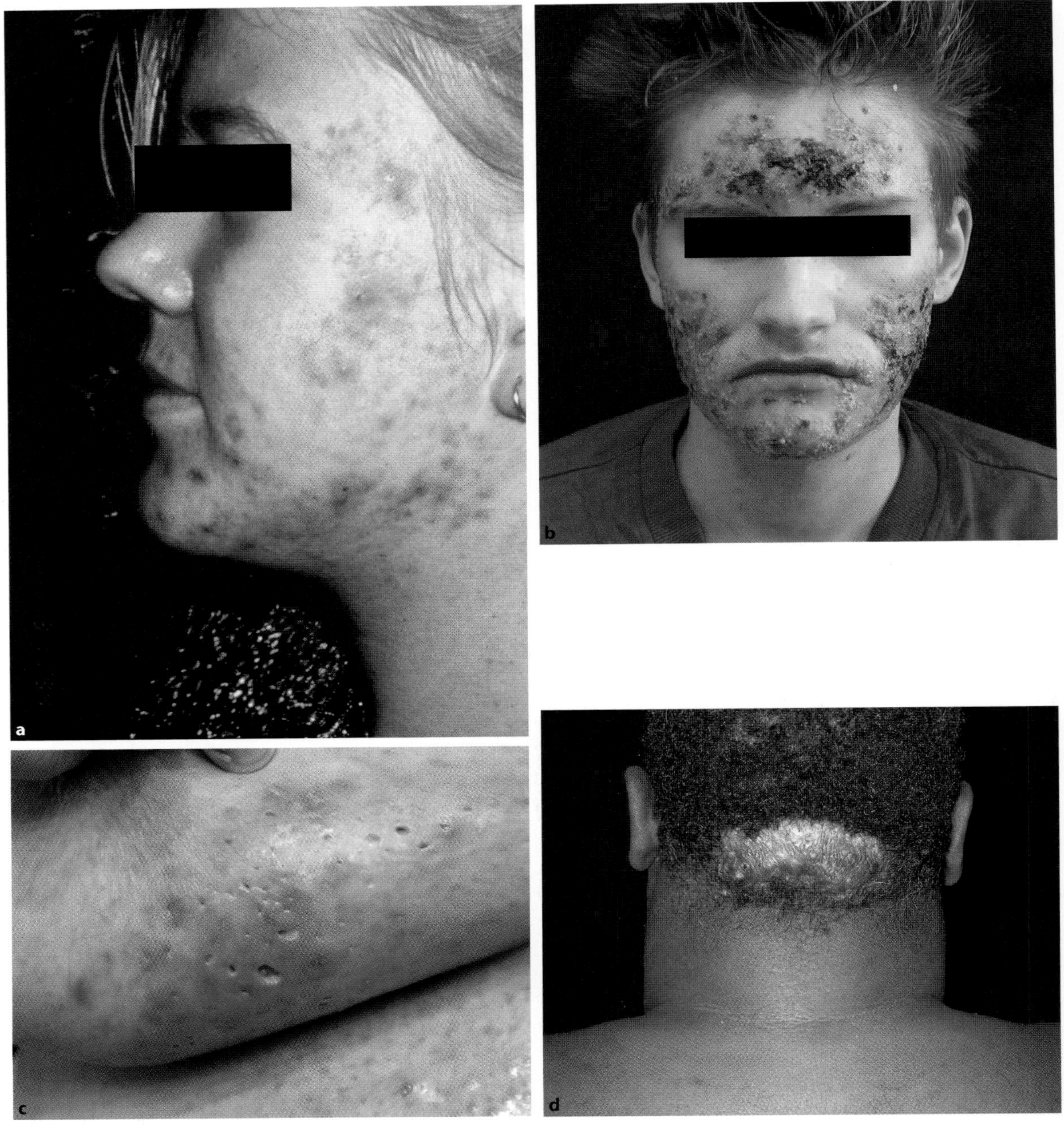

Fig. 2.3 **a** Facial acne conglobata with depressive disorder and impaired coping. The patient also felt pronounced helplessness due also to stigmatization. **b** A 25-year-old patient with acne fulminans and depression. **c** Acne inversa. **d** Folliculitis nuchae sclerotisans

tients with so-called persistent acne (acne after the 25th year of life). Our own studies in Giessen, Germany, show that exhaustion and gastrointestinal complaints occur more often in acne patients than in healthy controls. Insecurity and sensitivity are elevated, and the patients denigrate their own attractiveness.

Patients with acne have fewer dates, participate less in athletic activities, are more often unemployed, and have more emotional comorbidities. Acne is increasingly experienced as a disfiguring disease. The actual problem is not the disease itself, but the handling by the patients, who usually suffer emotionally from reduced self-esteem, social detriment, and reduced quality of life. Studies have shown that severe facial acne results in professional detriment; in one study, 68.3% of the patients reported psychological rejection (Niemeier et al. 2002).

Emotional comorbidity. A psychosomatic comorbidity is found in about 30% of all acne patients (Gupta and Gupta 1998). Depressions are present in acne patients, but in some studies not more frequently than in healthy persons (Gupta and Gupta 1998; Niemeier et al. 2002). Some studies refer to possible suicidal tendency, especially in male patients with acne conglobata and patients with body dysmorphic disorder (Cotterill and Cunliffe 1997). Anxiety disorders are considerably more frequent than in other chronic diseases.

Social anxieties and feeling of helplessness may lead to anxiety disorders and depression in acne patients.

Likewise, the differential diagnosis should rule out social phobia and sexual disorders (Gieler 1992). Inadequate knowledge and explanation of eliciting factors make this problem worse.

Quality of life. There is considerable detriment to the quality of life for acne patients in the psychological and social areas, comparable to those with other serious physical diseases such as diabetes, rheumatism, or asthma (Niemeier 2002). Acne is also comparable to other chronic skin diseases with respect to detriment to quality of life.

Stress. According to several studies, 60–78% of acne patients report exacerbation of their acne in subjectively experienced stress. Two experimental studies have demonstrated the increased occurrence of pustulae under academic examination conditions (Lorenz et al. 1953; Scholz 1987).

Compliance and coping. Acne patients' subjective concept of their disease influences their expectations of treatment and their compliance (Koo 1995; Niemeier et al. 1998). The most important psychological problem is poor compliance, which results from an unfavorable conviction regarding the pathogenesis, unfavorable expectations of therapy, and an unfavorable doctor–patient relationship. The latter was confirmed by a survey of 3,162 patients (Korczak 1989).

Only 17% of the acne patients questioned were undergoing medical treatment. Nearly half of these patients were dissatisfied with treatment or believed that the doctor didn't understand their problems, or they had the impression of receiving too little information from the doctor. They also usually felt that their problems were not taken seriously. After improvements in dermatologist – patient communication, 66% of the dermatologists reported improved patient compliance.

Summary of the Emotional Symptomatics in Acne Vulgaris

- The acne patient's subjective experience of disease does not correlate with the objective medical findings.
- Acne patients are often noncompliant.
- Acne patients often present with depressive and sociophobic tendencies.
- Acne patients have the highest known suicide rates in dermatology (in particular, adolescent males with acne conglobata).
- Self-esteem and disease coping are often impaired in these patients.

Psychological studies. Apart from generally applicable questionnaires on quality of life, depression, anxiety, and other psychological changes, several validated questionnaires are available that provide data specifically on acne patients: the Dermatological Life Quality Index, the Acne Disability Index, Skindex (skin-disease-specific quality of life), the MHF, the Social Phobia Scale, and the DCQ (questionnaire dealing with appearance).

Differential diagnosis. Careful differential-diagnostic determination of a body dysmorphic disorder and paraartefacts in the sense of acne excoriée des jeunes filles, which may be associated with the presentation of acne, is especially important, also with respect to initiating adequate therapy.

Dermatological therapy. In principle, therapy is dependent on the severity, skin type, gender, age, concurrent illnesses, and degree of acne manifestation. Nowadays a number of topical acne therapies exist that show keratolytic and antimicrobial efficacy. There are also topical sebosuppressives and anti-inflammatory interventions and a number of combination therapeutics.

Antibiotics (tetracycline, doxycycline, clindamycin, trimethoprim- sulfamethoxazole), isotretinoin, and spironolactone are especially used for systemic therapy. In Canada and Europe, antiandrogens (ciproterone acetate, chlormadinoacetate, dienogest) are also available.

Other procedures include ultraviolet light therapy, intralesional corticosteroid injections, cryotherapy, laser therapeutic procedures, chemical peeling and surgical therapy (especially for acne inversa or keloidal scars), and injection of filling substances in atrophic scars.

Psychotherapy. From a psychosomatic point of view, four problem areas in acne can be identified, making different psychotherapeutic approaches necessary:

- Adolescent acne (relative indication for psychotherapy in the case of comorbidities)
- Persistent acne after age 25 (relative indication in the case of comorbidities)
- Acne excoriée (psychotherapy usually necessary)
- Body dysmorphic disorder (psychotherapy always necessary)

Adolescent Acne and Persistent Acne After Age 25

The emotional components should be taken into consideration in the diagnosis of adolescent acne and especially in persistent acne after age 25, and the patient's problems should be addressed as part of psychosomatic primary care. Every kind of acne has a subjective influence on the patient's coping with the disease, quality of life, and preexisting emotional comorbidities. In dermatological practice, measures against emotional detriment should be included in the diagnostic consultation.

Therapeutic Recommendations for Treating Acne (Stangier 1987)

- Provide information about the cause and course of the disease (psychoeducation)
- Attend to the patient's subjective conception/misconception of the disease
- Understand the burden of the skin disease
- Be alert to signs of serious emotional disorders, including depression, social anxieties, and suicidal tendencies
- Address emotional changes during therapy
- Cooperate with specialist psychotherapists

Psychosomatic overdiagnosis ("psychologization") of the patient must be as carefully avoided as failure to recognize psychosomatic conflicts. To date, there are no studies on the effectiveness of psychotherapy in acne. According to expert opinion, adjuvant psychotherapy is indicated in depressive consequential reactions, social phobia, and body dysmorphic disorder.

! The question of when psychotherapy is indicated in acne depends on the comorbidity of emotional disorders.

Compliance improvement plays a central role in doctor–patient communication because therapy is often inadequate in acne. To improve compliance, the doctor should initially provide only three important bits of information about acne therapy:

1. How to apply it
2. How often to apply it
3. What to do if problems arise

Ideally, the patient should repeat all instructions in his or her own words and be allowed time to ask questions. It is important to promote nonverbal contact (the doctor should make eye contact!) and to use the patient's language.

Acne Excoriée/Body Dysmorphic Disorder

If acne excoriée or body dysmorphic disorders is present, specific measures are urgently indicated as part of psychosomatic primary care or specialist psychotherapy. It is essential to cooperate with a suitable therapist with basic dermatological knowledge. A detailed presentation of the psychotherapy is found in the chapters on paraartefacts and body dysmorphic disorders.

Psychopharmaceuticals. There is no general indication for psychopharmacological therapy in acne. Accompanying adjustment disorders, depressive disorders, and anxiety disorders should be accessible to psychopharmacological treatment.

Individual case reports have shown good success with selective serotonin reuptake inhibitors (SSRIs) including sertraline (Koo and Ng 2002) and olanzapine (Gupta and Gupta 2001) for accompanying depression in the management of acne excoriée.

References

Cotterill JA, Cunliffe WJ (1997) Suicide in dermatological patients. Br J Dermatol 137(2): 246–250

Gieler U (1992) Akne und Psyche. In: Friederich HC (Hrsg) Praxis der Akne-Therapy. Wissenschaftliche Verlagsgesellschaft, Stuttgart, S 57–88

Gupta MA, Gupta AK (1998) Depression and suicidal ideation in dermatology patients with acne, alopecia areata, atopic dermatitis and psoriasis. Br J Dermatol 139: 846–850

Gupta MA, Gupta AK (2001) Olanzapine may be an effective adjunctive therapy in the management of acne excoriée: a case report. J Cutan Med Surg 5(1): 25–27

Koo J (1995) The psychosocial impact of acne: patients' perceptions. J Am Acad Dermatol 32: 26–30

Koo JY, Ng TC (2002) Psychotropic and neurotropic agents in dermatology: unapproved uses, dosages, or indications. Clin Dermatol 20(5): 582–594

Korczak D (1989) Psychische Situation der Akne-Patienten. Persönlichkeitsstruktur und Arzt-Patient-Beziehung. Fortschr Med 107: 309–313

Lorenz TH, Graham DT, Wolf S (1953) The relation of life-stress and emotions to human sebum secretion and to the mechanism of acne vulgaris. J Lab Clin Med 41: 11–28

Niemeier V, Kupfer J, Demmelbauer-Ebner M, Stangier U, Effendy I, Gieler U (1998) Coping with acne vulgaris. Evaluation of the chronic skin disorder questionnaire in patients with acne. Dermatology 196(1): 108–115

Niemeier V, Kupfer J, Gieler U (2002) Acne is not a trivial disease! Psychosomatic aspects in routine therapy. Psychosom Dermatol 3: 61–70

Scholz O (1987) Stress und Akne. Dtsch Med Wschr 112: 516–520

Stangier U (1987) Einstellung zur Akne und psychische Krankheitsverarbeitung – Ansätze für eine verbesserte Aknetherapy. Ärztl Kosmetol 17: 407–408

Further Reading

Aktan S, Ozmen E, Sanli B (2000) Anxiety, depression and nature of acne vulgaris in adolescents. Int J Dermatol 39: 354–357

Alt C (1988) Symptomwahrnehmung. Symptomerleben, Körpererleben und Kontaktverhalten bei Jugendlichen mit Akne. Roderer, Regensburg

Arnold LM, Auchenbach MB, McElroy SL (2001) Psychogenic excoriation. Clinical features, proposed diagnostic criteria, epidemiology and approaches to treatment. CNS Drugs 15(5): 351–359

Cunliffe WJ (1986) Acne and unemployment. Br J Dermatol 115: 386

Cunliffe WJ, Hughes BR (1991) Treatment of the depressed and dysmorphophobic acne patient. Clin Exp Dermatol 16(3): 210–211

Kent A, Drummond LM (1989) Acne excoriée – a case report of treatment using habit reversal. Clin Exp Dermatol 14: 163–164

Koblenzer CS (2001) The use of psychotropic drugs in dermatology. Dermatol Psychosom 2: 167–176

Lucas CJ, Ojha A (1963) Personality and acne. J Psychosom Res 7: 41

Motley RJ, Finlay AY (1992) Practical use of disability index in the routine management of acne. Clin Exp Dermatol 17: 1

Panconesi E, Hautmann G (1998) Psychotherapeutic approach in acne treatment. Dermatology 196(1): 116–118

Polenghi MM, Zizak S, Molinari E (2002) Emotions and acne. Dermatol Psychosom 3: 20–25

Zaghloul SS, Cunliffe WJ, Goodfield MJD (2002) Compliance in acne is highly correlated to psychological well-being and self presentation. Br J Dermatol 147(suppl 62): 43

Psoriasis Vulgaris

AD –
HcN – } Corner
PV –

Definition. Psoriasis vulgaris (ICD-10: L40.0, F54) is a chronic inflammatory papulosquamous genodermatosis that may proceed in various forms. Among these are psoriasis vulgaris, pustular psoriasis, psoriasis arthropathica, and the often infection-associated guttate psoriasis.

Occurrence/prevalence. Psoriasis is the second most frequent skin disease following eczema, with a worldwide incidence between 1% and 4%.

The prevalence of psoriasis in Germany and in the Caucasian population in the United States is cited as 1.3%, and is 0.97% for mulattos in South America (Rassner 1980). The sometimes considerable differences in the population as well as genetic and environmental influences on the disease are responsible for the observed variability in prevalence.

Pathogenesis. An immunological genesis is in the foreground of discussions of pathogenesis, so the term genetically determined immune dermatosis can be used. It is characterized by a greatly increased transit time from the basal cell layer to the stratum corneum.

Meanwhile, numerous findings have made it plausible that psychosocial factors may exert a modulating influence on the immunological processes via close anatomical and functional bonds between the central nervous system (CNS) and the immune system (Farber et al. 1986). Patients often report deterioration of the psoriasis after stress.

Psychoendocrinological studies with measurement of adrenalin excretion in urine showed an elevation in the psoriasis group compared with healthy controls (Arnetz et al. 1985).

Moreover, a stress-induced elevation of CD-8-positive and CD-11-positive T lymphocytes was demonstrated in psoriasis patients (Schmid-Ott 1998; Kapp 1993).

Similar to AD, endocrinological and immunological reactions can apparently be triggered by stress. Here, too, neuropeptides play a central key role and may explain the stress vulnerability.

Clinical findings. Papulosquamous lesions are the hallmark of this condition, as well as prominent erythema. Additionally, pustules, joint involvement, and rheumatic complaints may predominate, depending on the clinical forms (Fig. 2.4).

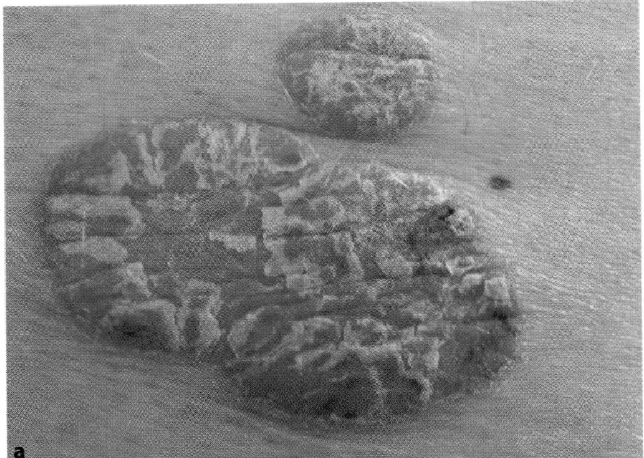

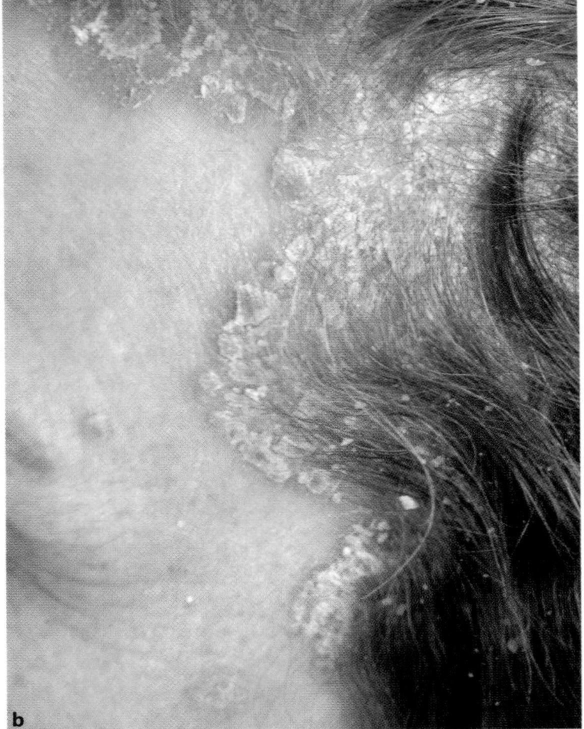

Fig. 2.4 a Psoriasis vulgaris in a 44-year-old woman with pronounced depression and Köebner phenomenon. **b** Psoriasis vulgaris with stigmatization

Emotional symptomatics. Psoriasis vulgaris can be triggered by emotional factors.

Stress. It is clear that stress and emotional burdens may trigger psoriasis episodes. Among these may be such diverse stress factors as shock of accident, war experiences or being drafted for military service, death of a near relative, or even fear of an examination (Koblenzer 1988; Borelli 1967).

Using the methods of life-event research, various teams have examined whether patients with psoriasis had experienced more stressful life events during a certain time prior to the outbreak of their disease than a comparable group of control persons with healthy skin. Thirth-nine percent of the psoriasis patients remembered experiencing a stressful event during the period 4 weeks before the onset of their disease versus only 10% in the control group (Seville 1978). According to information from more than 2,000 patients in a retrospective questionnaire study (Farber et al. 1968), psoriasis tended to occur or become worse in about 40% of the patients in times of emotional stress; 21% of those questioned denied such a relationship; and the rest of the patients were not sure about such a connection.

On the other hand, chronic everyday stress situations and annoyances ("daily hassles") appear to be more burdensome and decisive than the so-called critical life events (Gupta and Gupta 1995).

In a 20-week prospective study of psoriasis patients using a multivariate method, positive correlations were found between the severity of the psoriasis and psychological stress (Gaston et al. 1987). The authors recommend introducing stress reduction training in psoriasis therapy.

Taking psychoneuroimmunological pathogenesis concepts into account, it appears that there is a group (cluster) of stress responders among psoriasis patients, in whom the psychological factor of stress plays a particular role in eliciting an episode.

Psychodynamic view of psoriasis. Psoriasis is a multifactorial disease, but the patients' personality structures do not differ from those in other control groups (Welzel-Ruhrmann 1995).

Overall, psoriasis patients do not show any clear tendencies to neurotic developments or personality disorders, but rather a specific emotional maladaption.

Among psoriasis patients, from a psychodynamic point of view, disorders of self-esteem are more frequently diagnosed, which serve as a defense against feelings of inferiority, desire for regression, and depression. The "scaly armor" also serves as protection against inner vulnerability in this concept (Gieler 1986).

Depressive and compulsive character structures and experience reactions are often demonstrated in psoriasis patients; these may have arisen either premorbidly or as a consequence of the disease. Psychosocial disorders occupy a considerable disease value in a cluster of patients with psoriasis.

Thus, some authors assume the importance of psychodynamic processes as a decisive factor in symptom formation, with an underlying conflict in connection with the defense of symbiotic desires as the main symptom, which leads finally to a somatic purging of aggressive impulses (Schur 1993). The proven inhibition of aggression appears to be characteristic of psoriasis; the ability to cope with disease is considerably limited.

Coping with disease. Psoriasis has a decisive disease value because of the burden of outward appearance, especially in the patient's conviction that he or she is disfigured (stigmatization; Fig. 2.4b).

For the patient, another stress factor arises in that the eliciting of a disease episode is neither predictable nor controllable.

Resignation in this chronic disease often makes the patient feel helpless and depressed. Because it is a chronic disease, there is danger of identifying with the disease and experiencing oneself only as sick in all areas of life. On the other hand, denial of the disease's importance and the unrealistic hope of finally obtaining help is often found as a coping mechanism, which is supposed to protect against helplessness and depression.

The usually late onset of psoriasis is important in coping with the disease. Clinical experience has shown that the secondary coping with disease depends particularly on existing social contacts at the time of first manifestation, including sexual relationships, the individual's professional life, and periods of disability.

In general, the older the patients are at the onset of their disease, the better they are integrated into their environments, the better their secondary coping with disease, and the less likely they will experience disfiguration problems.

In addition to disease-specific stress situations, disease-related interpersonal conflicts are also seen, which arise in part from the groundless fear of contagion of the healthy person and fear of the psoriasis patient him- or herself (refer to the information on skin diseases and sexuality in Chap. 5).

Disrupted partnership relationships and problems with alcohol and depression are repeatedly reported. The increased occurrence of alcoholism, obesity, depression (Gupta et al. 1994; Gupta and Gupta 1998), and suicide that is repeatedly conspicuous among psoriasis patients is often seen in connection with the severity of the conflict-laden coping with disease, which may have arisen premorbidly or as a consequence of the disease.

Quality of life. Stigmatization due to the disease is in the foreground of coping with the disease, along with clearly increased limitations in the quality of life. This can be demonstrated using special questionnaires on coping with disease and quality of life.

Insults and rejection, and avoiding these in places such as swimming pools and saunas and in sports and partnerships, including sexual relations, occupy an important place in patients' lives, and patients with psoriasis repeatedly have to decrease their activities.

Differential diagnosis. Other papulosquamous skin diseases such as pityriasis rosea, pityriasis rubra pilaris, or parapsoriasis and cutaneous T-cell lymphoma must be ruled out, especially in the guttate forms of psoriasis.

Dermatological therapy. An immunological genesis predominates in psoriasis. Therefore, immunosuppressive local and systemic therapy approaches show very good rates of treatment success (Lebwohl and Tan 1998). Dermatological treatment comprises a number of immunomodulating therapy schemes, including topical steroids, vitamin D analogs, phototherapy, systemic immunosuppression (for example, methotrexate and cyclosporin), and the more recent "biological" therapies.

Psychotherapy. Psychotherapy should be considered, especially in chronic forms of psoriasis and for stress responders. The group of stress responders in psoriasis should be identified, diagnosed, and given adequate therapy under psychotherapeutic guidelines. Initiation of psychotherapy in psoriasis also depends decisively on the comorbidities. Depending on the severity of emotional symptoms, a stepwise plan may be meaningful. Patients with elevated stress levels especially show increased itching and higher depression scores, so symptomatic therapy with antihistamines and relaxation techniques, particularly autogenic training, is indicated for these patients (Fortune et al. 2002).

Individual studies on behavior therapy measures reveal these to be advantageous. To these can be added psychoeducation and special training measures to improve compliance and coping in everyday life, usually as group therapy. Patients who participate in a program with autogenic training show fewer recurrences. These programs focus on coping with disease, including measures to improve the quality of life. Only a few single case reports are available on psychodynamic approaches (Schur 1993; Koblenzer 1995).

Stepwise Plan for Psoriasis

1. Psychosomatic primary care
2. Psychoeducation
3. Relaxation therapy, concentrative movement therapy, mindful stress reduction, hypnosis
4. Improvement of compliance
5. Strengthened disease coping
6. Coping in everyday life
7. Group therapy
8. Psychotherapy/psychopharmaceuticals (depending on the dominant comorbidity)

Alcohol dependency must be diagnosed and treated. Finally, self-help is of central importance in coping with psoriasis. Coping strategies for everyday living and self-help concepts can often be learned. The concept of the duo formula should not be underestimated. In this concept, a newly afflicted or greatly burdened patient finds help in talking with a dermatologist and with a patient who has a lot of experience with the disease.

Psychopharmaceuticals. Concurrent therapy with psychopharmaceuticals may have a stabilizing influence in pronounced depressive disorder, anxiety disorder, of other comorbidities.

References

Arnetz BB, Fjellner B, Eneroth P, Kallner A (1985) Stress and psoriasis: psychoendocrine and metabolic reactions in psoriatic patients during standardized stressor exposure. Pychosom Med 47: 528–541

Borelli S (1967) Psyche und Haut. In: Gottron HA (Hrsg) Handbuch der Haut- und Geschlechtskrankheiten; Ergänzungsband 8, Springer, Berlin, S 464–466

Farber EM, Nickoloff BJ, Recht B, Fraki JE (1986) Stress, symmetry, and psoriasis: possible role of neuropeptides. J Am Acad Dermatol 14: 305–311

Farber EM, Bright RD, Nall ML (1968) Psoriasis. A questionnaire survey of 2144 patients. Arch Dermatol 98: 248–259

Fortune DG, Richards HL, Kirby B, Bowcock S, Main CJ, Griffiths CE (2002) A cognitive-behavioural symptom management programme as an adjunct in psoriasis therapy. Br J Dermatol 146(3): 458–465

Gaston L, Lassonde M, Bernier-Buzzanga J, Hodgins S, Crombez JC (1987) Psoriasis and stress: a prospective study. J Am Acad Dermatol 17: 82-86

Gieler U (1986) Mein Schuppenpanzer schützt mich! Persönlichkeitsbild und Körperbeschwerden bei Psoriasis-Patienten. Z Hautkr 61: 572–576

Gupta MA, Gupta AK (1995) The psoriasis life stress inventory: a preliminary index of psoriasis-related stress. Acta Derm Venereol 75: 240–243

Gupta MA, Gupta AK (1998) Depression and suicidal ideation in dermatology patients with acne, alopecia areata, atopic dermatitis and psoriasis. Br J Dermatol 139: 846–850

Gupta MA, Gupta AK, Schork NJ, Ellis CN (1994) Depression modulates pruritus perception: a study of pruritus in psoriasis, atopic dermatitis, and chronic idiopathic urticaria. Psychosom Med 56: 36–40

Kapp A (1993) Die Rolle von Zytokinen für die Pathogenese der Psoriasis. Hautarzt 44: 210–207

Koblenzer CS (1988) Stress and the skin: significance of emotional factors in dermatology. Stress Med 4: 21–26

Koblenzer CS (1995) Psychotherapy for intractable inflammatory dermatoses. J Am Acad Dermatol 32: 609–612

Lebwohl M, Tan MH (1998) Psoriasis and stress. Lancet 351: 82–82

Rassner G (1980) Psoriasis. In: Korting G (Hrsg) Dermatologie in Praxis und Klinik, Bd II, Thieme Stuttgart, S 10.1–10.25

Schmid-Ott G, Jacobs R, Jaeger B, Klages S, Wolf J, Werfel T, Kapp A, Schuermeyer T, Lamprecht F, Schmidt RE, Schedlowski M (1998) Stress-induced endocrine and immunological changes in psoriasis patients and healthy controls: a preliminary study. Psychother Psychosom 67: 37–42

Schur M (1993) Zur Metapsychologie der Somatisierung – dargestellt am Beispiel analytischer Untersuchungen von Hautkranken. In: Overbeck G, Overbeck A (Hrsg) Seelischer Konflikt und körperliches Leiden, 5. Aufl. Klotz, Eschborn, S 83–142

Seville R (1978) Psoriasis and stress. Br J Dermatol 97: 297–302

Welzel-Ruhrmann C (1995) Psychologische Diagnostik bei Hauterkrankungen. Verhaltensmod Verhaltensmed 16: 311–335

Further Reading

Augustin M, Zschocke I, Lange S, Seidenglanz K, Amon U (1999) Lebensqualität bei Hauterkrankungen: Vergleich verschiedener Lebensqualitätsfragebögen bei Psoriasis und atopischer Dermatitis. Hautarzt 50: 715–722

Glinski W, Brodecka H, Glinska-Ferenz M, Kowalski D (1994) Increased concentration of beta-endorphin in sera of patients with psoriasis and other inflammatory dermatoses. Br J Dermatol 131: 260–264

Huckenbeck-Goedecker B, Schroepl F (1988) Verhaltenstraining für Psoriasis-Patienten – Ein Beitrag zur Vorbeugung von Rezidiven? In: Romkopf G, Fröhlich WD, Lindner I (Hrsg) Forschung und Praxis im Dialog. Entwicklungen und Perspektiven. Bericht über den 14. Kongress für Angewandte Psychologie, Bd 2, Deutscher Psychologen Verlag, Bonn, S 189–194

Lange S, Zschocke I, Langhardt S, Amon U, Augustin M (1999) Effekte kombinierter therapeutischer Maßnahmen bei Patienten mit Psoriasis und atopischer Dermatitis. Hautarzt 50: 791–797

Price ML, Mottahedin I, Mayo PR (1991) Can psychotherapy help patients with psoriasis? Clin Exp Dermatol 16(2): 114–117

Zachariae R, Oster H, Bjerring P, Kragballe K (1996) Effects of psychologic intervention on psoriasis: a preliminary report. J Am Acad Dermatol 34: 1008–1015

Alopecia Areata

Definition. Alopecia areata (ICD-10: L63, F54 or F43.2) is usually a nonscarring circular area of hair loss on the scalp, in the beard area, or other haired parts of the body. It occurs acutely.

Occurrence. Alopecia areata is observed worldwide. In dermatological practice, the diagnosis is made in up to 2% of patients and in inpatient dermatology hospitals in 1–4%. The prevalence in the United States is 0.1–0.2% of the total population.

The cause of the disease is unclear. Autoimmune impairments are considered among the promoting factors, in addition to heredity.

Autoimmunological aspects are presently in the foreground of the disease hypothesis. Excretion of neuropeptides, possibly also in connection with life events and stress, appears to play a further role, also in plausibly explaining the influence of psychosocial disorders (Koblenzer 1987; Panconesi 1984).

Clinical findings. There are usually circular, hairless areas with maintained follicle openings. The clinical presentation ranges from minimal variants to total head hair loss in alopecia totalis or total hair loss on the entire body in alopecia universalis. Several convex, arch-shaped, limited bald spots the size of a hand may form by further spread and confluence (Fig. 2.5).

Emotional Symptomatics

Severe life events and stress can be demonstrated in connection with alopecia areata.

In a study using a standardized life-event inventory (Perini et al. 1984) in 48 patients with alopecia areata and 30 patients with fungal infections (control group), a significant occurrence of life events was determined in the alopecia areata group.

In another study of 73 patients, clear stress factors could be revealed in the patients' environments in 41 cases (de Weert et al. 1984). The authors found serious behavioral problems in the 15 children examined. In 23%, the authors found that acute emotional trauma had existed even before the onset of alopecia. In summary, subgroups of stress responders and those with emotional disorders should be identified and treated under biopsychosocial aspects in alopecia areata.

Stressful life events appear to frequently precede alopecia areata. Coping with the alopecia often leads to anxious and depressive reactions.

Several studies have shown that the association between psychiatric diseases and alopecia areata is clearly elevated. Colon et al. (1991), for example, demonstrated that 74% of 31 examined patients with alopecia areata had a preceding psychiatric diagnosis (depressions were especially frequent), and the authors concluded that these patients have a higher risk for psychiatric diseases. This was also confirmed by other authors (Attah-Johnson and Mostaghimi 1995).

Koo et al. (1994) demonstrated in 294 patients with alopecia areata that depressions, fears, social phobias, and paranoid states were significantly more frequent than in the general population.

In addition, the quality of life for the affected patients is greatly impaired.

Diagnostics. Psychometric questionnaires should be used as appropriate to record information on depression, anxiety, and quality of life (Finlay 1997).

Differential diagnosis. The differential-diagnostic delineation from trichotillomania may be very difficult in some cases. Differentiation is also important for initiating the corresponding adequate therapeutic concepts. For this reason, a trichogram should always be performed.

Normally, 80% of hair roots are found in the so-called anagen stage, in which the roots are firmly attached to the root sheath, and 20% in the telogen stage, in which the roots push up to the skin surface to fall out. In alopecia areata, there are mostly telogenic hairs. In trichotillomania, by contrast, the anagenic proportion predominates in the hair-root status, as the telogen hairs have already been pulled out. A biopsy is useful to differentiate between these two afflictions.

Dermatological therapy. In the majority of cases, the disease tends to spontaneous healing. In individual cases, especially in those of prepuberty onset, there is total and permanent hair loss (alopecia areata totalis).

No causal therapy is known. Patients will respond to high doses of systemic corticosteroids; however, the lesions will recur once these are discontinued. The use of contact sensitization therapy is effective in many cases. Similarly, patients sometimes respond to phototherapy.

The high rate of spontaneous remissions should be taken into account and then accompanied by appropriate bland local therapy.

Psychotherapy. There is as yet no scientific proof that psychotherapeutic procedures have any definite influence on hair growth in alopecia areata.

Based on available data, the identification, diagnostics, and therapy of stress-vulnerable and depressive disorders or adjustment disorders as part of psychosomatic primary care take first priority in alopecia areata.

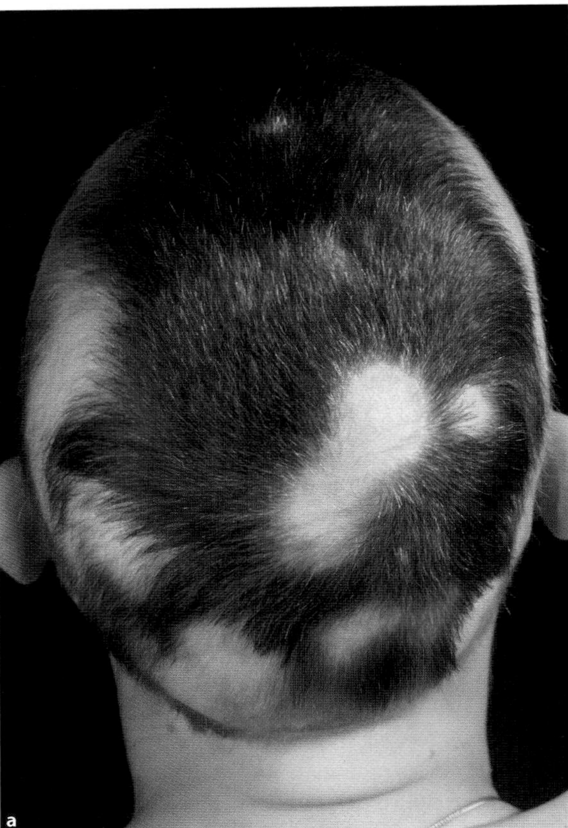

Stepwise Plan for Alopecia Areata

1. Psychosomatic primary care
2. Identification of stress responders
3. Disease coping
4. Relaxation therapy
5. Psychoeducation
6. Psychotherapy (depending on the dominant comorbidity)
7. Psychopharmaceuticals

Central to therapy, strengthening of active coping, sometimes with supportive psychotherapy and initiation of relaxation therapies, has proven beneficial. Especially in women, serious adjustment disorders due to sudden hair loss may be a psychotherapeutic challenge (Fig. 2.5b, c).

Teshima et al. (1991) demonstrated the effectiveness of psychotherapeutic relaxation techniques under immunological control of lymphocyte subsets and beta-endorphin in five of six cases and confirmed the success of hair growth by means of a 6-month catamnesis. A single case comparison between 7 months without treatment and 7 months under psychotherapeutic treatment revealed new hair growth (Putt et al. 1994), even though a spontaneous remission cannot be completely ruled out in this case.

As part of more in-depth psychosomatic exploration, the topics of shame, sociophobic tendencies, and depression should also be addressed.

There are only single case reports on successful psychodynamic therapy (Koblenzer 1987; Willenberg 1987). The indication depends on the comorbidities present. The

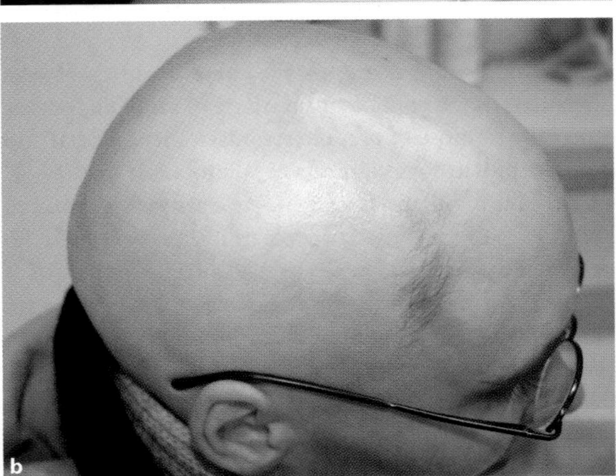

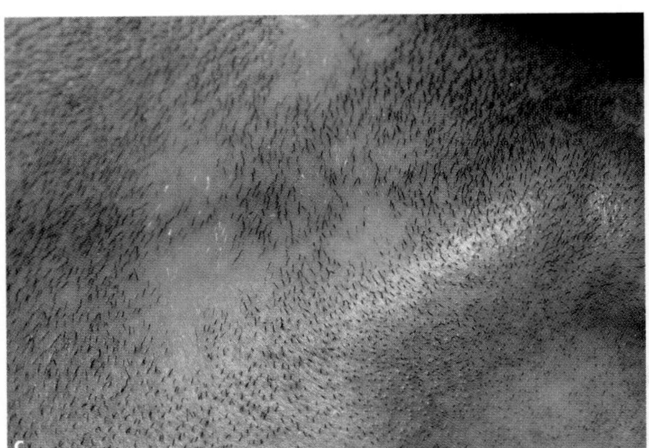

Fig. 2.5 **a** Alopecia areata in a 28-year-old woman with adjustment disorder. **b** Alopecia subtotalis with adjustment disorder. **c** Alopecia barbae with adjustment disorder

quality of life of the affected patients is greatly impaired. In this aspect, psychotherapy as focal therapy may possibly clearly reduce suffering and improve the quality of life.

Psychopharmaceuticals. Double-blind, placebo-controlled studies with psychopharmaceuticals (imipramine) document the positive effects of this therapy (Perini et al. 1994).

References

Attah-Johnson FY, Mostaghimi H (1995) Co-morbidity between dermatologic diseases and psychiatric disorders in Papua New Guinea. Int J Dermatol 34: 244–248

Colon EA, Popkin MK, Callies AL, Dessert NJ, Hordinsky MK (1991) Lifetime prevalence of psychiatric disorders in patients with alopecia areata. Compr Psychiatry 32: 245–251

Finlay AY (1997) Qualitiy of life measurement in dermatology, a practical guide. Br J Dermatol 136: 305–314

Koblenzer CS (1987) Alopecia areata, telogen effluvium, and hirsutism. In: Psychocutaneous disease. Grune & Stratton, Orlando, pp 248–263

Koo JY, Shellow WV, Hallman CP, Edwards JE (1994) Alopecia areata and increased prevalence of psychiatric disorders. Int J Dermatol 33: 849–850

Panconesi E (1984) Stress and skin diseases: Psychosomatic dermatology. In: Parish LC (ed) Clinics in Dermatology 2. Lippincott, Philadelphia

Pericin T, Kündig TM, Trüeb RM (1996) Trichotillomanie in Verbindung mit Alopecia areata. Z Hautkr 71: 921–924

Perini G, Veller-Fornasa C, Cipriani R, Bettin A, Zecchino F, Peserico A (1984) Life events and alopecia areata. Psychother Psychosom 41: 48–52

Perini G, Zara M, Cipriani R, Carraro C, Preti A, Gava F, Coghi P, Peserico A (1994) Imipramine in alopecia areata. A double-blind, placebo controlled study. Psychother Psychosom 61: 195–198

Putt SC, Weinstein L, Dzindolet MT (1994) A case study: massage, relaxation, and reward for treatment of alopecia areata. Psychol Rep 74: 1315–1318

Teshima H, Sogawa H, Mizobe K, Kuroki N, Nakagawa T (1991) Application of psychoimmunotherapy in patients with alopecia universalis. Psychother Psychosom 56: 235–241

Weert J de, Temmerman L, Kint A (1984) Alopecia areata: a clinical study. Dermatologica 168: 224–229

Willenberg H (1987) Zur Psychotherapy der Alopecia universalis. In: Spezialisierung und Integration in Psychosomatik und Psychotherapy. Springer, Berlin, S 418–426

Further Reading

Beard H (1986) Social and psychological implications of alopecia areata. J Am Acad Dermatol 14: 697–700

Egle UT, Tauschke E (1987) Die Alopecie – ein psychosomatisches Krankheitsbild? Psychother Psychosom Med Psychol 37: 31–35

Harrison PV, Stephanek P (1991) Hypnotherapy for alopecia areata. Br J Dermatol 124: 509–510

Madani S, Shapiro J (2000) Alopecia areata update. J Am Acad Dermatol 42: 549–566

Steen P van der, Boezeman J, Duller P, Happle R (1992) Can alopecia areata be triggered by emotional stress? An uncontrolled evaluation of 178 patients with extensive hair loss. Acta Derm Venereol 72: 279–280

Terashima Y, Ichikawa T, Suzuki T, Koizumi J (1989) An adult case of psychogenic alopecia universalis. Jpn J Psychiatry Neurol 43: 585–589

Zalka AD, Byarlay JA, Goldsmith LA (1994) Alopecia a deux: simultaneous occurence of alopecia in a husband and wife. Arch Dermatol 130: 390–392

Perianal Dermatitis (Anal Eczema)

Anal eczema is primarily characterized by dermatitis in a specific localization.

Definition. Perianal dermatitis is a subacute to chronic eczema (ICD-10: L23–L30, F54) around the anus, accompanied by pruritus. The genesis of anal eczema is multifactorial.

Pathogenesis. Perianal dermatitis is considered a collective term that may denote several underlying diseases. Thus, anal eczema is not a disease *sui generis*, but its occurrence is accompanied by various dermatological, allergological, infectious, compulsive, or emotional disorders of usually artificial maintenance.

Thus, primarily or dispositionally, a malformation with infundibuliform anus, hyperhidrosis, or hypertrichiosis may dominate, or acquired hemorrhoids, anal fissures, anal fistulas, various infections such as yeast infections, proctitis, colitis, condylomata acuminata, urinary incontinence, and benign or malignant neoplasms including rectal carcinoma must be considered. Moreover, parasitic infections must be ruled out.

Irritative toxic eczema, atopic dermatitis, psoriasis inversa, or allergic contact eczema are decisive as specific dermatoses. In addition, damage from corticosteroids or nutrition-related irritations from chili, citrus fruits, or other foods, as well as systemic diseases such as diabetes mellitus, lymphoma, leukemias, or ulcerating colitis may play a role.

Clinical findings. Predominant are various forms of acute to subacute dermatitis ranging to chronic forms with macerative erosive intertrigo in the perianal area, as well as lichenified chronic eczemas, which may show sharp or polycyclic delineated edges in contact allergic

2

superimposition. Anal eczema is characteristically accompanied by itching (Fig. 2.6).

Sometimes there is also proctalgia fugax, an anorectal neuralgia in which the individual experiences attacks of sharp, cramplike pains in the rectum, lasting up to 30 min, which usually occur at night (Sect. 1.3.4).

Emotional symptoms. In studies of pruritus ani of unclear origin, Laurent et al. (1997) demonstrated differences in the areas of depression and hypomania. Thus far, the database is rather disappointing, although experience shows that patients with anal eczema form a group of problem patients usually with depression or personality disorders, in whom compulsive symptoms are relevant. From a psychodynamic point of view, anal eczema is often related to problems in impulse dynamics.

Coping with the disease by limiting lifestyle and quality of life should be clarified with respect to anxiety, depression, and social withdrawal.

In pruritus ani with multifactorial triggers, the itching–scratching cycle has a further central importance. Scratching leads to irritation, excoriation, and subsequently to eczematization with superinfection, which elicits excessive treatment or anal hygiene with resultant renewed severe itching.

Differential diagnosis. The underlying diseases cited for the pathogenesis must first be ruled out in the differential diagnosis; anal eczema is an epiphenomenon or collective term. Other specific dermatoses such as psoriasis inversa, allergic contact eczema, and intertriginous candidiasis must be considered.

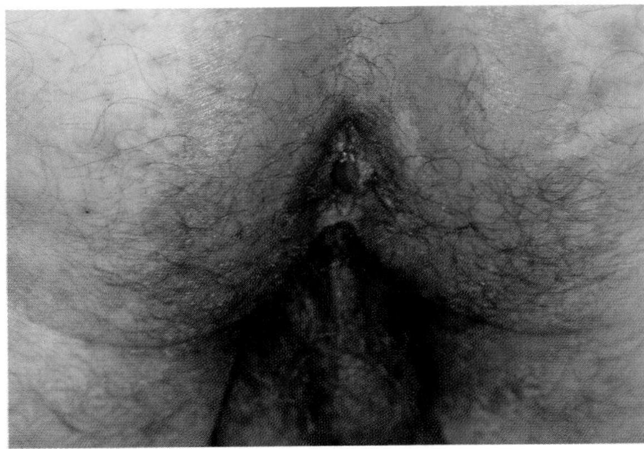

Fig. 2.6 Chronic anal eczema in a patient with depressive-compulsive personality disorder and hemorrhoids

Dermatological therapy. Therapy should be undertaken according to the underlying organic disease, including allergen avoidance and prevention of additional iatrogenic damage. Long-term local corticosteroid use is contraindicated.

Psychotherapy. No studies are available on the efficacy of psychotherapy. Individual cases successfully treated with deep-psychological procedures have been described.

Behavior therapy to break the itching–scratching cycle predominates, but relaxation measures such as autogenic training and progressive muscle relaxation are also used.

Stepwise Plan for Anal Eczema

1. Psychosomatic primary care
2. Psychoeducation
3. Relaxation therapy
4. Motivation psychotherapy
5. Behavior therapy (itching–scratching cycle)
6. Psychodynamic psychotherapy
7. Psychopharmaceuticals (SSRIs)

Frequently, the patient is not motivated to undergo more in-depth psychotherapy. Especially if the impulse-dynamic conflicts are addressed awkwardly or too early, the result may be termination of the doctor–patient relationship and perhaps even derogatory accusations. Presenting the case in Balint groups may be helpful for the doctor dealing with such difficult patients.

Psychopharmaceuticals. The underlying compulsive disorder or depressive disorder may support a treatment attempt with SSRIs. However, there are not yet any studies on this.

Reference

Laurent A, Boucharlat J, Bosson JL, Derry A, Imbert R (1997) Psychological assessment of patients with idiopathic pruritus ani. Psychother Psychosom 66(3): 163–166

Further Reading

AWMF (1999) Analekzem. http://www.AWMF-Leitlinien.de

Blecher T, Korting HC (1995) Tolerance to different toilet paper preparations: toxicological and allergological aspects. Dermatology 191: 299–304

Cohen R, Roth FJ, Delgado E et al. (1969) Fungual flora of the normal human small and large intestine. New Engl J Med 280: 638–641
Groot AC de, Baar TJM, Terpstra H, Weyland JW (1991) Contact allergy to moist toilet paper. Contact Dermatitis 24: 135–136
Doucet P (1988) Pruritus ani. Int J Psychoanal 69: 409–417
Helle S (1973) Pruritus und Eczema ani bei Candidiasis. Phlebol Proktol 2: 41–43
Neri J, Bardazzi F, Marzaduri S, et al (1996) Perianal streptococcal dermatitis in adults. Br J Dermatol 135: 796–798
Schneider KW (1976) Zur Behandlung von Hefen bei perianaler Dermatitis. Phlebol Proktol 5: 160–165
Schultz-Amling W, Köhler-Weisker A (1996) Pruritus ani. In: Gieler U, Bosse KA (Hrsg) Seelische Faktoren bei Hautkrankheiten, 2. Aufl. Huber, Bern, S 105–112
Wein S, Blecher P, Ruzicka T (1994) Die Rolle der Atopie in der Pathogenese des Analekzems. Z Hautkr 69: 113–119
Wienert V (1996) Analekzeme. Coloproctology 18: XII–XVI

Dyshidrosiform Hand Eczema (Dyshidrosis)

Definition. In dyshidrosiform eczemas (ICD-10: L-3–L30, F54), there are usually recurrent, itching blisters that appear periodically on the hands and feet.

Pathogenesis. Skin changes in connection with dyshidrosis form a polyetiological group of diseases. Predominant are an atopic diathesis, hyperergic id reactions (fungi, bacteria), or medication-allergic reactions. Furthermore, there are subgroups of patients who characteristically present with dyshidrosiform eczemas that can be triggered by situations of psychosocial stress.

Clinical findings. Dyshidrosiform eczema is seen most often on the hands and feet. The maximal variant of dyshidrosis presents with large blisters, which are also called cheiropompholyx when on the hands or podopompholyx when on the feet (Fig. 2.7).

Emotional symptoms. Dyshidrosiform hand eczema may be triggered by emotional factors.

Stress. In half of the cases, patients with dyshidrosiform hand eczema report that stress has an influence on the course of the disease.

A detailed variance analysis has shown that a high subjective stress vulnerability is associated with greater severity of the dyshidrosis, increased itching, higher depression scores, and more frequent life events. This was demonstrated especially in young patients, who additionally reported increased helplessness (Niemeier et al. 2002).

Personality type. Kellum (1975) was able to determine a certain personality type in dyshidrosiform hand eczema, characterized as overly conscientious, serious persons who are responsible at all levels. Their lives are well-organized, and they work efficiently and precisely and pay attention to details. Their days are highly structured with many appointments. They expect too much of their own performance and are pitiless in their dealings with themselves. Tension results from the excessive performance that they demand of themselves. Feelings of inferiority and incompetence arise from the inevitable failure to meet their excessive expectations. These people feel guilty, frustrated, and angry.

Psychodynamic concepts. In their study of 20 young women, Hansen et al. (1981) identified dyshidrosiform hand eczema as an expression event in the form of a pregenital conversion. The patients showed increased inhibited aggression and felt dependent and controlled, but they also showed a tendency to want to control relationships. They appeared to present their dependency conflicts in symbolized form with their hands, which became manifest at a point at which they wanted to take life into their own hands, but independent acts were hindered by their desire to be dependent.

Psychotherapy. Therapy should first be done as part of psychosomatic primary care. Relaxation therapies are appropriate for patients with pronounced stress induction. Dependency conflicts can be thematized as part of a deep-psychological focal therapy.

Psychopharmaceuticals. Initially, antihistamines according to the stepwise plan (Chap. 15, section on antihistamines)—nonsedating or sedating antihista-

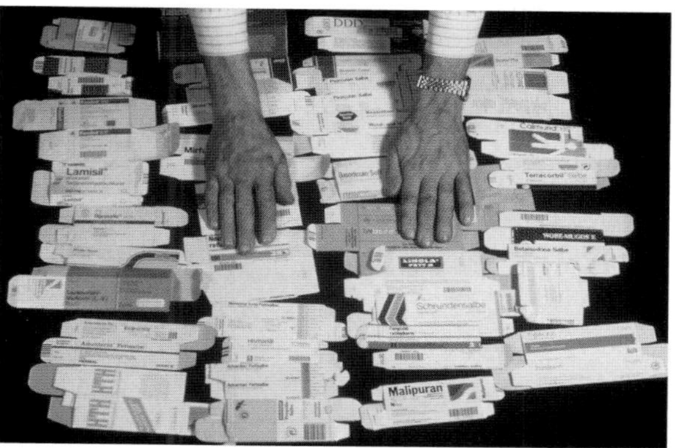

Fig. 2.7 Allergic contact eczema and compulsive disorder; collection of external medications applied

2

mines such as hydroxyzine or doxepin—can be recommended.

References

Hansen O, Kuchler T, Lotz GR, Richter R, Wilckens A (1981) Es juckt mich in den Fingern, aber mir sind die Hände gebunden. Z Psychosom Med Psychoanal 27(3): 275–290

Kellum RE (1975) Dyshidrotic hand eczema. A psychotherapeutic approach. Cutis 11: 875–878

Niemeier V, Nippesen M, Kupfer J, Schill WB, Gieler U (2002) Psychological factors associated with hand dermatoses: which subgroup needs additional psychological care? Br J Dermatol 146(6): 1031–1037

Further Reading

Stangier U, Gieler U (2000) Hauterkrankungen. In: Senft W, Broda M (Hrsg) Praxis der Psychotherapy, 2. Aufl. Thieme, Stuttgart, S 566–581

Herpes Genitalis/Herpes Labialis

The drastic increase in viral infections will be a paramount medical as well as psychosocial challenge in the coming years (Stanberry et al. 1999).

The increasing prevalence of sexually transmitted viral diseases that are not required to be reported, including herpes simplex virus (HSV), human papilloma virus (HPV), and human immunodeficiency virus (HIV), will result in a "new venereology" compared with the classical venereal diseases (syphilis, gonorrhea; Fig. 2.8).

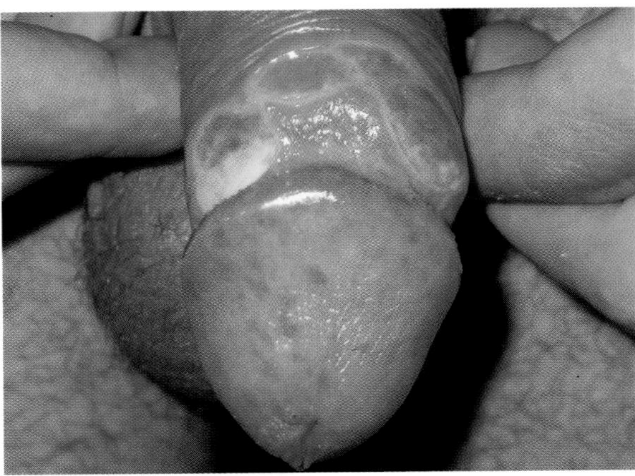

Fig. 2.8 Herpes simplex

Prevalence/incidence. The seroprevalence for HSV-1 is 88% and for HSV-2 is 13% in the German population. In selected collectives (HIV-positive patients), the prevalence of HSV-2 is as high as 48% (Adler and Meheust 2000; Wutzler et al. 2000).

Clinical findings. HSV infections (HSV-1, HSV-2) are characterized by painful blisters and erosions – which are recurrent in 40% of cases – that occur around the lips (usually HSV-1) and genitals (usually HSV-2).

In adolescents, there may be sexual transmission; in children, transmission may be due to contaminated hands. Sexual abuse must also be taken into consideration.

Emotional symptoms. Disgust and stressful situations have been described as emotional elicitors in the recurrent courses of herpes labialis and genitalis. Often there are depressive disorders and detriment to quality of life.

Herpes Labialis (ICD-10: B00.1, F54)

Immunological dysregulations and clinical symptoms were demonstrated by stress induction in patients with recurrent courses of herpes infections (Bonneau et al. 1991).

! HSV-1 recurrences may be elicited by emotional stress (disgust and stress) in a subgroup of patients with corresponding anamnesis. Patients often report depressions and detriment to quality of life.

In a stress experiment with corresponding exposition, patients with anamnestic disgust of unclean objects showed clearly reproducible HSV-1 symptoms and elevated concentrations of tumor necrosis factor-alpha compared with a control group (Buske-Kirschbaum et al. 2001).

Special signal molecules, especially epinephrine, interleukin-6, cAMP, glucocorticoids, and prostaglandins, are more frequently found during acute and chronic stress and have been identified as possible effectors of herpes virus reactivation in clinical recurrence (Sainz et al. 2001). Taking offense is more frequent, and the estimation of personal success in achieving socially desirable goals correlates negatively with the onset of herpes recurrences.

Herpes Genitalis (ICD-10: A60.0, F54)

Patients with herpes genitalis infections have social isolation, anxiety, proximity–distance conflicts, feelings of hopelessness, overconscientiousness, reduced self-esteem, and resultant flight in the face of an imminent sexual relationship (Cassidy et al. 1997).

To this are added insults from rejection by the partner and a narcissistic rage based on the fantasy of transmitting the disease to the partner. Central to this is the fear of further recurrences in chronic courses and the attendant frequent depressive disorders.

Deep-psychological concepts discussed in connection with recurrence may reveal that an emotional experience of physical or moral uncleanness preceded the onset or recurrence of the disease. Moreover, the conscious or unconscious drive to avoid an imminent sexual contact, which is internally undesired or impermissible, may elicit recurrences. The emotional situation is partly similar to the sexual incapacity of impotence (Dimitrov 1973).

In connection with a herpes genitalis infection, there is both primary and secondary sexuality avoidance, limited communication structures, and withdrawal, so the manner in which the disease was coped with after the first infection is in the focus of the chronic course.

Coping with the disease. Recent studies confirm that the recurrence frequency of herpes genitalis infections depends especially on how the patient copes with the disease (Lynch 1998).

! Positive coping, along with subjective relief and reduction of fear and depression, lowers the frequency of recurrence of herpes genitalis disease.

Psychotherapy. In addition to an indication-appropriate effective antiviral therapy, today's therapy concepts must promote individual coping strategies to reduce the recurrence frequency of genital herpes simplex infections.

Attention must be paid to the following:

- Measures for psychoeducation, also within psychosomatic primary care, have proven beneficial in providing knowledge about the disease and supporting better coping with the disease (Connor-Greene 1986).
- Based on available data, it may be assumed that stress-reducing relaxation procedures such as autogenic training may contribute to the reduction and prevention of further recurrences (Koehn et al. 1993).
- Behavior therapy models, including group therapy in large specialized treatment centers, led to a reduction in recurrences and helped patients cope with their disease (McLarnon and Kaloupek 1988; Hoon et al. 1991).
- When differential diagnosis rules out medical-somatic factors, the doctor should check for comorbidities such as depression, anxiety, or unresolved conflicts. Indications for psychotherapy or psychopharmacological treatment arise primarily from the comorbidities of the diagnosed emotional disorders.

References

Adler MW, Meheust AZ (2000) Epidemiology of sexually transmitted infections and human immunodeficiency virus in Europe. J Eur Acad Dermatol Venereol 14(5): 370–377

Bonneau RH, Sheridan JF, Feng N, Glaser R (1991) Stress-induced suppression of herpes simplex virus (HSV)-specific cytotoxic T lymphocyte and natural killer cell activity and enhancement of acute pathogenesis following local HSV infection. Brain Behav Immun 5: 170–192

Buske-Kirschbaum A, Geiben A, Wermke C, Pirke KM, Hellhammer D (2001) Preliminary evidence for herpes labialis recurrence following experimentally induced disgust. Psychother Psychosom 70(2): 86–91

Cassidy L, Meadows J, Catalan J, Barton S (1997) Are reported stress and coping style associated with frequent recurrence of genital herpes? Genitourin Med 73(4): 263–266

Connor-Greene PA (1986) The role of conseling in the treatment of genital herpes. J Am Coll Health 34(6): 286–287

Dimitrov CT (1973) Psychische Faktoren bei Herpes simplex recidivans genitalis. Z Psychosom Med Psychoanal 19(3): 279–287

Hoon EF, Hoon PW, Rand KH, Johnson J, Hall NR, Edwards NB (1991) A psycho-behavioral model of genital herpes recurrence. J Psychosom Res 35(1): 25–36

Koehn K, Burnette MM, Stark C (1993) Applied relaxation training in the treatment of general herpes. J Behav Ther Exp Psychiatry 24: 331–341

Lynch PJ (1998) Psychiatric, legal, and moral issues of herpes simplex infections. J Am Acad Dermatol 18(1Pt2): 173–175

McLarnon LD, Kaloupek DG (1988) Psychological investigation of genital herpes recurrence: prospective assessment and cognitive-behavioral intervention for a chronic physical disorder. Health Psychol 7(3): 231–249

Sainz B, Loutsch JM, Marquart ME, Hill JM (2001) Stress-associated immunomodulation and herpes simplex virus infections. Med Hypotheses 56(3): 348–356

Stanberry L, Cunningham A, Mertz G, Mindel A, Peters B, Reitano M, Sacks S, Wald A, Wassilew S, Woolley P (1999) New developments in the epidermiology, natural history and management of genital herpes. Antiviral Res 42(1): 1–14

Wutzler P, Doerr HW, Färber I, Eichhorn U, Helbig B, Sauerbrei A, Brandstadt A, Rabenau HF (2000) Seroprevalence of herpes simplex virus type 1 and type 2 in selected German populations – revalence for the incidence of genital herpes. J Med Virol 61: 201–207

Further Reading

Cohen F, Kemeny ME, Kearney KA, Zegans LS, Neuhaus JM, Conant MA (1999) Persistent stress as a predictor of genital herpes recurrence. Arch Intern Med 159(20): 2430–2436

Doward LC, McKenna SP, Kohlmann T, Patrick D, Thorsen H (1998) The international development of the quality of life measure for recurrent genital herpes. Qual Life Res 7(2): 143–153

Glaser R, Kiecolt-Glaser JK (1997) Chronic stress modulates the virus-specific immune response to latent herpes simplex virus type I. Ann Behav Med 19(2): 78–82

Luborsky L, Mintz J, Brightman VJ, Katcher AH (1976) Herpes simplex virus and moods: a longitudinal study. J Psychosom Res 20: 543–548

Spencer B, Leplege A, Ecosse E (1999) Recurrent genital herpes and quality of life in France. Qual Life Res 8(4): 365–371

Stock C, Guillen-Grima F, Mendoza JH de, Marin-Fernandez B, Aguinaga-Ontoso I, Kramer A (2001) Risk factors of herpes simplex type 1(HSV-1) infection and lifestyle factors associated with HSV-1 manifestations. Eur J Epidemiol 17(9): 885–890

Hyperhidrosis

Definition. Hyperhidrosis (ICD-10: R61.0, F54) denotes an increase in secretion by sweat glands that exceeds the normal temperature regulation. The diagnosis must be reached by a sweat test, with gravimetric measurement if possible. There are two types of hyperhidrosis: primary and secondary.

Prevalence/incidence. Primary hyperhidrosis, also called essential hyperhidrosis, primarily affects the hands, feet, or axillae, with an estimated prevalence of between 0.5% and 1% of the population.

Pathogenesis. Genetic factors are considered to predominate in primary hyperhidrosis. The onset is usually in adolescence and is potentiated multifactorially by high temperatures, emotional burdens, and other stress burdens and nervousness. Elevated sympathetic activity may lead to increased sweating in people who are easily excitable.

In secondary hyperhidrosis, generalized hyperhidrosis is usually observed, and hyperthyroidism, diabetes mellitus, neoplasias (pheochromocytoma), infections, or elevated catecholamine excretion play a central role. Medical administration of beta blockers, sympathomimetics, and, especially, antidepressants (SSRIs) can also cause generalized (secondary) hyperhidrosis, as can foods with particularly sharp spices, coffee, chocolate, or the like. Gustatory hyperhidrosis syndrome is a special form that was described by Frey.

Emotional symptoms. Hyperhidrosis is a multifactorial dermatosis that may be potentiated by psychic emotional stress factors (Sect. 1.3.3).

Characteristically, patients with hyperhidrosis have anxiety disorders (fear of sweating) as well as depressive disorders and sociophobias. The concept of sweating for fear is common even in everyday jargon, but a conspicuously high comorbidity of emotional disorders was found in a single study (Ruchinskas et al. 2002).

Hyperhidrosis in the context of a body dysmorphic disorder, especially botulinophilia or delusion of body odor, is particularly problematic, so a more detailed presentation of these is given in the appropriate chapters. The differential diagnosis between the delusion of body odor and fishy-odor disease (trimethylaminuria) must be considered.

Problem Area: Hyperhidrosis (Possible Emotional Symptoms)

- Somatopsychic adjustment disorder
- Anxiety disorder
- Body dysmorphic disorder
- Somatoform autonomic function disorder
- Botulinophilia
- Body odor delusion

Psychotherapy. Psychotherapy depends on the dominant emotional disorder. It is important to clarify the suspected differential diagnostics as early as possible.

In somatopsychic adjustment disorders, thematization of the underlying conflict situation is usually possible within psychosomatic primary care. Stress burdens or stress vulnerability may occupy a central position, for which the initiation of relaxation therapy shows good therapeutic response, as well as in combination with psychopharmaceutical therapy if depressive or anxiety disorders are present.

Body dysmorphic disorders, including the special form of botulinophilia, are usually much more difficult to treat due to low patient motivation.

The therapeutic consequences must be determined individually and may comprise psychodynamic psychotherapy, behavior therapy, or psychopharmacological treatment strategies (refer to the stepwise plan for body dysmorphic disorders in Sect. 1.3.2).

In the foreground of the therapeutic strategy are treatment with psychopharmaceuticals (neuroleptics) in the delusional type of body odor delusion and adequate psychotherapy in the nondelusional type.

Dermatological therapy. Tap-water iontophoresis, aluminum chloride salts (Drysol), beta-receptor blockers, and sedatives are used as local therapeutics and systemic anticholinergics. Therapy with botulinus toxin and operative measures including sweat gland suction, sweat gland curettage, excision (large-area skin removal), and endoscopic thoracic sympathectomy are among the invasive interventions.

Psychopharmaceuticals. Therapy with psychopharmaceuticals depends on the dominant emotional disorder and the resultant target symptomatics. Differentiation must be made between delusional and nondelusional disorders.

SSRIs (fluoxetine, sertraline, paroxetine, citalopram) show good efficacy in treating somatoform disorders (body dysmorphic disorder) and have been used with promising results. Taking the comorbidities into account, a combination therapy or monotherapy with anxiolytics, for example, may be indicated.

The benzodiazepine alprazolam has proven effective for moderate-length treatment of acute stress-dependent hyperhidrosis with anxiety disorders, states of tension, and excitation.

Reference

Ruchinskas RA, Narayan RK, Meagher RJ, Furukawa S (2002) The relationship of psychopathology and hyperhidrosis. Br J Dermatol 147(4): 733–735

Further Reading

Lerer B, Jacobowitz J, Wahba A (1980) Treatment of essential hyperhidrosis by psychotherapy. Psychosomatics 22: 536–538

Special Forms

Bromhidrosis

Definition. Bromhidrosis(ICD-10: F22.8, L75.0, L75.1) is characterized by an unpleasant odor development of physiological sweat, caused by bacterial decomposition.

Prevalence/incidence. Only single case reports are available at present.

Clinical findings. Often there is no pathological skin finding. An attempt to objectify the sweat reaction can be made by eliciting sweating by athletic activity or sauna, whereby the changes appear more clearly.

If mycological or bacterial colonization is suspected, an appropriate cultivation with proof of pathogen is always required to be able to treat specifically if appropriate.

The diagnosis should always include clarification of possible delusional phenomena.

Chromhidrosis

In chromhidrosis (ICD-10: L57.1), colored sweat is secreted, especially from the apocrine glands in the axillae. Causally, discoloration of the sweat is explained by an increase in lipofuscin. In eccrine chromhidrosis, substances usually ingested exogenously and excreted via the sweat glands are decisive. It must be delineated differential-diagnostically from pseudochromhidrosis, in which sweat discoloration is caused by bacterial pigments.

Trichobacteriosis Palmellina

Secondarily, infections and a penetrating odor may occur as a result of bacterial decomposition of the sweat (bromhidrosis). Frequently the sweat is decomposed by corynebacterium, and odor-active substances are formed, with an unpleasant, rancid-sour odor.

Around the axillary hairs, especially in hyperhidrosis, there are yellowish-white, reddish, or black coatings in the area of the terminal hair growth, which are hard to remove. The hair looks encrusted or covered with hoarfrost. The skin changes are accompanied by an acrid odor.

Regarding etiopathogenesis, corynebacteria, which belong to the normal site flora of the skin, may result in high germ counts and clinically visible coating in areas of hair on the head, axillae, pubis, and trunk, especially in cases of deficient hygiene and hyperhidrosis.

Symptomatically, there is often a genuine bromhidrosis, which is actually present in this case and must be differential-diagnostically delineated from the presumed, sometimes delusional bromhidrosis.

Pitted Keratolysis

In pitted keratolysis, there may be dimple-like defects in the horny skin caused by diphteroids (corynebacteria) in the mechanically burdened areas.

Emotional symptoms. The main problem for patients with bromhidrosis or chromhidrosis lies in mastering their handling of the disease when dermatological measures bring no improvement. Their perception of the changes may lead to changes in social behavior similar to those seen with acne (see section on acne).

The psychopathological diagnosis should always include the possibility of a delusional development within schizophrenia or an isolated delusional perception.

More frequent than physiological elicitation is a bromhidrosis or chromhidrosis that is perceived only subjectively and is sometimes attributed to environmental toxins. This cannot, however, be objectified.

The changes that are subjectively perceived as "troublesome," and which cover a spectrum from ignorance of these changes to uncorrectable delusional assumptions, must be delineated from these physiological variants of human sweating.

Psychogenic eliciting of increased chromhidrosis has thus far been described in only one case report of a patient undergoing psychotherapy (Köpp and Pawlofsky 1988).

Differential diagnoses. The delusional disorder in the framework of schizophrenia or an isolated delusional perception may predominate, whereby the bromhidrosis or chromhidrosis occurs as a concurrent disorder.

Therapy. Therapy consists of adequate body hygiene using cleansing detergents and deodorants, frequent changes of clothing, and avoidance of synthetic materials. Local therapy is performed with appropriate antibiotics or antimycotics to reduce the growth of the corresponding pathogens. Solutions with 10–20% aluminum trichloride hexahydrate are used to reduce sweat. Regular, but not too intensive, use of water without additives is a prerequisite. Therapies with capsaicin or even excision of the affected sweat gland area have been described.

Strengthening of positive coping with the disease has proven beneficial. Relaxation procedures are certainly indicated to reduce the sweat reaction.

Psychosomatic primary care and psychoeducative measures may be initially successful in some cases of presumed bromhidrosis or chromhidrosis (somatoform disorder).

An indication for expert psychotherapy depends on the comorbidities present with the psychosocial disorder. Only one case report is currently available (Köpp and Pawlofsky 1988) on psychodynamic procedures. Behavior therapy measures in the sense of cognitive restructuring or social training may be indicated.

A neuroleptic (see Chap. 15) may be necessary in a delusional disorder.

Reference

Köpp W, Pawlofsky C (1988) Chromhidrosis – ein Fallbericht. In: Schüffel W (Hrsg) Sich gesund fühlen im Jahre 2000. Springer, Berlin, S 441–444

Further Reading

Cilliers J, Beer C de (1999) The case of the red lingerie – chromhidrosis revisited. Dermatology 199(2): 149–152

Kreyden OP, Heckmann M, Peschen M (2002) Delusional hyperhidrosis as a risk for medical overtreatment: a case of botulinophilia. Arch Dermatol 138(4): 538–539

Park DH (1999) Treatment of axillary bromhidrosis with superficial liposuction. Plast Reconstr Surg 104(5): 1580–1581

Schwarz T, Neumann R, Duschet P, Bruckler B, Klein W, Oppolzer G, Bardach H, Gschnait F (1989) Apocrine chromhidrosis. Hautarzt 40(2): 106–109

Shelly WB, Hurley JJ (1954) Localized chromidrosis; a survey. AMA Arch Derm Syphilol 69: 449–471

Thami GP, Kanwar AJ (2000) Red facial pseudochromhidrosis. Br J Dermatol 142(6): 1219–1220

Hypertrichosis

Hypertrichosis (ICD-10: L68, F54) is important for dermatologists, especially in the framework of esthetic medicine, in hormone disorders, in genodermatoses (Rubinstein–Taybi syndrome), and as a side effect of certain medications (cyclosporine). We refer the reader here to the detailed presentation in the chapter on body dysmorphic disorders (Sect.1.3.2).

Lichen Planus

Definition. Lichen planus (ICD-10: L43, F54) is a noninfectious, sometimes severely pruritic skin disease with lichenoid papules and characteristic mucosal changes.

Prevalence/incidence. Lichen planus occurs relatively often (Nasemann 1980). In Germany, the rate of disease in the population is 0.2%. The disease peaks between the ages of 25 and 29.

Pathogenesis. The origin of lichen planus is unclear. Numerous findings indicate that immunological factors occupy a decisive place in the pathogenesis. This is supported on the one hand by the characteristic immunofluorescence phenomenon, which can be proven, and on the other by the good therapeutic response to immunomodulating/immunosuppressing therapies.

Traditionally, lichen planus is usually included among the so-called psychosomatic dermatoses (Veltman and Weitz 1966).

Clinical findings. Lichenoid papules and characteristic netlike mucosal changes are predominant in lichen planus. Moreover, hyperkeratotic and ulcerating forms up to the bullous variants also occur. An exanthematic course can often be observed (Figs. 2.9, 2.10).

Emotional symptoms. Large studies have revealed that the skin changes occurred in some patients after serious life events (Veltman and Weitz 1966).

A typical emotional or personality disorder could not be demonstrated either primarily or secondarily.

It appears that emotional instability predominates as a characteristic in patients with lichen planus (Obermayer 1955), and the patients often report that they are tense, overworked, and anxious and that they worry excessively (Tompkins 1955). There appears to be a pronounced reciprocity between psychological factors and activity of the adrenergic system in patients with lichen planus (Puchalski 1986).

As with other chronic skin disease, the development of depressive reactions, psychosocial withdrawal, and/or addictions in impaired coping are observed in lichen planus.

Overall, the patients often appear to be thin-skinned and emotionally unstable or nervous.

Dermatological therapy. Immunosuppressing therapies show very good treatment results. Phototherapy is usually very effective.

Psychotherapy. Deep-psychological, psychodynamic, or behavior therapy procedures are indicated if the patient has a relevant emotional comorbidity or impaired coping and if there is appropriate motivation for therapy.

Psychopharmaceuticals. No specific studies or experiences have been reported on psychopharmacotherapy in lichen planus.

References

Nasemann T (1980) Lichen ruber planus und seine Varianten. In: Korting GW (Hrsg) Dermatologie in Praxis und Klinik, Bd II, Thieme, Stuttgart

Obermayer M (1955) Psychocutaneous medicine. Thomas, Springfield, IL

Puchalski Z (1986) Angststruktur und Parameter von Katecholaminen bei Patienten mit Rosazea, Alopecia areata und Lichen ruber planus. Z Hautkr 61: 137–145

Tompkins J (1955) Lichen planus: a statistical study of forty-one cases. AMA Arch Derm Syphilol 71: 515–519

Veltman G, Weitz R (1966) Über die Bedeutung psychosomatischer Einflüsse für die Entstehung des Lichen ruber planus. Hautarzt 17: 7–16

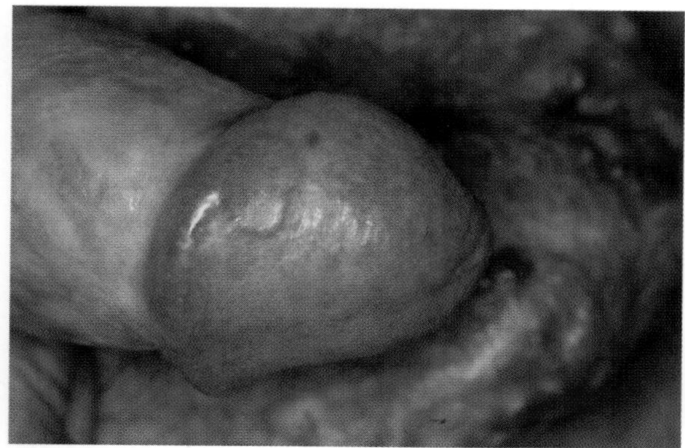

Fig. 2.9 Lichen planus of the glans penis in a patient with guilt complex after adultery. The skin lesions occurred 3 weeks after unprotected sex

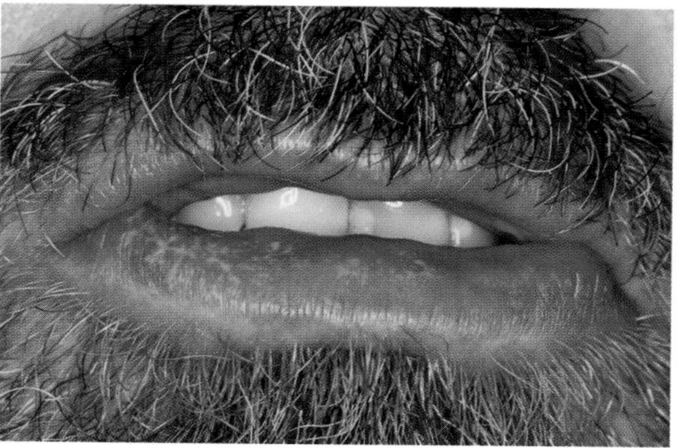

Fig. 2.10 Lichen planus: the same patient as in Fig. 2.9 with lip lesion, which he interpreted as symbolic causality after oral sex

Lupus Erythematodes

Definition. Lupus erythematodes is an inflammatory autoimmune disease that may manifest in various courses and clinical presentations.

Clinical findings and classification. In principle, differentiation can be made between two main forms of lupus erythematodes, which differ in severity and extent of symptoms: chronic discoid lupus erythematodes (CDLE; ICD-10: L93, F54) and systemic lupus erythematodes (SLE; ICD-10: M32, F54).

The mainly cutaneous form of CDLE is characterized by chronic, sharply delineated papulosquamous plaques, which heal with atrophy.

The severe form of SLE is a generalized rheumatic autoimmune disease with characteristic malar erythema, alopecia, oral ulcerations, and the facultative affliction of all organs, especially joints, nephritis, and CNS involvement. The initial symptom may be fatigue and general malaise, which should not be misinterpreted as psychogenic.

Pathogenesis Humoral and cellular immunity are impaired, resulting in the production of circulating autoantibodies. Immunocomplexes accumulate in the vascular walls and, depending on the form, cause vascular inflammation and deposition in target organs, including the skin. The clearance of circulating complexes is also impaired.

The course, which usually waxes and wanes, may be triggered by various elicitors, such as ultraviolet light exposure, medications, and hormonal factors, as well as emotional stress.

Emotional symptoms. A connection between an episode of lupus erythematodes and life events is often observed. Stress, depression, anxiety, and daily hassles may influence the severity of symptoms and the daily fluctuation of the complaints (Adams et al. 1994; Wekking et al. 1991). Foremost among the psychosomatic problems are ability to cope with the disease, hopelessness, and marked detriment to quality of life (Adams et al. 1994).

Adjustment disorders may cause reactive depressive symptoms when the disease activity increases and cause detriment to the quality of life (Fig. 2.11).

Thus, stress-dependent adjustment disorders may result in a vicious cycle in the later course by leading to deterioration in the symptoms of the disease, which in turn leads to more stress. Deficient compliance in depressive disorders can also promote progression of the disease due to omitted therapy.

Emotional Problem Areas in Lupus Erythematodes

- Primary trigger factors
  - Psychosocial burdens
  - Life events
  - Daily hassles
- Reactive adjustment disorders
  - Anxiety disorders
  - Depressive disorders
  - Problems in coping with the disease
- Direct inflammatory CNS involvement
  - Organic psychosyndrome
  - States of confusion (psychoses)
  - Convulsions
  - Parkinson-like symptomatics

Of all the collagenoses, SLE most frequently shows CNS involvement. Counting mild cognitive disorders, emotional disorders occur in more than 90% of those afflicted (Haupt 2004). In every 2nd–5th case, more or less severe states of confusion, psychoses, anxiety disorders, depressive disorders, and convulsions arise.

Dermatological therapy. Depending on the severity of the lupus erythematodes, nonsteroidal antirheumatics, antimalarials, glucocorticosteroids, or immunosuppressives are used. By improving the disease activity, these also result in stabilizing the reactive emotional disorders.

Psychotherapy. Foremost is treatment within psychosomatic primary care. There are often problems of compli-

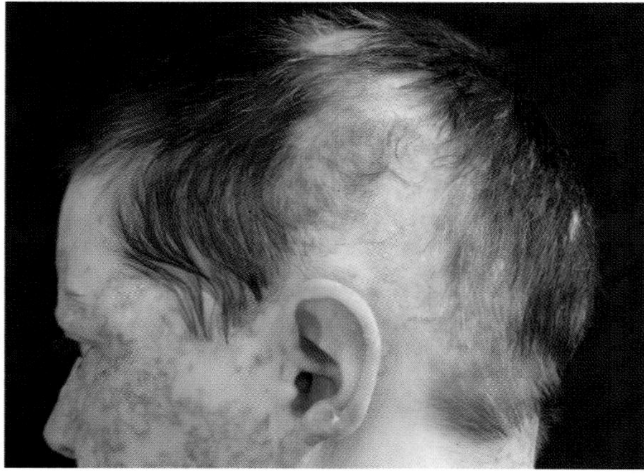

Fig. 2.11 Scarring alopecia in lupus erythematodes

ance with respect to inadequate protection against light and the resultant episodes due to sunlight exposure. Supportive promotion of positive coping is often necessary. Overcoming chronic pain may present an interdisciplinary challenge, especially in SLE.

There are individual reports of successful psychotherapy. The indication should be based on the dominant comorbidity and must be determined individually.

Stepwise Plan for Lupus Erythematodes

1. Improvement of compliance
2. Improvement of coping with disease
3. Dealing with pain (SLE)
4. Coping in everyday life
5. Psychosomatic primary care
6. Group therapy
7. Possibly, psychotherapy/psychopharmaceuticals

Participation in a self-help group may aid in coping with the disease. Psychiatric treatment may be necessary if the patient has suicidal tendencies or has attempted suicide, as well as in brain-organic psychosyndromes or transitional syndromes including delirium (Matsukawa et al. 1994).

Psychopharmaceuticals. The CNS may be involved in systemic forms. Psychoses have been described in single cases with central involvement of lupus erythematodes, and these require appropriate medication in cooperation with a psychiatrist.

References

Adams SG, Dammers PM, Saia TL, Brantley PJ, Gaydos GR (1994) Stress, depression, and anxiety predict average symptom severity and daily symptom fluctuation in systemic lupus erythematosus. J Behav Med 17(5): 459–477

Matsukawa Y, Sawada S, Hayama T, Usui H, Horie T (1994) Suicide in patients with systemic lupus erythematosus: a clinical analysis of seven suicidal patients. Lupus 3(1): 31–35

Wekking EM, Vingerhoeb AJ, Dam AP van, Nossent JC, Swaak AJ (1991) Daily stressors and systemic lupus erythematosus: a longitudinal analysis, first findings. Psychother Psychosom 55(2–4): 108–113

Further Reading

Brody S (1956) Psychological factors associated with disseminated lupus erythematosus and effects of cortisone and ACTH. Psychiatr Q 30(1): 44–60

Haupt M (2004) Psychische Störungen bei rheumatischen Erkrankungen am Beispiel des Systemischen Lupus Erythematodes (SLE). Z Rheumatol 63(2): 122–130

O'Connor JF (1959) Psychoses associated with systemic lupus erythematosus. Ann Intern Med 51: 526–536

Malignant Melanoma

Definition and prevalence. Malignant melanoma is a malignant melanocytic neoplasia that is increasingly affecting populations with skin types 1 and 2 worldwide.

Pathogenesis. Psychosocial factors alone cannot cause malignant melanoma. Stress and the resultant immunosuppression are probably not sufficient to cause tumor induction.

Clinical findings. Clinically and histologically, there are four main types: superficial spreading melanoma, nodular melanoma, acral lentiginous melanoma, and lentigo maligna melanoma. In addition, there are special forms such as amelanotic melanoma and desmoplastic melanoma.

Emotional symptoms. Central factors in malignant melanoma consist of coping with the disease and, especially, fear, particularly when social support is lacking in the patient's environment (Fig. 2.12).

In a study of 2,173 patients, the metastasis-free long-term survival time in malignant melanoma was associated with an effective coping style (Drunkenmölle et al. 2001). Early consultation with the dermatologist and performance of consistent therapy are part of coping. Thin melanomas have a better prognosis.

As a result of a tumor disease, one-third of the patients may develop considerable psychosocial stress and adjustment disorders (Augustin et al. 1997; Derogatis et al. 1983). Affective disorders occur in a considerable number of patients.

Active coping is also a prognostically important factor for the course of the disease.

Psychotherapy. Unfortunately, there is only one psychosomatic long-term study on malignant melanoma.

In a landmark, but not yet reproduced, study (Fawzy et al. 1993), in addition to tumor therapy according to

2

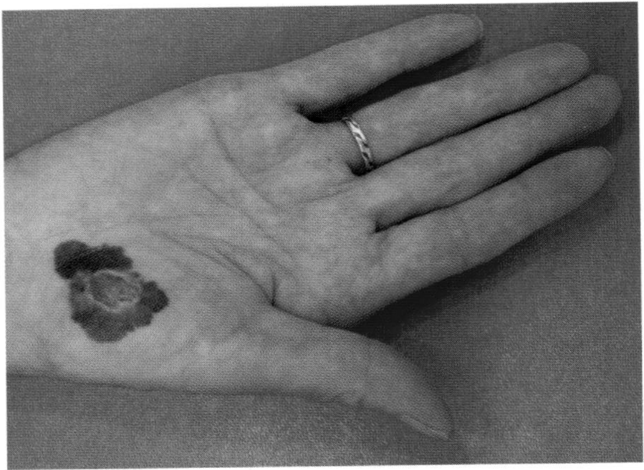

Fig. 2.12 Melanoma considered as a spiritual sign

guidelines, a positive effect of group interventions comprising the following three components was found for patients with malignant melanoma, similar to that for patients with AD and psoriasis:
1. Group psychotherapy
2. Stress management (relaxation procedures)
3. Health training

The treated group had more favorable affects and more active coping strategies. Moreover, the patients had significantly lower depression values and less fatigue.

The follow-up study performed 6 years later (Fawzy et al. 1993) revealed that significantly more patients in the control group had died than in the intervention group. These favorable effects were only observed, however, in the group with medium-risk melanoma (tumor diameter 1.5–4 mm, with no distant metastases).

In a recently published follow-up, no significant differences were observed when comparing the groups after 10 years (Fawzy et al. 2003).

Summary. It can be determined from the database that in a subgroup of patients with tumor-related psychosocial problems, psychosomatic concepts should be considered an integrated component in oncological dermatology, especially malignant melanoma. An appropriate offer should be made. Patients with tumor diseases usually desire a detailed, empathic discussion with the doctor responsible for long-term treatment and only seldom want purely psychological care.

Malignant melanoma should be accompanied by supportive psychosomatic primary care and, if appropriate, focal group psychotherapy. The question of when individual psychotherapy is indicated depends on the comorbidity of emotional disorders.

Relaxation procedures, patient information, and group therapies are helpful for reducing perioperative tension and strain; moreover, they are effective in reducing the side effects of chemotherapy and immunotherapies. They are also helpful in reducing the patient's fear if the tumor actually progresses or if the patient is afraid it will progress.

Psychopharmaceuticals. Psychopharmaceuticals can be used beneficially in tumor-related depression and also tumor therapy depression (interferon). Anxiolytics and adequate pain therapy should be used generously.

Zolpidem and zopiclon have been found beneficial in the therapy of insomnias in this connection. SSRIs, especially escitalopram (Lexapro) and paroxetine, have been found particularly effective for treating depression induced by interferon-alpha. Sometimes these are also used as prophylaxis if indicated by the anamnesis or conditions.

References

Augustin M, Zschocke I, Dieterle W, Schöpf E, Muthny FA (1997) Bedarf und Motivation zu psychosozialen Interventionen bei Patienten mit malignen Hauttumoren. Z Hautkr 5(72): 333–338

Derogatis L, Morrow G, Fetting J, Penman D, Piasetsky S et al. (1983) The prevalence of psychiatric disorders among cancer patients. JAMA 249: 751–757

Drunkenmölle E, Helmbold P, Kupfer J, Lübbe D, Taube KM, Marsch C (2001) Metastasenfreies Langzeitüberleben bei malignem Melanom ist mit effektivem Copingstil assoziiert. Z Hautkr 76(suppl 1): 47

Fawzy FI, Canada AL, Fawzy NW (2003) Malignant melanoma: effects of a brief, structured psychiatric intervention on survival and recurrence at 10-year follow-up. Arch Gen Psychiatry 60(1): 100–103

Fawzy FI, Fawzy NW, Hyun CS, Elashoff R, Guthrie D, Fahey JL, Morton DL (1993) Malignant melanoma. Effects of an early structured psychiatric intervention, coping, and affective state on recurrence and survival 6 years later. Arch Gen Psychiatry 50(9): 681–689

Further Reading

Bonci F, Salimbeni G, Gandini D, Massei A, Conte PF (1995) Evaluation of the psychological health in melanoma patients treated with alpha-interferon. Melanoma Res 5(suppl 1): 20–21

Brandberg Y, Mansson-Brahme E, Ringborg U, Sjoden PO (1995) Psychological reactions in patients with malignant melanoma. Eur J Cancer 31A(2): 157–162

Brown JE, King MT, Butow PN, Dunn SM, Coates AS (2000) Patterns over time in quality of life, coping and psychological adjust-

ment in late stage melanoma patients: an application of multilevel models. Qual Life Res 9(1): 75–85
Cassileth BR, Lusk EJ, Tenaglia AN (1982) A psychological comparison of patients with malignant melanoma and other dermatologic disorders. J Am Acad Dermatol 7(6): 742–746
Fritzsche K, Struss Y, Stein B, Spahn C (2003) Psychosomatic liaison service in hematological oncology: need for psychotherapeutic interventions and their realization. Hematol Oncol 21(2): 83–89
Schafer M, Schwaiger M (2003) Incidence, pathoetiology and treatment of interferon-alpha induced neuro-psychiatric side effects. Fortschr Neurol Psychiatr 71(9): 469–476
Söllner W, Mairinger G, Zingg-Schir M, Fritsch P (1996) Krankheitsprognose, psychosoziale Belastung und Einstellung von Melanompatienten zu unterstützenden psychotherapeutischen Maßnahmen. Hautarzt 47: 200–205
Spiegel D, Bloom J, Kraemer H, Gottheil E (1989) Effects of psychosocial treatment on survival of patients with metastatic breast cancer. Lancet 14: 888–891
Temoshok L, Heller B, Sagebiel R, Blois M, Sweet D, DiClemente R, Gold M (1985) The relationship of psychosocial factors to prognostic indicators in cutaneous malignant melanoma. J Psychosom Res 29(2) 139–153
Zschocke I, Augustin M, Muthny FA (1996) Krankheitsverarbeitung bei Patienten mit malignem Melanom in verschiedenen Krankheitsphasen. Psychomed 8: 83–88

Perioral Dermatitis

Perioral dermatitis (ICD-10: L71.0, F54) mainly affects women between 30 and 45 years of age.

Pathogenesis. The multifactorial genesis of perioral dermatitis can be elicited by the application of topical corticoids or cosmetics, as well as by infections and hormone disorders. Histologically, there are hyperproliferation of the follicle epithelium and lymphohistiocytic infiltrates. Furthermore, there is a tendency to recurrence, chronicity, and resistance to the usual treatments for acne or rosacea.

Steroid applications usually lead to prompt improvement but also to immediate recurrence upon their withdrawal (rebound), which should be generally avoided.

Clinical findings. Perioral dermatitis is characterized by the episodic occurrence of small, inflamed papules on spotty or diffusely reddened skin, usually in the perioral region. It sometimes also affects the periorbital area (periorificial dermatitis).

Perioral dermatitis is very similar to acne but can be differentiated because it has a typical localization. In contrast to acne, it is characterized by papules without comedones.

Emotional symptoms. Perioral dermatitis is a considerable cosmetic impairment for the person afflicted. Only a few older studies have been published on the emotional symptomatics of perioral dermatitis.

Hornstein (1976) published one of the few biopsychosocial articles on perioral dermatitis and concluded that it is a so-called primary psychosomatic disease. Patients with perioral dermatitis present with the following special characteristics of personality structure and social habits:

Psychosomatic Factors of Perioral Dermatitis (Hornstein 1976)

- The disease affects mostly women, especially those who are sexually mature.
- These are usually particularly well-groomed, emotionally differentiated women with high social claims or in higher professional or social positions.
- Most of the patients show increased vegetative lability in their history or clinical symptoms, such as hypotensive symptom complex, tendency to obstipation, headache, or insomnia. The list of medications taken is usually impressive.
- The dermatitis is limited to or accentuated in the centrofacial, usually perioral, region.
- The skin events often occur in irregular episodes, sometimes in critical connection with conflict situations or persistent stress in the individual's partnership or profession.

Psychological test results show clear evidence of emotional immaturity with relatively high intelligence; disorders in interpersonal contacts, counteracted by rational attempts at adjustment; and a tendency for "hysterieform" behavior (Hartung and Lehrl 1976).

Deep-psychological concepts. From a deep-psychological point of view, the fundamental disorder of most patients with perioral dermatitis lies in pronounced narcissism, which has arisen due to a deficient, more than normally attentive, incompetent, or even missing father figure with resultant compensation mechanisms of idealization. The compensation or overcompensation of the unconscious conflict and impulse failure explain the positive traits cited (independence, activity, success, etc.). The disease episode, with its topographically repulsive character, should protect the person from further, deeper disappointments.

From both the degree of symptom severity and the different life histories, it appears that there are two types of patients. On the one hand is the passive type with more pronounced skin symptoms, who was often completely without a father in childhood, has less possibility of compensating for partnership problems in a profession, and has somatic concept of illness and fewer vegetative secondary symptoms. On the other hand is the active type with less severe skin symptoms, a father who was present during childhood, compensation possibilities in a profession where identification and narcissism can often be enjoyed, acceptance of emotional components, greater pressure of suffering, and a shorter healing time.

Both types usually have idealized father figures as partners and are repeatedly disappointed with the man's reality, which leads either to frequent partner change or to very dissatisfying long-term relationships. The dermal symptoms arise when the labile equilibrium is threatened. In the active-type patient, the eliciting situation is often found in the professional area.

! Emotional eliciting factors in older studies were seen in self-esteem problems and in connection with difficulties in realizing the patient's own demands for autonomy.

Psychotherapy. Hornstein (1976) concludes that this is a so-called primary psychosomatic disease that is accessible to short-term therapy in which unresolved conflicts are worked out.

References

Hartung ML, Lehrl S (1976) Psychological findings in a group of patients with perioral dermatitis. Z Psychosom Med Psychoanal 22(1): 110–114

Hornstein OP (1976) Development of the psychosomatic concept of perioral dermatitis. Z Psychosom Med Psychoanal 22(1): 93–98

Further Reading

Stangier U, Gieler U (2000) Hauterkrankungen. In: Senft W, Broda M (Hrsg) Praxis der Psychotherapy, 2. Aufl. Thieme, Stuttgart, S 566–581

Progressive Systemic Scleroderma

Definition. Sclerodermas are diseases of the connective tissue, characterized by excessive proliferation of fibroblasts. They are chronic, progressive diseases that lead to fibrosis and sclerosis of the skin and internal organs. They are subdivided into progressive systemic scleroderma (ICD-10: M34, F54), circumscript scleroderma (ICD-10: L94.0, F54), and overlapping syndromes.

Incidence/prevalence. Sclerodermas are rather rare and very difficult to determine diagnostically, especially in the early stages. Progressive systemic scleroderma (PSS) is a rare disease with an estimated annual incidence of 10–20 per 1 million inhabitants and a prevalence of about 500 per million (Medsger 2003). Women are considerably more often afflicted than men, in a ratio of 3–4:1. The disease peak is between the 3rd and 4th decades of life, with men being afflicted somewhat earlier.

Pathogenesis. The etiopathogenesis of PSS is largely unclear. Genetically, there is a predisposition coupled to the human leukocyte antigens DR5, DR1, and DR3. In PSS, there is pathologically elevated collagen synthesis due to the proliferation of fibroblasts. The proof of autoantibodies is also important. Scleroderma is an autoimmune disease that presents both vascular involvement and inflammatory reaction, which manifests in the skin, lungs, heart, kidneys, and gastrointestinal tract.

In addition to a genetic disposition, the interaction of the immune system with numerous exogenic substances appears to play a role. According to today's knowledge, it is assumed that vascular changes, impaired collagen metabolism, and impaired immunoregulation are involved in the pathogenesis.

Clinical findings. PSS is a chronic systemic disease of the connective tissue with a usually progredient course, leading to advancing fibrosis and sclerosis of the skin and internal organs. The first typical symptoms of PSS are edema of the hands, Raynaud's phenomenon, and pain in the terminal phalanx and joints.

The Raynaud phenomenon is cited as an early symptom that occurs in about 90% of scleroderma patients. This phenomenon consists of vascular spasms in the hands, which especially occur following cold exposure. The fingers become white due to contraction of the blood vessels as a sign of reduced perfusion. When perfusion resumes, there is usually pain, followed by swelling, hardening, and a shrinking and tightening of the tissue (sclerosis). Fingertip necrosis occurs in some patients, which may lead to amputation.

The advancing sclerosing in the patient's face results in a loss of mimicry and an immobile facial expression.

The organ involvements are numerous, may lead to serious complications, and make the seriousness of the disease clear. Changes in the esophagus occur in most scleroderma patients in the early phase of the disease. Involvement of the lungs is quite frequent, at 40–60%. Affliction of the sclerotically changed kidney manifests as limited filtering function and may make dialysis necessary in severe cases. Involvement of the cardiac muscle may lead to limited function and to cardiac arrhythmias. The musculature of scleroderma patients is rarely affected, occurring in only 6–12%; nonetheless, two-thirds of the patients develop rheumatic complaints that are very similar to chronic polyarthritis.

Scleroderma patients complain of general symptoms such as pain, shortness of breath, and exhaustion.

Emotional effects of the disease. The following are cited as concrete problems with the disease: pain, a chronic progradient course of the disease, danger of death, lack of performance capacity, decreasing mobility, loss of attractiveness, necessity of informing others about the disease, loss of the accustomed roles in the individual's profession and family. Anxiety, social withdrawal, depression, and helplessness in dealing with the disease occur as emotional secondary factors. Angelopoulos et al. (2001) demonstrated that a connection exists between the number and intensity of daily stressors and the extent of physical and social detriment. With increasing stressors, there was functional limitation of the extremities and a decrease in social activities, as well as an increase in anxiety and depression values.

! Vicious cycle: pain and depression

Pain and depression are the most important psychosomatic aspects in the diagnosis and treatment of patients with PSS. They also lead to problems coping with the disease and limit the patient's quality of life. Fatigue due to time-consuming treatment methods frequently leads to exhaustion and depression.

Psychosomatic Problems in Scleroderma

- Hopelessness of ever coping with the disease
- Vicious cycle of pain and depression
- Negative social reactions of family members and relatives
- Marked detriment to quality of life

The chronic progressive course is especially stressful for the patient because the final degree of impairment cannot be predicted. The patients tend at first to deny and repress the symptoms of the disease, which characteristically gives rise to impairment in compliance and coping with the disease. In the clinical practice, it is often conspicuous how long the patients wait to first consult a dermatologist compared with patients in other disease groups; they sometimes wait until the disease has already reached an advanced, extensive stage.

Coping with disease. Psychosocial variables play an essential role in coping, especially in diseases involving chronic pain. Differentiation must be made between active and passive coping in connection with coping strategies (see the section on coping in Chap. 12).

In passive coping, the control is transferred to others, and pain influences all areas of the patient's life; thus, helplessness and hopelessness occur. Unfavorable coping can, in turn, be a cofactor in exacerbation of the symptoms, especially by potentiating the experience of pain or by limiting functioning.

In active coping, the patients attempt to control their pain, use their own resources, and participate actively in daily life. On the other hand, overgeneralizations and catastrophizing tendencies lead to emotional and physical dysfunction.

Dermatological therapy. Therapy for PSS is based on administration of immunosuppressives, anti-inflammatory and vasoactive agents, and antifibrotic substances. Physiotherapeutic measures are performed in parallel. The basis of therapy is usually physical treatment with heat and physiotherapeutic measures.

Psychotherapy. So far, only a few studies have been done on the efficacy of psychological therapy procedures.

Seikowski et al. (1995) examined the influence of hypnosis and autogenic training on Raynaud symptomatics and coping with the disease. There was a significant increase in finger temperature. Long-term effects could not, however, be demonstrated for either the Raynaud episodes or for the psychosomatic complaint status.

Teaching relaxation exercises and imaginative techniques as well as giving information on disease-relevant topics has been found to be therapeutically successful in patients with chronic diseases.

The efficacy of programs focused on dealing with pain has been confirmed (Jungnitsch and Kohler 1997). The pain can be viewed as a stressor, and dealing with the pain is considered a problem-solving process in the broadest sense.

! Initiation of measures comprising multimodal behavior therapy elements for coping with pain and the disease take precedence in scleroderma.

Stepwise Plan for Progressive Systemic Scleroderma

1. Psychosomatic primary care
2. Psychoeducation (information about the disease, coping in everyday life)
3. Strengthening of coping (coping with pain)
4. Improvement of compliance
5. Pain therapies (including pain medications)
6. Relaxation therapy
7. Group therapy
8. Psychotherapy (behavior therapy)
9. Beware of suicidal tendencies
10. Psychopharmaceuticals

Based on the difficulties that scleroderma patients express regarding dealing with pain and coping with the disease, a behavior therapy model may be applied as a psychological treatment program. In addition to cognitive procedures (diversionary techniques, mediation of coping strategies and problem-solving strategies for dealing with stress in everyday life, new points of view and techniques for dealing with pain, information about the disease) and behavior-oriented procedures (reduction of pain-promoting behaviors and avoidance behavior, promotion of social activities and social competence), relaxation methods should also be considered because they are a physiological counterweight to excitation from pain and tension.

Finally, in connection with depression and single case reports, evidence of suicidal tendency should definitely be taken seriously and, if necessary, psychiatric cotreatment instituted (Cotteril and Cunliffe 1997).

References

Angelopoulos NV, Drosos AA, Moutsopoulos HM (2001) Psychiatric symptoms associated with scleroderma. Psychother Psychosom 70: 145–150

Cotteril JA, Cunliffe WJ (1997) Suicide in dermatological patients. Br J Dermatol 137: 246–250

Jungnitsch G, Kohler H (1997) Indication and limits to behavioral therapy for patients with chronic pain. Schmerz 11(5): 314–321

Medsger TA Jr (2003) Natural history of systemic sclerosis and the assessment of disease activity, severity, functional status, and psychologic well-being. Rheum Dis Clin North Am 29(2): 255–273

Seikowski K, Weber B, Haustein UF (1995) Zum Einfluß der Hypnose und des autogenen Trainings auf die akrale Durchblutung und die Krankheitsverarbeitung bei Patienten mit progressiver Sklerodermie. Hautarzt 46: 94–101

Prurigo

Definition. Prurigo diseases (ICD-10: L28.1–L28.2, F54) overall are a heterogeneous group of diseases comprising prurigo simplex acuta (ICD-10: L28.2), prurigo simplex subacuta (ICD-10: L28.2), prurigo simplex chronica (ICD-10: L28.2), and prurigo nodularis Hyde (ICD-10: L28.1).

Clinical findings. The clinical presentation is characterized according to the disease entity: in prurigo simplex acuta by the predominance of urticarial seropapulae; in prurigo simplex subacuta and chronica by sometimes coarse papulae, excoriations, hyperpigmentations, and depigmentations; and in prurigo nodularis Hyde primarily by nodes and pigmented edges (Fig. 2.13).

The skin lesions are often scratched until they bleed, especially in prurigo simplex subacuta.

Differential diagnosis. Based on the varied presentation, the differential diagnosis ranges from infectious dermatoses such as varicella to autoimmune dermatoses and others. There is often a multifactorial genesis, especially in prurigo simplex subacuta, so an investigation should be done for metabolic diseases such as diabetes mellitus, hepatic disease, pregnancy, uremia, or even a paraneoplastic genesis.

Emotional symptoms. No generally typical personality for prurigo has been identified (Seikowski and Frank 2003), but a frequency of critical life events is noticeable. One-third of the patients are completely emotionally healthy. An often episodic, mentally triggerable itching is typical. Psychosocial stress contributes to the onset of prurigo in about 33% of patients (Rowland-Payne et al. 1985). Disease coping is often deficient, and depressive disorder is often present as a comorbidity. The itching may become unbearable and lead in a crisis to the danger of suicide (Braun-Falco et al. 1996).

Diagnostics should especially address coping mechanisms, taking the stress of suffering due to the disease and the disease model into account.

Dermatological therapy. Eradication of the possible cause is important. Antihistamines, local therapy and phototherapy are used.

Psychotherapy. Relaxation procedures, behavior therapy (e.g., diversion, cognitive restructuring), and psychodynamic psychotherapy have proven beneficial for treatment in cases of chronification and noncompliance. Discussion with the doctor, corresponding to psychosomatic primary care and psychoeducation, help provide information and knowledge and sensitize for possible relationships between emotional stress and itching. Using the visual analog scale and keeping an itching diary have proven helpful.

Relaxation techniques such as autogenic training and progressive muscle relaxation have proven beneficial in practice for improving itching control and breaking the itching–scratching cycle, as well as for achieving inner calm. Similarly, biofeedback can be useful.

Deep-psychological therapies are indicated, especially in cases of depressive disorder. Prurigo simplex subacuta patients are often elderly and seldom have the indication and motivation for deep-psychological long-term therapy, but it should be considered because of its proven efficacy.

Psychopharmaceuticals. With corresponding comorbidity of depression or anxiety disorders, doxepin, which has a good itch-relieving effect, should be administered. Antihistamines alone are often ineffective. The stepwise plan for therapy is presented in detail in Chap. 15 concerning antihistamines and doxepin.

References

Braun-Falco O, Plewig G, Wolff HH (1996) Dermatologie und Venerologie, 4. Aufl. Springer, Berlin

Rowland-Payne CM, Wilkinson JD, McKee PH, Jurecka W, Black MM (1985) Nodular prurigo – a clinicopathological study of 46 patients. Br J Dermatol 113: 431–439

Seikowski K, Frank U (2003) Role of psychosomatic factors in the development and course of prurigo simplex subacuta. Dermatol Psychosom 4: 72–78

Further Reading

Rechenberger I (1979) Prurigo bei Atopie. Materialien zur Psychoanalyse und analytisch orientierten Psychotherapy 5: 67–96, Universität Düsseldorf

Rosacea

Definition. In rosacea (ICD-10: L71, F54) there is centrofacial erythema with teleangiectasias, papulopustules, or even sebaceous gland hypertrophies leading to nose involvement (rhinophyma).

Pathogenesis. Rosacea is a multifactorial skin disease in which genetic factors, vascular impairment, sebaceous gland hyperplasia, inflammatory influences, and emotional stress may contribute to the genesis (Fig. 2.14).

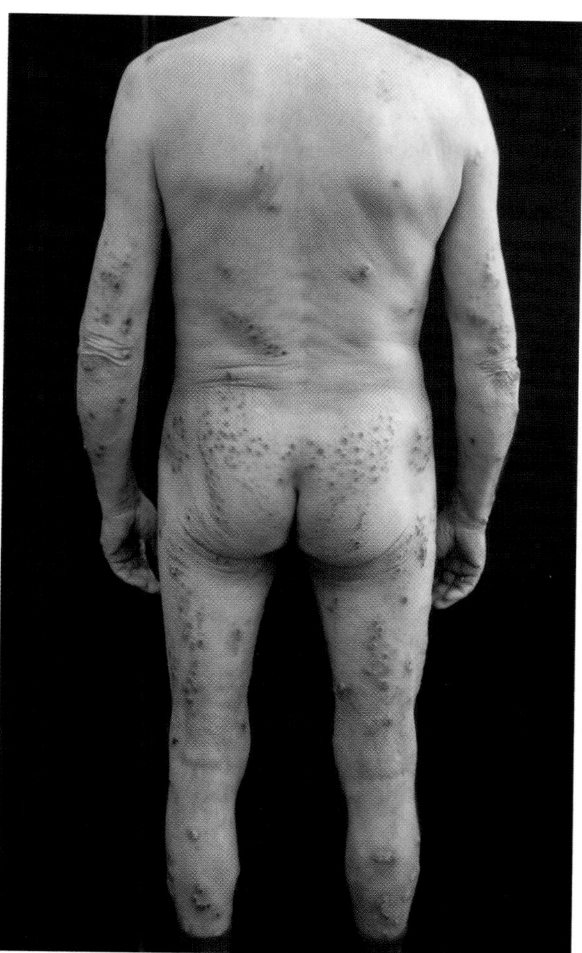

Fig. 2.13 Prurigo in depression

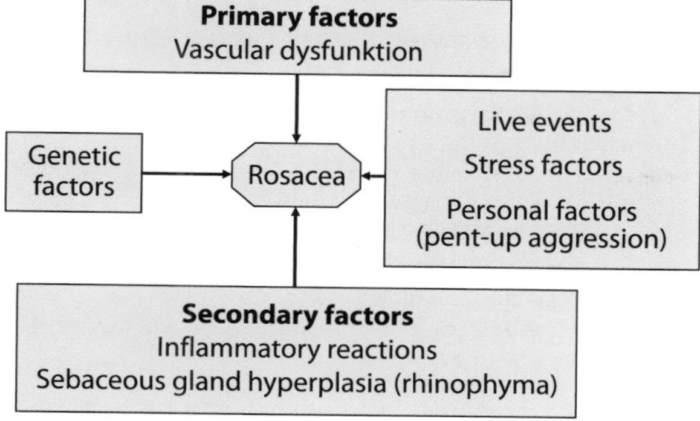

Fig. 2.14 Multifactorial pathogenesis of rosacea

Clinical findings. The presentation of rosacea is classified according to three degrees of severity: rosacea erythematosa, rosacea papulopustulosa, and hyperplastic rosacea. Other special forms are differentiated.

Classification of Rosacea

1. Rosacea erythematosa
   - This type mainly involves persistent erythema and teleangiectasias in the areas of the nose, lips, cheeks, and forehead.
2. Rosacea papulopustulosa
   - In this type, there are often isolated or grouped erythematous papules, papulopustules, or edematous swelling with a centrofacial focus.
3. Glandular hyperplastic rosacea (phymatous rosacea: rhinophyma, gnatophyma, metophyma, and otophyma)
   - This form of rosacea is characterized by thickened, irregular hardening of the skin surface on the nose, chin, forehead, cheeks, or ears, with sebaceous gland hypertrophy and increased connective tissue. A massive increase in volume may be present with inflammatory infiltrates.
4. Special forms of rosacea
   - Ocular rosacea: Blepharitis, iridocyclitis, iritis, or keratitis is present in this form of rosacea. The eye complications are not coupled to the presentation of the skin changes but may precede them.
   - Lupoid or granulomatous rosacea: Disseminated tuberculoid efflorescences develop on the foundation of rosacea.
   - Steroid rosacea: If patients with rosacea are treated over longer periods with steroids, steroid atrophy may develop as well as rebound phenomena with markedly increased erythema and subsequent pustules.
   - Rosacea conglobata: Confluent hemorrhagic and abscessing nodes and plaques similar to acne conglobata are present.
   - Rosacea fulminans: This type has a severe, rapidly progressing course with significant signs of inflammation. A variant is termed lupus miliaris disseminatus faciei.

Emotional symptoms. Psychodynamic aspects in rosacea may arise, especially with increasing vasodilatation due to affective regulation disorders. These lead to further potentiation of vasoactive reactivity by means of inhibited aggression and social anxieties, and to a latent erythrophobia (Garnis-Jones 1998) that in turn stimulates sebaceous gland activity. Emotionally stressful situations would then act to strengthen the pathogenetic development and additionally magnify the patient's anxieties and problems.

! Emotional stress may lend a somatic expression in rosacea via vasoactive reactivity and sebaceous gland activity.

Other connections were identified very early (Klaber and Wittkower 1939) to feelings of disgust and shame, usually coupled with sexual problems and social anxiety.

Compared with patients in other groups, psychological studies in patients with rosacea have revealed a weak ego, autoaggression, tendency to self-accusation, excessive feeling of responsibility for oneself and others, low tolerance for frustration, and a great discrepancy between what the person is and what he or she wishes to be. The measured forms of anxiety – both situational fear and anxiety as a personality trait – had the highest values in rosacea patients. The autoaggression, according to the researchers, coupled with the low frustration tolerance and the deficient personality integration, is interrelated with the feeling of personal menace.

Moreover, stress from the disease is also important due to the stigmatization associated with the disease (Blount and Pelletier 2002; Fried 2002; Koblenzer 1987). Rhinophyma is also called cauliflower nose and bulb nose and is often called alcohol nose in the vernacular and related incorrectly to excessive alcohol consumption. Rosacea is often associated with social anxieties (Koblenzer 1987) and, especially, impaired contacts. Rosacea may also potentiate already existing premorbid social anxieties of the patient, in whom the skin disease then leads to further social withdrawal and isolation (Fig. 2.15).

Quality of life in rosacea. The quality of life of rosacea patients is limited (Staudt et al. 2002). Although the limitations appear to be considerably less than those for patients with AD, psoriasis, or acne, they are real and must be taken into account.

Differential diagnoses. Beside the anxiety disorders, depressions, social phobias, and personality disorders must be differential-diagnostically clarified as comorbidities in rosacea patients, since these require different therapeutic regimens.

Forms of body dysmorphic disorders (ICD-10: F 45.2) must also be ruled out in rosacea, in which the patient's subjective suffering and the impairment that can be objectively recorded by the dermatologist can vary considerably.

Psychotherapy. According to current knowledge, psychotherapy should always be undertaken in rosacea when the patient has developed clear social anxieties, when the emotional stress of the rosacea becomes worse, when it has led to depression or anxieties, or when a body dysmorphic disorder is present with considerable discrepancy between objective findings and subjectively experienced severity.

Although there are no controlled studies on psychotherapy in rosacea to date (Fried 2002), stabilization with respect to quality of life and coping appears possible by both psychodynamic therapy and behavior therapy (Ryzhkova and Liagushkina 1978).

Psychopharmaceuticals. There is no experience on the psychopharmacological therapy of rosacea. The guidelines for emotional comorbidities apply.

References

Blount BW, Pelletier AL (2002) Rosacea: a common, yet commonly overlooked, condition. Am Fam Physician 66: 435–440

Fried RG (2002) Nonpharmacologic treatment in psychodermatology. Dermatol Clin 20: 177–185

Garnis-Jones S (1998) Psychological aspects of rosacea. J Cutan Med Surg 2(suppl 4): 4–16

Klaber R, Wittkower E (1939) The pathogenesis of rosacea: a review with special reference to emotional factors. Br J Dermatol 51: 501–524

Koblenzer C (1987) Psychocutaneous disease. Grune & Stratton, Orlando, pp 230–237

Ryzhkova EI, Liagushkina MP (1978) Comprehensive therapy of rosacea (a clinical and morphological study). Vestn Dermatol Venerol 6: 16–22

Staudt A, Ring J, Schäfer T (2002) Deutsches Instrument zur Erfassung der Lebensqualität bei Hauterkrankungen (DIELH) – Analyse nach Erkrankungsgruppen und Domänen. Allergo J 11: 445–456

Further Reading

Cohen CG, Krahn L, Wise TN, Epstein S, Ross R (1991) Delusions of disfigurement in a woman with acne rosacea. Gen Hosp Psychiatry 13: 273–277

Fox RH, Goldsmith R, Kidd DJ (1962) Cutaneous vasomotor control in the human head, neck and upper chest. J Physiol 161: 298–312

Jansen T, Plewig G (1997) Die chronisch-progrediente Gesichtsdermatose Rosazea. Dtsch Ärztebl 94: C84–C90

Marks R 1(968) Concepts in the pathogenesis of rosacea. Br J Dermatol 80: 170–177

Plesch E (1951) A Rorschach study of rosacea and morbid blushing. Br J Med Psychol 24: 202–205

Puchalski Z (1984) Angststruktur und Parameter von Katecholaminen bei Patienten mit Rosacea, Alopecia areata und Licher ruber planus. Z Hautkr 61: 137–145

Sobye P (1950) Aetiology and pathogenesis of rosacea. Acta Derm Venereol 30: 137–158

Whitlock FA (1961) Psychosomatic aspects of rosacea. Br J Dermatol 73: 137–148

Seborrheic Dermatitis

Prevalence/incidence. There are only a few individual publications on the psychosomatic relationships to seborrheic dermatitis. This is surprising, given the relatively high prevalence of this dermatosis.

Definition and clinical findings. Seborrheic dermatitis is characterized by an erythematous, sometimes reddish-brown inflammation and greasy yellow scaling, which appears mostly in the seborrheic areas of the hairline, retroauricular, anterior sweat furrow, and nasolabial folds. On occasion, other seborrheic areas such as the central chest, back, and genitals are involved (seborrheic balanitis).

Pathogenesis. Yeasts (Pityrosporon) appear to be of importance, and the disease tends to responds to antimycotic therapy.

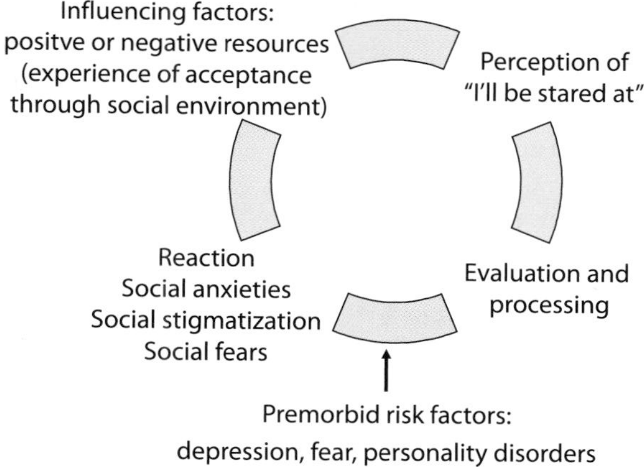

Fig. 2.15 Disfiguration problem in rosacea

2

Emotional symptoms. It has been demonstrated that emotional triggering occurs in about 40% of patients with seborrheic dermatitis (ICD-10: L21, F54). Stress factors also may influence the severity of disease. Itching and burning are rare but may be potentiated by psychosocial conflicts and situations of tension. In addition, comparable to perioral dermatitis, a vicious cycle develops between the external therapy and triggering of the disease.

Due to the facial localization, the disfiguration problems must be emphasized because sociophobic tendencies, communication impairments, and avoidance and social withdrawal may result.

Psychotherapy. Care is generally given as part of medical psychosomatic primary care and psychoeducation. Compliance appears to be very good compared with other facial dermatoses in men and women.

Psychotherapy may be meaningful if disfiguration problems and the related psychosocial disorders arise.

Psychopharmaceuticals. There is no general indication for psychopharmacological therapy.

Further Reading

Griesemer RD (1978) Emotionally triggered disease in dermatology practice. Psychiatr Ann 8: 49–56

Ulcers of the Leg (Venous Stasis)

In leg ulcers, there are some special findings such as artificial maintenance and "social ulcer," so this dermatosis must be considered under multifactorial aspects.

Definition. Leg ulcer (ulceration of the lower calf; ICD-10: L97, F54) is a loss of substance due to local circulation impairment.

Prevalence/incidence. Leg ulcers are frequently seen, with 1–1.5 million sufferers in the German-speaking region. The prevalence is about 1% and is age-related, being 4–5% in the elderly.

Pathogenesis. Leg ulcers develop because of local circulation impairments, usually due to venous insufficiency (80–90%) and less often to arterial occlusive disease. The genesis is, however, multifactorial overall, with a bacterial infection, vasculitic component, postthrombotic syndrome or trauma, and neurogenic disorders being additional factors. Emotional factors in the elicitation of leg ulcers apply mainly to an artificial genesis.

Clinical findings. Depending on the pathogenesis, ulcerations are variably configured and of different localizations, usually on the distal internal aspect of the lower calf. Very large ulcers may affect the entire lower calf, and there is almost invariably pyodermic superinfection. The course may last for decades and be severely painful.

Emotional symptoms. Psychosocial factors of leg ulcers particularly affect the individual's quality of life and compliance. One central aspect of the disease is the pain-magnifying cycle of fear and depression, which can be observed as a challenge in coping. Anxious patients with chronic wounds suffer greater pain. The stress from the disease with respect to limitations in quality of life is dependent on the stage. The patients understandably feel limited in their activities and worry more about their health.

Focus: Leg Ulcers

- Pain and depression/anxiety
- Quality of life
- Social ulcer/compliance
- Artefact/malingering

On the other hand, the secondary profit from disease that arises in many patients is especially problematic and must be taken into account in the treatment. The disease ("social ulcer") also represents a possibility to establish contact with the environment, including caregivers, especially in old age. In individual cases, an artificial genesis or even malingerings may be decisive factors in the onset or maintenance of the ulceration.

Psychotherapy. Support of active coping takes first place here. Psychosomatic primary care, psychoeducation, psychopharmaceuticals, or psychotherapy may be meaningful in light of psychopathological comorbidity. Several studies confirm that improved training in independent care of the wound may improve the person's quality of life (Augustin and Maier 2003).

Psychopharmaceuticals. Drug therapy is indicated if emotional comorbidities are present.

Reference

Augustin M, Maier K (2003) Psychosomatic aspects of chronic wounds. Dermatol Psychosom 4: 5–13

Further Reading

Augustin M, Dieterle W, Zschocke I, Brill C, Trefzer D, Peschen M, Schöpf E, Vanscheidt W (1997) Development and validation of a disease-specific questionnaire on the quality of life of patients with chronic venous insufficiency. Vasa 26(4): 291–301

Blättler W, Davatz U (1993) Zur Psychogenese vermeintlich venös bedingter Beinbeschwerden. Phlebologie 22: 57–60

Erickson CA, Lanza DJ, Karp DL, Edwards JW, Seabrook GR, Cambria RA, Freischlag JA, Towne JB (1995) Healing of venous ulcer in an ambulatory care program: the roles of chronic venous insufficiency and patient compliance. J Vascular Surg 22(5): 629–636

Flett R (1994) Psychological aspects of chronic lower leg ulceration in the elderly. West J Nurs Res 16(2): 183–192

Moffatt CJ, Dorman MC (1995) Recurrence of leg ulcers within a community ulcer service. J Wound Care 4(2): 57–61

Urticaria

Definition. Urticaria (ICD-10: L50.0, L50.3, L50.8, ggf. F54) is defined by the occurrence of wheals – transient edemas of the upper dermis – that are associated with erythema and pruritus and resolve within 24 h. The wheals are sometimes accompanied by angioedemas, which heal more slowly and last up to 72 h.

Occurrence. Urticaria, with a prevalence of 7–15% of the population, is one of the most common skin diseases (Czarnetzky 1986). It is assumed that every 4th person will be affected by urticaria at least once during his or her life.

Pathogenesis. The pathomechanism is based essentially on a release of so-called mediator substances (histamine, prostaglandin, leukotrienes, serotonin, etc.) from mast cells (Gauger et al. 2000). These cause vasodilatation, increased vascular permeability, leakage of plasma from the vessels into the skin tissue, and elicitation of itching. Among the numerous eliciting factors are physical influences (cold, heat, pressure), allergens (foods, medications), and nonallergic factors (such as medication intolerance). In 50–65% of cases, however, no elicitor can be identified and no cause can be found despite thorough examination. This is then termed chronic idiopathic urticaria.

Clinical findings and differential diagnosis. Urticaria is a heterogeneous spectrum of skin diseases, differentiated by duration, frequency, and cause. The thorough differential diagnosis also includes diseases that are considered for historical reasons as belonging to the group of urticarial diseases (Fig. 2.16).

Classification of Urticaria (ICD-10: L50.0, F54; Zuberbier et al. 2003)

A. Depending on the course of the disease
   - Acute/spontaneous urticaria (<6 weeks' duration)
   - Recurrent/chronic continuous urticaria (>6 weeks' duration)

B. After physical elicitors
   - Urticaria factitia (ICD-10: L50.3, F54)
   - Delayed pressure urticaria
   - Cold urticaria
   - Heat urticaria
   - Light urticaria
   - Vibration urticaria/angioedema

C. Other forms of urticaria
   - Cholinergic urticaria (ICD-10: L50.5, F54)
   - Adrenergic urticaria
   - Nonphysical contact urticaria
   - Aquagenic urticaria
   - Light urticaria

D. Diseases belonging to urticaria for historical reasons
   - Urticarial vasculitis
   - Urticaria pigmentosa
   - Familiar cold urticaria
   - Hereditary angioedema

Aquagenic urticaria, which is also characterized by pinhead-size wheals, must be differentiated from cholinergic urticaria. The skin changes are elicited by contact with water, whereby the water possibly releases an allergen from the corneal layer of the epidermis and diffuses it in the dermis, so this is not a real "water allergy."

Urticarial vasculitis must be considered when the individual lesions last more than 48 h. A particular variant is hypocomplementemic urticarial vasculitis. These conditions are usually associated with the presence of SLE.

Emotional symptoms. Urticaria is a multifactorial disease. Clinical experience has shown a clear possibility of psychosomatic triggering in a subgroup of patients with

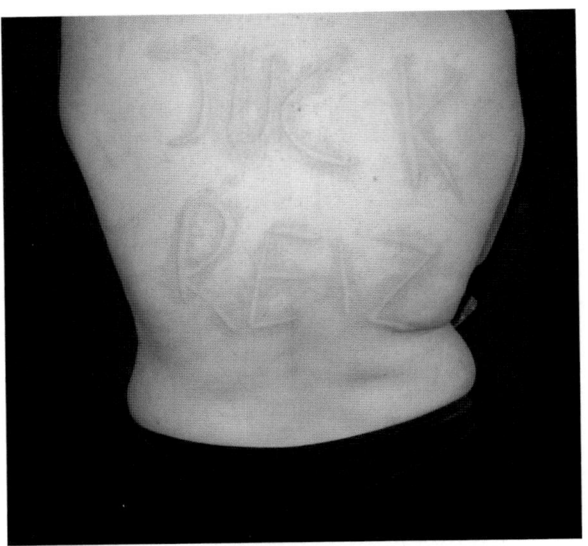

Fig. 2.16 A 34-year-old woman with urticaria factitia (dermographism) with pronounced itching (itching–scratching cycle). (In German, *Juckreiz*, translated as pruritus.) Posttraumatic stress disorder after car accident

reproducible, stress-dependent acute urticaria. It has been found that remembering a trauma during psychotherapy can lead to an episode of acute urticaria (Brosig et al. 2000). Moreover, cholinergic urticaria especially can be elicited under emotional stress in a particular patient group.

It is more difficult to make statements about the chronic forms of urticaria. There is apparently no typical psychosomatic urticaria personality, but there is a subgroup in whom psychosocial factors are decisive.

Stress. The results of various studies using psychometric test procedures, clinical interviews, and prospective time-series analyses of connections between urticaria and emotional stress do not indicate a general consideration of chronic urticaria in the sense of a psychosomatic disease, but they suggest the formation of subgroups with stress-dependent pathogenesis (stress responders versus nonstress responders; Stangier and Gieler 2000; Sheehan-Dare et al. 1990; Leuschner et al. 1994).

Stress factors play a central role in the subgroup of stress responders in urticaria. Pathogenetically, acute and acute-recurrent stress situations and unresolved conflicts often lead to stress reactions in urticaria, which can then lead to increased histamine release via neuropeptides or psychoneuroendocrinological factors. Time-series analytical studies have demonstrated the relationship between emotional stress and urticaria, as well as the reverse influence.

Psychological Aspects of Urticaria

- Elevated stress reactivity:
  The likelihood of reacting to stressful interpersonal situations with increased excretion of mediator substances and intense emotional reactions; a subgroup of stress-dependent urticaria appears to exist
- Unfavorable strategies of coping with stress:
  Reactions to emotionally stressful situations that are not directed at active coping (positive coping with disease)
- Elevated anxiety and depression:
  Situation-independent personality traits, usually accompanying chronic physiological activation

Deep-psychological concepts. The attempt to identify general and universally valid characteristic personality traits, such as latent aggression, anxiety, or depression, in all patients with urticaria by means of questionnaires or clinical interviews has produced only inconsistent results. However, simultaneous dermatological-psychosomatic diagnostics appear essential, especially in identifying a subgroup (cluster) of patients with increased depression (Hein et al. 1996).

In scientific investigations, patients with urticaria often show inhibition of aggression. Anger or rage is hardly expressed. In opposition to this is the marked need for recognition in the environment (Gupta and Gupta 1996). Characteristic of patients with urticaria may be their interpersonal relationships, in which they feel helplessly at the mercy of and dependent on the partner, whom they experience as powerful and limiting to their own independence.

Psychodynamically, attention should be paid to a somatization of separation and dependency conflicts (autonomy conflict). Some urticaria patients present with symbolic conversion symptoms.

Koblenzer summarized the deep-psychological constellations in chronic urticaria as follows (Koblenzer 1987):

Deep-Psychological Concepts in Chronic Urticaria

- Patients find themselves in situations from which they see no escape.
- These are often ambitious people who want to reach their goals at any price.
- The patients are caught in a conflict in which the desire for love and recognition is frustrated by sexual taboos. The symbolic sexual meaning of tumescence and detumescence in the swelling and abating of the wheals may fit in this context.
- Patients who attempt to protect themselves from strong dependency desires and to control their anxiety by excessive activity develop urticaria when this possibility is blocked. There is often an unconscious enmity.
- Patients bear resentment because they truly are or subjectively feel unjustly treated, but they cannot express their hostility openly.
- Anxiety, depression, and compulsive disorders are often characteristic of patients with chronic urticaria.

Diagnostic questionnaires. The Giessen Complaint Sheet (Gießener Beschwerdebogen) and the Giessen test are examples of psychometric tests to measure stress reactivity and the tendency to depressive moods and anxiety (Hein et al. 1996).

An urticaria diary is helpful for disclosing unclear relationships between possible emotional stress and the skin lesions.

Psychotherapy. Psychotherapy is meaningful in urticaria only for patients in the subgroup of psychosomatic urticaria. A clear indication, taking comorbidities into account, is important from the start.

For this reason, Bone (1992) developed diagnostic criteria for the psychotherapeutic treatment of urticaria.

Because conflicts with anger and rage are frequently a characteristic trait of patients with urticaria, the psychotherapeutic approach should be attempted in this situation and is usually promising. Emotionally unresolved rage affects can be made clear in the psychotherapeutic setting and worked out both interactionally and by interpretation. Focal psychotherapy and short-term psychotherapy that address a possible eliciting event have proven especially beneficial in urticaria. As a supplement, relaxation procedures and methods of coping with stress appear to help these patients (Bone 1992).

Diagnostic Criteria of Emotional Urticaria According to Bone (1992)

- Elevated anxiety
- Low ego strength
- Lack of assertive capacity
- Stressful childrearing behavior by the parents
- Marked stress burden on the patient
- Tendency to psychosomatic reactions
- Wheals, mainly at night and in the evening
- Inability of an emotional co-involvement to be ruled out by other urticaria causes
- Patient's belief that the urticaria is emotionally elicited

Antihistamines and psychopharmaceuticals. In acute urticaria, emergency treatment with antihistamines (H1 and H2 blockers) and corticosteroids is sometimes indicated. Short-term therapy is often sufficient.

The long-term course of chronic-recurrent urticaria is more problematic and needs to be differentiated from the acute form. Other therapeutic concepts are required here because of the long-term side effects of corticosteroids.

In the foreground initially is therapy with nonsedating antihistamines, and in a further step, the use of sedating antihistamines.

This process often does not control the episode, so a third step using sedating antihistamines (hydroxyzine) or a tricyclic antidepressant (doxepin) is necessary (Chap. 15). On many occasions the physician will need to combine agents belonging to different groups of antihistamines.

Stepwise Plan for Urticaria

- Acute urticaria
  - Emergency antihistamines (H1 and H2 blockers), corticosteroids
- Chronic recurrent urticaria
  - Step 1: Nonsedating antihistamines
  - Step 2: Sedating antihistamines
  - Step 3: Tricyclic antidepressants (doxepin)

Sometimes combination therapies are required, in which sedating medications are administered in the evening and nonsedating medications during the day.

The tricyclic antidepressant doxepin shows the best long-term success in both prurigo diseases and cholinergic urticaria with depression. It can successfully break through the itching–scratching or itching–depression cycle. The tricyclic antidepressant opipramol (Insidon) not available in USA is used often in Germany for anxiety, tension, depressive moods, and vegetative organ complaints and additionally has an antipruriginous effect.

References

Bone HG (1992) Psychische Faktoren bei chronischer Urtikaria. Eine Literatureübersicht und Untersuchung an 53 ambulanten Patienten. Dissertation, Universität Münster

Brosig B, Niemeier V, Kupfer J, Gieler U (2000) Urticaria and the recall of a sexual trauma. Dermatol Psychosom 1: 72–75

Czarnetzky B (1986) Urticaria. Springer, Berlin

Gauger A, Ring J, Abeck D (2000) Puzzling urticaria. Allergies, pseudo-allergy, bacteria, fungi, parasites? MMW Fortschr Med 142(43): 41–44

Gupta MA, Gupta AK (1996) Psychodermatology: an update. J Am Acad Dermatol 6: 1030–1046

Hein UR, Henz BM, Haustein UF, Seikowski K et al. (1996) Zur Beziehung zwischen chronischer Urtikaria und Depression/Somatisierungsstörung. Hautarzt 47: 20–23

Koblenzer C (1987) Psychocutaneus disease. Grune & Stratton, Orlando

Leuschner G, Köstler E, Baunacke A, Roch R, Seebach C (1994) Belastungserleben, Entwicklungssituation und Persönlichkeit bei 100 Patienten mit chronischer Urtikaria. Z Hautkr 69(11): 749–753

Sheehan-Dare RA, Henderson MJ, Cotterill JA (1990) Anxiety and depression in patients with chronic urticaria and generalized pruritus. Br J Dermatol 123: 769–774

Stangier U, Gieler U (2000) Hauterkrankungen. In: Senft W, Broda M (Hrsg) Praxis der Psychotherapy, 2. Aufl. Thieme, Stuttgart, S 566–581

Zuberbier T, Aberer W, Grabbe J, Hartmann K, Merk H, Ollert M, Ruëff F, Wedi B, Wenning J (2003) Diagnostik und Therapy der Urtikaria: Leitlinie der DDG. JDDG 1: 655–663

Further Reading

Gieler U, Stangier U (1995) Dermatologie. In: Uexküll T von et al. (Hrsg) Psychosomatische Medizin, 5. Aufl. Urban & Schwarzenberg, München

Henz BM, Zuberbier T (1998) Causes of urticaria. In: Henz BM, Zuberbier T, Grabbe J, Monroe E (eds) Urticaria. Clinical, diagnostic and therapeutic aspects. Springer, Berlin, pp 19–38

Juhlin L (1981) Recurrent urticaria: clinical investigation of 330 patients. Br J Dermatol 104: 369–381

Rechenberger I (1976) Tiefenpsychologisch ausgerichtete Diagnostik und Therapy von Hautkrankheiten. Verlag für Medizinische Psychologie, Vandenhoeck & Ruprecht, Göttingen, S 64–77

Shertzer CL, Lookongbill DP (1997) Effect of relaxation therapy and hypnotizability in chronic urticaria. Arch Dermatol 123: 913–916

Stangier U, Kolster B, Schlicht C, Krause W, Gieler U (1993) Psychoendokrine und subjektive Reaktionen von Urtikaria Patienten unter standardisierten Stressbedingungen. In: Hauterkrankungen in psychologischer Sicht. Jahrbuch der Medizinischen Psychologie, Bd 9, S 192–209

Vitiligo

Definition. Vitiligo is a macular depigmentation of the skin, mucosa, or hair with destruction of melanocytes.

Prevalence/incidence. It is assumed that about 1% of the population, regardless of gender, race, or educational level, develops vitiligo.

Pathogenesis. Stress can be demonstrated as an elicitor in a subgroup of patients with vitiligo (ICD-10: L80, F54). An influence of immune function via neuropeptides may have a central psychosomatic key function.

The opioid peptides such as alpha-MSH, beta-endorphin, and metenkephalin may be important stress-dependent messenger substances in the pathogenesis of vitiligo.

Special importance is ascribed to natural killer cell activities, which are upregulated during stress and can then affect melanocytes.

Clinical findings. In vitiligo, there are focal or expansive, generalized, variously sized, sharply delimited, irregular depigmented areas of skin (Figs. 2.17, 2.18).

Emotional symptoms. One-third of all vitiligo patients report a history of "stress." Various psychosocial models for the pathogenesis of vitiligo exist, but to date they have not been reproducibly verified.

In psychological studies, vitiligo shows an association with elevated anxiety scores, reduced self-esteem, and elevated psychiatric morbidity. In longer-lasting disease, elevated depression scores have been demonstrated depending on the duration of disease (Gieler et al. 2000).

An adjustment disorder plays a particular role due to stigmatization because of the disease. Among these are depressive disorders, sociophobias, and withdrawal tendencies.

Dermatological therapy. The treatment of vitiligo is still unsatisfactory. The first consideration is cosmetic covering and light protection to prevent both burns of the unprotected areas without melanocytes and tanning of

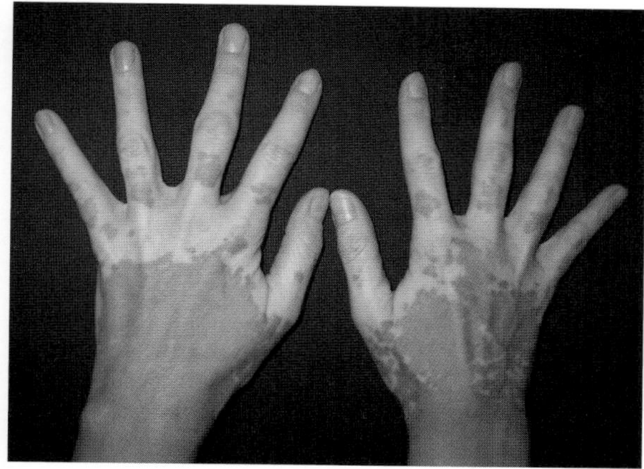

Fig. 2.17 Woman with vitiligo and adjustment disorder and pronounced helplessness. She especially suffered from stigmatization because of visible areas on her hands

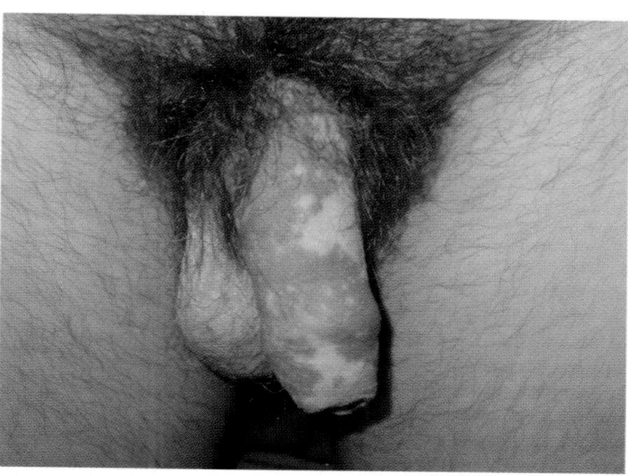

Fig. 2.18 Vitiligo and sexual partnership problems (adjustment disorders)

the unaffected areas with conspicuous transition to the depigmented lesions.

Other procedures comprise photochemotherapy (PUVA), UVB or phenylalanine combined with UVA exposure (PAUVA therapy) or transplantation, as well as local therapies with immunosuppressives such as tacrolimus.

Psychotherapy. Psychotherapeutic interventions often focus on coping with the disease. Strengthening of positive coping is initially part of psychosomatic primary care. In later therapy, group discussions and additional relaxation therapies have been found beneficial in working against withdrawal tendencies or sociophobia. Focal therapies may be necessary, especially in chronic courses with pronounced depressive disorders or sociophobias.

Psychopharmaceuticals. Antidepressants with additional anxiolytic components may be indicated in individual cases. No detailed studies on the psychopharmacological therapy of vitiligo are presently available.

Reference

Gieler U, Brosig B, Schneider U, Kupfer J, Niemeier V, Stangier U, Küster W (2000) Vitiligo – coping behavior. Dermatol Psychosom 1: 6–10

Further Reading

Firooz A, Bouzari N, Fallah N, Ghazisaidi B, Firoozabadi MR, Dowlati Y (2004) What patients with vitiligo believe about their condition. Int J Dermatol 43(11): 811–814

Mattoo SK, Handa S, Kaur I, Gupta N, Malhotra R (2002) Psychiatric morbidity in vitiligo: prevalence and correlates in India. J Eur Acad Dermatol Venereol 16(6): 573–578

Njoo MD, Spuls PI, Bos JD, Westerhof W, Boosuyt MM (1998) Nonsurgical repigmentation therapys in vitiligo. Arch Dermatol 134: 1532–1540

Picardi A, Abeni D (2001) Can cognitive-behavioral therapy help patients with vitiligo? Arch Dermatol 137(6): 786–788

Picardi A, Pasquini P, Cattaruzza MS, Gaetano P, Melchi CF, Baliva G, Camaioni D, Tiago A, Abeni D, Biondi M (2003) Stressful life events, social support, attachment security and alexithymia in vitiligo. A case-control study. Psychother Psychosom 72(3): 150–158

3

Secondary Emotional Disorders and Comorbidities

In emotional disorders resulting from dermatoses, the skin disease is primary and the emotional disorders secondary. These are somatopsychic disorders in the classical sense.

Somatopsychic disorders occur especially in chronic skin diseases affecting exposed cutaneous areas, with limitations of self-esteem, self-image, and self-satisfaction, particularly when these limitations interfere in interpersonal relationships, giving rise to feelings of shame.

Focal Points of Somatopsychic Disorders

- General problem areas
  - Stigmatization
  - Disfiguration problems
  - Impaired coping
  - Impaired compliance
  - Limitation of quality of life/disability
- Comorbidities
  - Adjustment disorders
  - Anxiety disorder
  - Depressive disorder

In somatopsychic disorders, the dermatoses are often associated with disfiguration or take on a threatening character for the patient. Moreover, there are comorbidities with impairment of coping and compliance (Chap. 17) that become manifest with the occurrence of the skin conditions. However, clear-cut separation between the primary emotional disorders due to the dermatosis, premorbid, preexisting disorders, and additional reactive emotional diseases (adjustment disorders) cannot always be made under biopsychosocial aspects. In particular, preexisting predisposing factors, such as somatoform and affective disorders, anxiety disorders, and personality disorders, may play a decisive role as comorbidities in the manifestation of a somatopsychic disorder.

Affective disorders (6.3%), anxiety disorders (9%), and somatoform disorders (7.5%) are widespread in the German population and are the most important comorbidities.

A comparison between the new (former East German) and old federal states showed a lower prevalence rate of somatoform (5.46% vs. 7.96%) and affective disorders (4.82% vs. 6.65%) in the new states (Wittchen et al. 1999).

Differentiation is made between lesions that have existed since birth and those that have developed over the course of the person's life.

3

Significantly, congenital skin changes like hemangiomas or large nevi can usually be integrated into the personality, apparently because they are perceived in the mirror image before the ego develops, whereas later changes such as acne or psoriasis or changes arising from an accident, for example, often subjectively cause an exaggerated feeling of disfiguration. It is significant that the subjective perception of one's own appearance does not in any way correlate with the objective estimation of the health provider.

Differential diagnoses. In disfiguring skin diseases, the body dysmorphic disorder must be distinguished from "objective" (i.e., demonstrable) skin changes that are detrimental to appearance; these may, however, be associated with an adjustment disorder. Concurrent carcinophobia or hypochondria must be ruled out.

Clinical entities and dermatoses. The following overview differentiates those disfiguring or threatening dermatoses that may lead to secondary emotional disorders.

Dermatoses with Disfiguring or Threatening Character that May Lead to Secondary Emotional (Somatopsychic) Disorders

- Congenital disfiguring dermatoses (genodermatoses)
  - Ichthyoses
  - Epidermolyses
  - Lipomatoses
  - Phacomatoses (Klippel–Trenaunay syndrome, hemangioma, Schimmelpenning–Feuerstein–Mims syndrome, etc.)
- Acquired disfiguring dermatoses and sequelae
  - Infections
  - Autoimmune dermatoses
  - Trauma
  - Keloid
- Neoplasias (threatening dermatoses)
  - Benign neoplasias: nevocellular nevus, von Recklinghausen disease
  - Malignant neoplasias: carcinomas, ulcus terebrans, malignant melanoma

3.1 Congenital Disfiguring Dermatoses and Their Sequelae (Genodermatoses)

A number of genodermatoses, including ichthyoses, epidermolysis bullosa, neurofibromatosis, lipomatoses, and the Klippel–Trenaunay syndrome, may cause somatopsychic disorders (Fig. 3.1a, b). Very often, worried parents consult the doctor because the infant or child has a hemangioma. This condition may cause great concern, especially in a stigmatizing facial localization (Fig. 3.1b).

Genetically determined skin disease existing since birth along with physical disability is, on the other hand, often associated with a lack of compliance in diseases requiring control. This may include a lack of pressure due to suffering and relatively little or delayed seeking of medical diagnostics and therapy, or it may even extend to the development of avoidable and, by then, often extensive neoplasias in precancerous patients (Harth and Linse 2001).

Only a few detailed studies have been done on epidermolysis. Depending on the patient's age, the dystrophic forms of epidermolysis in particular are associated with delayed development. The psychosocial stress for the family is considerable, and family detachment problems are often the consequence. Younger epidermolysis patients especially show less emotional stress than patients with AD, which has been taken as evidence of displacement behavior. In later life, feelings of disfiguration and limitations in quality of life, which may also lead to social withdrawal, play a role.

Psychotherapy. Supportive psychotherapy is in first place, especially in connection with an unstable ego and self-esteem problems, and also as part of psychosomatic primary care for the entire family (family therapy). Psychoeducation with explanation of the disease is also helpful psychosomatic support for coping with the disease.

References

Harth W, Linse R (2001) Schimmelpenning–Feuerstein–Mims-Syndrom in Kombination mit einem primären Lymphödem und Basalzellkarzinomen. Akt Dermatol 27: 66–69

Wittchen HU, Müller N, Pfister H, Winter S, Schmidtkunz B (1999) Affektive, somatoforme und Angststörungen in Deutschland – Ergebnisse des bundesweiten Zusatzsurveys "Psychische Störungen." Gesundwesen 61(Sonderheft): 216–222

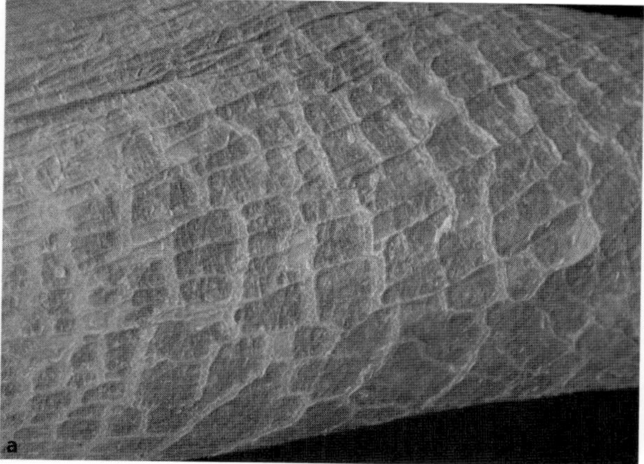

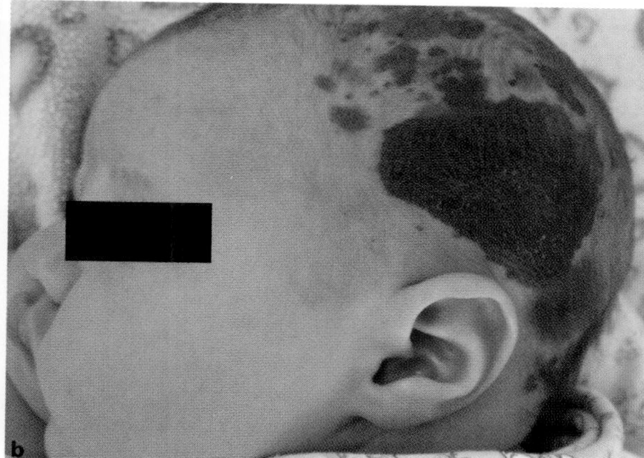

Fig. 3.1 **a** Ichthioses vulgaris. **b** Congenital nevus

3.2 Acquired Disfiguring Dermatoses and Their Sequelae

Infections, Autoimmune Dermatosis, Trauma

Acquired disfiguring dermatoses and their sequelae comprise the presentations after infections, destructive diseases, trauma with subsequent keloid formation, and sometimes serious courses of autoimmune diseases (Fig. 3.2).

Keloid formation is a particular therapeutic problem in aesthetic dermatology and may lead to adjustment disorders and impaired coping. There is often a difference between the subjective assessment of a scar and the objective findings. The presence of a body dysmorphic disorder must be included in the differential diagnosis.

Emotional symptoms. Disfiguring dermatoses lead in the majority of cases to adjustment disorders (Fig. 3.3). Anxiety and depression arise in differing degrees. Detriment to physical integrity is associated with limitations in quality of life and lifestyle and may be experienced as a vital threat.

Psychotherapy. Reports of individual cases are available demonstrating that supportive psychotherapy is meaningful within the framework of psychosomatic primary care, psychoeducation, and promotion of coping.

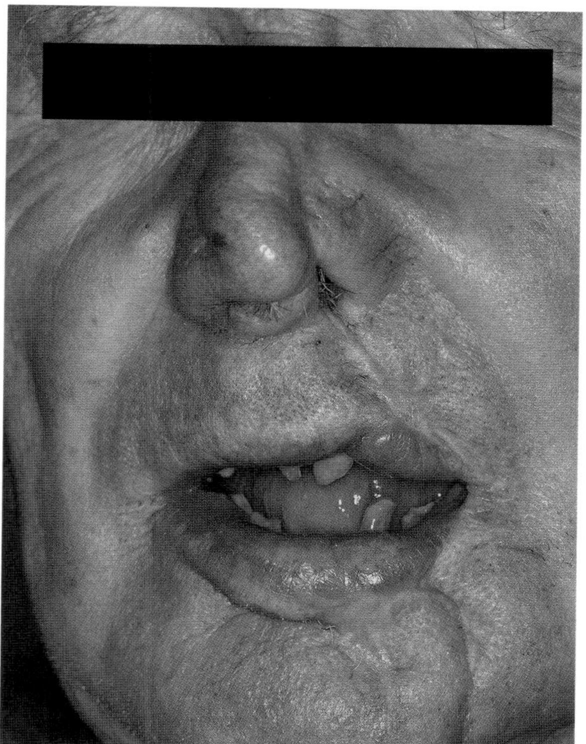

Fig. 3.2 Shrapnel injury from World War II

Neoplasias

Neoplasias are among the threatening dermatoses, especially if the course is metastatic and destructive, with a question of life or death for the patient.

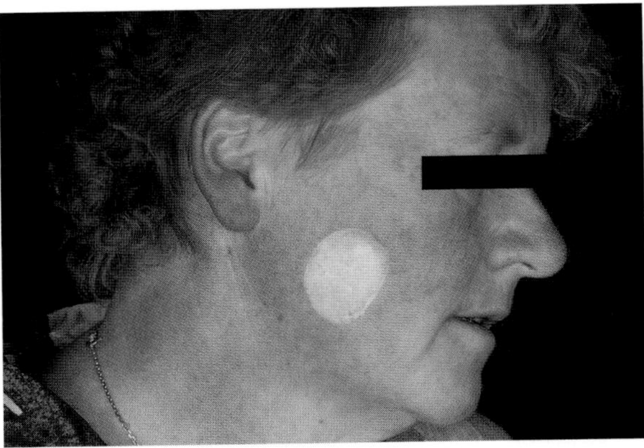

Fig. 3.3 Woman with postoperative adjustment disorder after treatment with full-skin transplantation in the face

Benign Neoplasias

Benign neoplasias that have a favorable somatic course, such as nevi, take on a threatening character only in the concurrent presence of an emotional disorder, such as carcinophobia or hypochondria. This may mean that the patient expresses unjustified or even masochistic wishes for surgery.

Denial of benign but rapidly growing neoplasias also plays a role. Surgical treatment in a late stage may be difficult, usually due to the size.

Malignant Neoplasias

Malignant neoplasias may lead to fear of tumor, fear of metastasis, fear of death, and fear of the consequences of extensive invasive therapies (see Chap. 8 on oncology).

Psychosomatic aspects of oncology that are especially problematic are anxiety disorders on the one hand and denial of the disease on the other.

Moreover, because of fear of the truth, neoplasias may be ignored and denied such that early consultation with the specialist is avoided or sought only in stages that are extensive and difficult to treat. Thus, carcinomas with local destructive growth may take on broad dimensions. Necessary therapy is postponed, especially in elderly patients, which is in part understandable (Figs. 3.4, 3.5).

Malignant melanoma treatment should be accompanied by psychoeducation and psychosomatic support as part of psychosomatic primary care. In cases of pronounced psychosocial detriment, group therapies should be considered for better active coping.

Psychopharmaceuticals may be beneficial in cases of tumor-related or tumor-therapy-related depression (interferon; see Chap. 8).

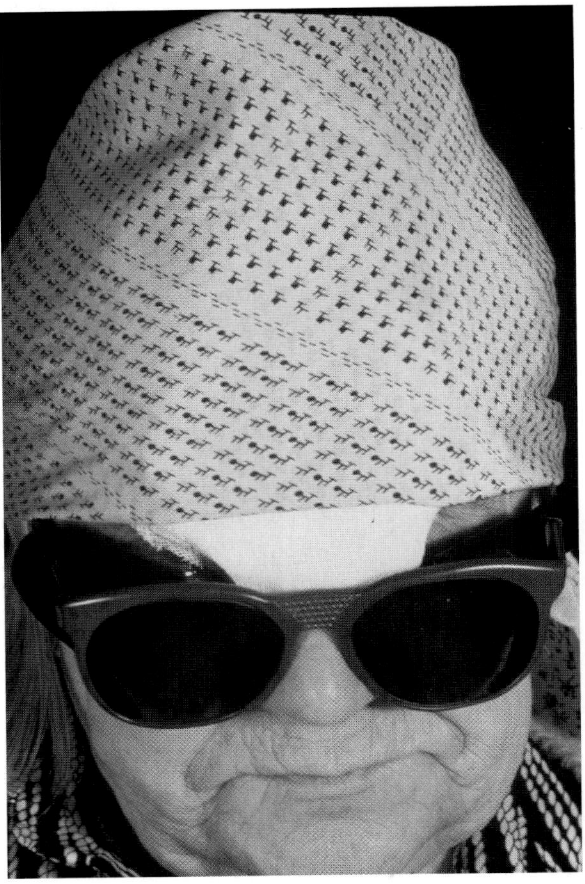

Fig. 3.4 Woman with various caps, sunglasses, and bandages to cover or hide ulcus terebrans

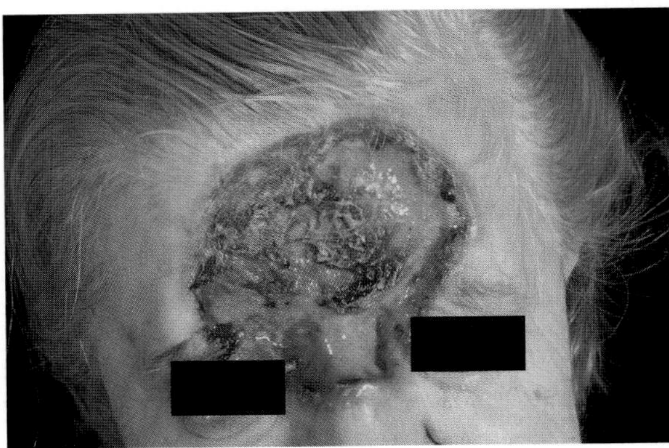

Fig. 3.5 Apparent ulcus terebrans: same patient as in Fig. 3.4 without covering

Further Reading

Frederikson M, Furst CJ, Lekander M, Rotstein S, Blomgrenz H (1993) Trait anxiety and anticipatory immune reactions in women receiving adjuvant chemotherapy for breast cancer. Brain Behav Immun 7: 79–90

Wendler M, Harth W, Linse R (2003) 12. Jahrestagung der Arbeitsgemeinschaft dermatologische Onkologie (ADO) der Deutschen Dermatologischen Gesellschaft 26. bis 28.09.03 in Erfurt. Akt Dermatol 29: 145–147

3.3 Comorbidities

Somatopsychic disorders often become manifest only in preexisting disposition to emotional disorders. If a latent emotional disorder becomes manifest during tumor disease or tumor therapy, this often means a serious complication for the course of treatment and for compliance and coping. Depression and anxiety disorders are especially to be watched for as comorbidities.

Comorbidity: Concurrent presence of an emotional disorder and a skin disease.

In this case, for example, the minimal symptoms of an existing depressive disorder may become considerably worse because of the additional somatic disease, and thus more serious adjustment disorders, depressive disorders, hypochondrias, anxiety disorders, sociophobias, compulsive disorders, or somatoform disorders may become manifest. It should be noted here that clear separation between secondary emotional disorders and already existing emotional disorders may not always be possible.

Comorbidities in Psychosomatic Dermatology

- Depressive disorders/hypochondrias
- Anxiety disorders/sociophobias
- Compulsive disorders
- Adjustment disorders
- Somatoform disorders

Somatoform disorders are discussed in detail in Sect. 1.3 and are therefore mentioned only briefly here.

3.3.1 Depressive Disorders

Patients with depressive disorders in dermatology present with increased itching, neurotic excoriations, suicidal thoughts, and hypochondriacal concepts about the skin disease.

Pathogenesis. There are various biomedicinal and psychosomatic concepts about the pathogenesis that indicate a multifactorial causality.

Genetic aspects are in the foreground of an inherited depressive disorder (endogenous depression). Transmitter/hormone and serotonin receptors in the synaptic cleft also appear to play a decisive role. The traditional differentiation between neurosis and psychosis has largely been omitted in the ICD-10 and replaced by the term "disorder." Affective disorders are viewed as transitions of depressive disorders of various degrees, a view that is supported, for example, by the fact that psychopharmaceuticals with antipsychotic effects may show good efficacy in depressions that were formerly classified as neurotic.

Classification and definition. The spectrum of depression ranges from mild, brief moods, such as normal reactions to grief (on the death of a partner, for example) up to the most severe psychotic disorders.

The concept of division into neurosis and psychosis was abandoned in favor of classification by severity because of the often fluent transition. The current classification comprises the disorders presented in Table 3.1.

Table 3.1 Overview of affective disorders, ICD-10: F3

ICD-10	Type of disorder
F30	Manic episode
F31	Bipolar affective disorder
F32	Depressive episode
F32.0	Mild depressive episode
F32.1	Moderate depressive episode
F32.2	Severe depressive episode
F33	Recurrent depressive disorders
	Seasonal affective disorders
F34	Persistent affective disorders
F34.0	Cyclothymia
F34.1	Dysthymia

Frequency. Depressions are common emotional disorders in the population, with a prevalence of 2–7%. The estimated incidence (new cases per year) for diagnosis of a depressive episode is one or two new disorders per 100 persons.

The probability of suffering depression during one's lifetime is up to 12% for men and up to 26% for women. Patients with depression present a high rate of comorbidities (75–90%).

Clinical presentation. Depressive disorders or episodes (ICD-10: F32) are a therapeutic problem in the dermatological practice, especially in combination with hypochondriacal somatoform disorders and somatized depression (Fig. 3.6).

In the specialty of dermatology, the following skin diseases in particular are characteristically often associated with depressive disorders.

Skin Diseases Frequently Associated with Depression

- Chronic recurrent urticaria
- Alopecia areata
- Psoriasis
- Acne vulgaris
- Pruritus/prurigo diseases

Moreover, in the case of multifactorial diseases there are coping difficulties that often have no correlation between the degree of depression and the severity of the clinical presentation, for example, in acne.

Emotional symptoms. Depressive disorders are characterized by main symptoms, common symptoms, and additionally by a characteristic (multiorganic) "somatic syndrome."

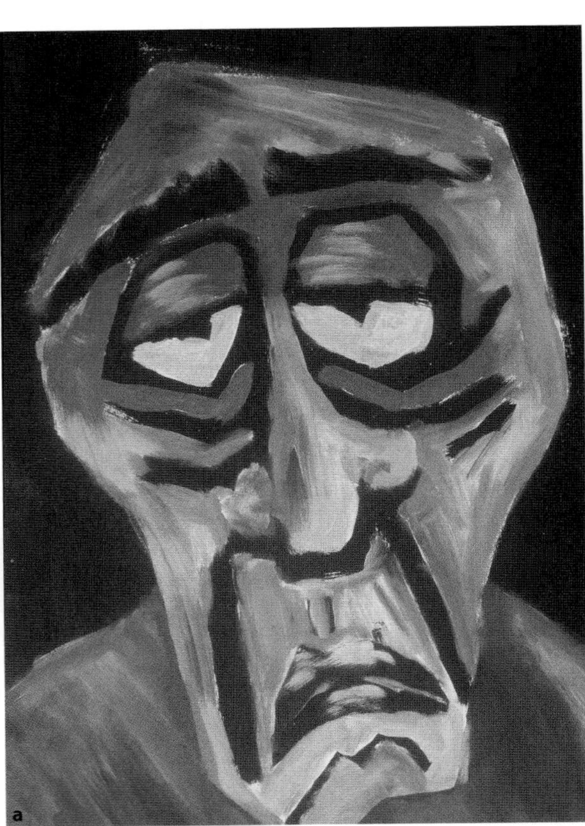

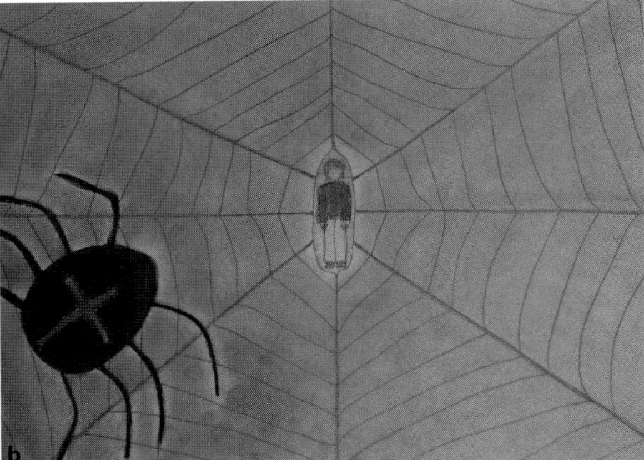

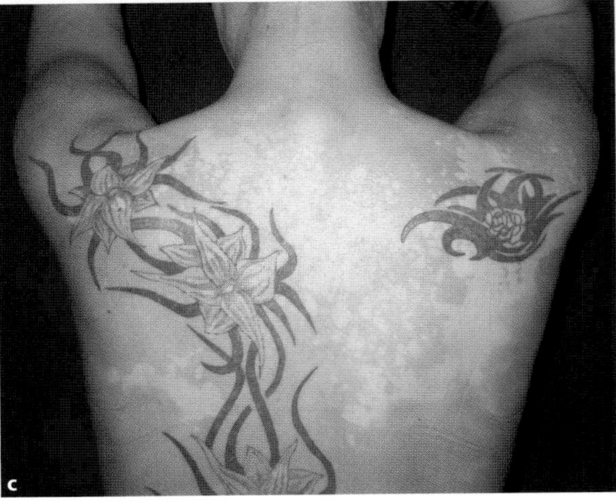

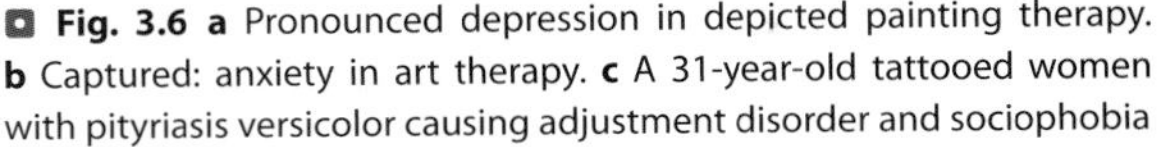

Fig. 3.6 a Pronounced depression in depicted painting therapy. **b** Captured: anxiety in art therapy. **c** A 31-year-old tattooed women with pityriasis versicolor causing adjustment disorder and sociophobia

In particular, the somatic substitution symptoms of the depression lead the patient to consulting a doctor to clarify a presumed serious disease.

Diagnostic Criteria of Depression (ICD10: F32)

- Main symptoms
  1. Depressive mood (unlike sadness)
  2. Loss of interest and enjoyment
  3. Reduced energy/increased fatigability/diminished activity
- Common symptoms
  1. Reduced concentration and attention
  2. Reduced self-esteem and self-confidence
  3. Ideas of guilt and unworthiness
  4. Bleak and pessimistic views of the future
  5. Ideas or acts of self-harm or suicide
  6. Disturbed sleep
  7. Diminished appetite

Some of the above characteristics may lead to a somatic syndrome, which is diagnostically important for the physician.

- Somatic syndrome
  - Loss of interest
  - Lack of emotional reactivity
  - Waking in the morning/depression in the morning
  - Marked loss of appetite
  - Weight loss
  - Marked loss of libido

Depressive moods, loss of interest, and reduced energy with often increased tiredness and limitation of activities are in the foreground of the affective disorders. Marked fatigue often occurs after only slight efforts. Suicidal thoughts are characteristic of serious depressive disorders, and the dermatologist should pay increased attention to them. Moreover, self-injuries and suicidal acts may be seen (Chap. 10).

Impairment of general well-being; gastrointestinal complaints, especially impaired appetite; insomnia; loss of libido; and increased pain are among the typical physical symptoms.

The classification of severity depends on the number of symptoms present (Table 3.2).

Persistent Affective Disorders

Patients with persistent mood disorders comprise one of the main disease groups in medicine in general and also in dermatology. Among the persistent affective disorders, the current classifications differentiate and specify (F34) the following:

- Cyclothymia (F34.0): persistent mood instability with numerous episodes of milder depression alternating with elevated moods
- Dysthymia (F34.1): chronic, persistent, mild depressive mood

For medicine in general, including dermatology, persistent dysthymia is of clinical relevance because it is often associated as a comorbidity with difficulties in treatment and coping.

Dysthymia

The essential characteristic of the dysthymic disorder (ICD-10: F34.1) is long-lasting depressive mood. Moreover, there is a loss of interest or loss of enjoyment of normally pleasant activities, as well as a lack of ability to react emotionally to them. For the specific subgroup of depression, refer to more detailed specialized textbooks and the ICD-10.

Differential diagnosis. Depressions have a high rate of comorbidities (75–90%). The occurrence is often concurrent with anxiety disorders, such as social anxiety,

Table 3.2 Severity of depression (depressive episodes)

Severity	Number of symptoms	ICD-10
Mild	Two main symptoms and two additional symptoms	ICD-10: F32.0
Moderate	Two main symptoms and three or four additional symptoms	ICD-10: F32.1
Severe	Three main symptoms and four or more additional symptoms	ICD-10: F32.2

panic disorders, generalized anxiety disorders and compulsive symptoms, eating disorders, substance abuse, insomnias, sexual disorders, somatoform disorders, and personality disorders.

In the case of these comorbid disorders, the question of whether the depression is primary or only secondary as a consequence of the other diseases can rarely be reliably answered. Classification is often made more difficult by the patient's subjective theory of disease. This applies especially to the affective disorders, for which the diagnostic criteria also include somatic criteria.

The need for therapy for a clinically relevant depressive disorder, however, is given for both primary and secondary genesis.

Furthermore, serious depressive disorders may be associated with psychotic symptoms. Among these are delusions and hallucinations and also depressive stupor, which makes the involvement of a specialist in psychiatry urgently necessary.

Further Reading

Böhme H, Finke J, Teusch L (1998) Effekte stationärer Gesprächspsychotherapie bei verschiedenen Krankheitsbildern: 1-Jahres-Katamnese. Psychother Psychosom Med Psychol 48: 20–29

Franz M, Janssen P, Lensche H, Schmidtke V, Tetzlaff M, Martin K, Woller W, Hartkamp N, Schneider G, Heuft G (2000) Effekte stationärer psychoanalytische orientierter Psychotherapie – eine Multicenterstudie. Z Psychosom Med Psychother 46(3): 242–258

Hautzinger M, Jong-Meyer R de (1996) Depression (Themenheft). Z Klin Psychol 25: 79–160

Gupta MA, Gupta AK (1998) Depression and suicidal ideation in dermatology patients with acne, alopecia areata, atopic dermatitis and psoriasis. Br J Dermatol 139: 846–850

Gupta MA, Gupta AK, Schork NJ, Ellis CN (1994) Depression modulates pruritus perception: a study of pruritus in psoriasis, atopic dermatitis, and chronic idiopathic urticaria. Psychosom Med 56: 36–40

Hashiro M, Okumura M (1997) Anxiety, depression and psychosomatic symptoms in patients with atopic dermatitis: comparison with normal controls and among groups of different degrees of severity. J Dermatol Sci 14: 63–67

Sandell R, Blomberg J, Lazar A, Carlsson J, Broberg J, Schubert J (2001) Unterschiedliche Langzeitergebnisse von Psychoanalysen und Psychotherapien. Aus der Forschung des Stockholmer Psychoanalyse- und Psychotherapieprojekts. Psyche 55: 270–310

Shuster S (1991) Depression of self-image by skin. Acta Derm Venereol Suppl (Stockh) 156: 53

Special Form: Season-Dependent Depression

One special form is seasonal affective disorder (SAD), which occurs with dependence on the time of year, mainly in the winter months. The diagnosis of SAD: seasonal affective depression (ICD-10:F33) has been defined, with the following diagnostic criteria (Kasper et al. 1988):

Diagnostic Criteria: Seasonal Affective Disorder (SAD)

- Depressive episodes in at least 2 consecutive years in the fall/winter with a mostly symptom-free or manic/hypomanic state in spring/summer.
- The following minor symptoms are characteristic but not obligatory:
  - Lack of energy
  - Increased need to sleep
  - Prolonged, nonregenerating sleep
  - Morning tiredness
  - Craving for carbohydrates
  - Increased appetite
  - Weight gain

Reference

Kasper S, Wehr TA, Rosenthal NE (1988) Saisonal abhängige Depressionsformen (SAD). Nervenarzt 59: 200–214

Further Reading

Meesters Y, Beersma DG, Bouhuys AL, Hoofdakker RH van den (1999) Prophylactic treatment of seasonal affective disorder (SAD) by using light visors: bright white or infrared light? Biol Psychiatry 46: 239–246

Partonen T, Lonnqvist J (1998) Seasonal affective disorder. Lancet 352: 1369–1374

Mixed Disorders/New Syndromes (Sisi Syndrome)

Depressive disorders and anxiety disorders are often found in combination, and they may partly be potentiated by cultural and social factors in western industrial countries.

This becomes clear by the description and inauguration of new, culture-dependent syndromes such as "Sisi syndrome." According to some authors, the diagnosis of a Sisi syndrome, launched by the media and the pharmaceutical industry, is not scientifically justified because of the lack of studies.

The name of the Sisi syndrome refers to the Austrian Empress Elisabeth. "Sisi" combated her depressions by engaging continuously in sports, maintaining a strict diet, and traveling. At the age of 25, the young woman often fled and traveled restlessly throughout the world. At a time when men preferred voluptuous forms, Sisi did everything she could to remain as thin as possible – finally, she weighed only 45 kg, although she was 1.72 m tall.

According to some authors, nearly one-third of all depressive disorders (dysthymias) can be ascribed to the "Sisi type." Patients in this subgroup are often restless and impulsively active. Sisi is the prototype of a patient who attempts to flee inner emptiness by means of feveris activity, extreme physical training, travel activities, search for meaning of life, pronounced beauty rituals, or strict diets. Characteristically, the patients have anxiety symptoms and disorders of affectivity, impulse, sleep, and eating behavior.

3.3.2 Anxiety Disorders

Anxiety is a state of worry and nervousness occurring in a variety of mental disorders, usually accompanied by physical symptoms. Anxiety disorders are especially found in conjunction with the skin diseases listed in the following overview.

Skin Diseases Frequently Associated with Anxiety Disorders

- Atopic dermatitis
- Nummular eczema
- Dyshidrosiform eczema
- Seborrheic dermatitis
- Acne vulgaris
- Rosacea
- Recurrent herpes simplex
- Metastasizing tumor diseases
- Allergological diseases

Classification. Anxiety disorders are basically differentiated into acute panic disorders, chronic persistent anxiety, and specific phobias (Table 3.3, Fig. 3.6 b,c).

Nonspecific diffuse anxiety disorders are not limited to a certain environmental situation. Differentiation is made between persistent fear (generalized anxiety disorder) and acute fear (panic), which may play a decisive role in allergic reactions in emergency care, as in undifferentiated somatoform idiopathic anaphylaxis (Sect. 4.1).

Another important position in dermatology is occupied by social phobias, also because of the visual exposure of a dermatosis or the resultant stigmatization. Social phobias are characteristically associated with pronounced avoidance behavior and social withdrawal.

Specific phobias refer to special situations (visit to the doctor, crowds of people) or objects (for example, arachnids).

Panic Disorders

Panic disorder (ICD-10: F41.0) is a clearly limited episode with intensive fear or discomfort in which sudden palpitations, a feeling of suffocation, chest pain, and dizziness occur. The essential characteristic is recurrent fear attacks (panic), which need not be limited to specific situations.

At least four of the following symptoms must occur abruptly and peak within 10 min.

Panic Disorder Symptoms

- Palpitations, pounding heart, or accelerated heart rate
- Sweating
- Tremors or shaking
- Feeling of shortness of breath or respiratory distress
- Feeling of suffocation
- Pains and feeling of tightness in the chest
- Nausea or gastrointestinal complaints
- Dizziness, insecurity, giddiness, or feeling close to fainting
- Derealization (feeling of unreality)
- Depersonalization (feeling of dissolution)
- Fear of losing control
- Fear of dying
- Paresthesias, numbness, or tingling
- Hot flashes or waves of coldness

Acute fear (panic) plays a decisive role in the practice in pseudoallergic reactions (Chap. 4).

Generalized Anxiety Disorders

Generalized anxiety (ICD-10: F41.1) is characterized by excessive fear and worry or fearful expectations that do not relate to a specific situation or object. It is a so-called

3

Table 3.3 Classification of anxiety disorders, ICD-10: F4

ICD-10	Type of disorder
F41.0	Panic disorder (acute fear)
F41.1	Generalized anxiety disorder (chronic persistent fear)
F41.2	Anxiety and depressive disorder mixed
F40.1	Social phobia
F40.2	Specific phobia
	Special eliciting situations
	Fear of objects
	Special form: iatrogenic phobia

free-floating fear that occurs on most days over a period of at least 6 months. The person has difficulty controlling the worries.

Definition. Anxiety and worry are characterized by fears, motor tension, and vegetative hyperexcitability, and at least three of the following six symptoms must have been present on most days during the preceding 6 months.

Anxiety Symptoms

- Restlessness or constant "readiness"
- Easily tired
- Difficulty concentrating
- Irritability
- Muscular tension
- Insomnia

Mixed Disorders

Phobias often occur not only monosymptomatically but in association with other disorders. Most frequently, there is a combination and interaction of anxiety and depressive disorders (ICD-10: F41.2). Elucidation of adjustment disorders is especially important in this connection.

Social Phobias

Social phobias (ICD-10: F40.1) are frequently encountered in dermatology and are associated with a pronounced avoidance behavior, especially when coupled with stigmatization. Proximity and distance conflicts are often apparent in patients with atopic dermatitis, psoriasis, and somatoform disorders (especially body dysmorphic disorder) and may develop into social phobias.

Social phobias often begin in youth and are centered around the fear of being closely observed by other individuals or groups. Social phobias are usually coupled with low self-esteem and fear of criticism. Direct eye contact is often very difficult for the affected patients.

The clinical symptoms of a social phobia are blushing, trembling hands, hyperhidrosis, nausea, and urinary urge. They finally lead to avoidance of certain social situations. In extreme cases, there is danger of psychosocial isolation and chronically impaired contact and relationships. Social phobias usually do not occur in isolation but within the group of depressive disorders.

Special Forms

Iatrogenic Fear

Specific phobias are characterized by clearly defined objects or situations, including fear of institutions (hospitals, dental practices) or medical treatments (operations, injections). The phobia may be fixated on the medical area and lead to pronounced avoidance behavior or rejection of necessary therapies, whereby required medical treatment is not performed. Differential diagnosis must rule out fear of illness (nosophobia), fear of disfiguration due to the intervention, and also, in individual cases, hypochondriacal disorders.

Further Reading

Charman C, Williams H (2003) The use of corticosteroids and corticosteroid phobia in atopic dermatitis. Clin Dermatol 21(3): 193–200

Patterson R, Walker CL, Greenberger PA, Sheridan EP (1989) Prednisonephobia. Allergy Proc 10(6): 423–428

Patterson R, Greenberger PA, Patterson DR (1991) Potentially fatal asthma: the problem of noncompliance. Ann Allergy 67(2 Pt 1): 138–142

3.3.3 Compulsive Disorders

The groups of compulsive disorders (ICD-10: F42) comprise disorders with predominant compulsive thoughts (ICD-10: F42.0) or compulsive acts (ICD-10: F42.1), which may also occur in various combinations (ICD-10: F42.2) (Table 3.4).

Compulsive thoughts are recurrent and persistent thoughts, impulses, or fantasies that are experienced as intrusive and inappropriate and which elicit pronounced fear and great discomfort.

Compulsive acts are repeated behaviors (such as hand washing or controlling the order of objects) or ideate acts (such as praying, counting, or repeating words) to which the person feels compelled as a reaction to a compulsive thought or because of rules that must be strictly followed. One characteristic dermatosis here is hand eczema secondary to repeated washing. The clinical diseases are presented in detail in Sect. 1.4.

These behaviors serve to prevent malaise or to reduce or avert feared events and situations, but they are in no realistic relationship to that which they attempt to neutralize or prevent.

A compulsive disorder is often present in body dysmorphic disorders whereby the patient spends hours in front of the mirror to control or influence his or her outward appearance. The similarity to depression and anxiety disorder is significant.

3.3.4 Stress and Adjustment Disorders

More or less serious stress and life events may elicit skin diseases such as acute urticaria or may lead to attacks and deterioration of chronic dermatoses (such as atopic dermatitis and psoriasis).

Table 3.4 Classification of compulsive disorders, ICD-10: F42

ICD-10	Type of disorder
F42	Compulsive disorders
F42.0	Compulsive thoughts
F42.1	Compulsive acts
F42.2	Mixed disorders

On the other hand, skin diseases themselves are stressful and may elicit emotional disorders (adjustment disorders).

Differentiation is made between acute stress disorders, posttraumatic stress disorders, and the group of adjustment disorders, for example, as a result of dermatoses (Table 3.5).

Adjustment disorders are observed especially often in dermatology.

Adjustment Disorders

Adjustment disorders (ICD-10: F43.2) occur after drastic life changes or stressful life events, as well as after serious physical disease. There is subjective suffering and emotional detriment, which hinder social functioning and performance. Adjustment disorders occur when a partner dies or there is death in the immediate family or an experience of separation. They are characterized by anxiety, depression, and social withdrawal.

! In dermatology, the following central mechanism and relationships can repeatedly be observed: illness – adjustment disorder – anxiety – depression – social withdrawal.

The emotional presentation of adjustment disorders is heterogeneous and characterized by brief depressive reactions (F43.20), longer depressive reactions (F43.21), and anxiety and depressive reactions as mixed symptomatics (F43.22).

Moreover, there are disorders of social behavior and disorders of emotional life. In dermatology, problems of coping and compliance also often play a decisive role (Fig. 3.6c).

Table 3.5 Classification of reaction to severe stress and adjustment disorders, ICD-10: F43

ICD-10	Type of disorder
F43.0	Acute stress reaction
F43.1	Posttraumatic stress disorder
F43.2	Adjustment disorders
F43.20	Brief depressive reaction
F43.21	Longer depressive reaction
F43.22	Anxiety and depressive reaction

A prerequisite is an individual disposition or vulnerability for the occurrence of adjustment disorders. Acute stress reactions (F43.0) and posttraumatic stress disorders (F43.1) occur without the necessity of predisposition.

Acute Stress Reactions/Posttraumatic Stress Disorder

The acute stress reaction shows considerable severity in immediate temporal sequence to traumatization (accident, crime, rape). The symptoms usually abate after a short period.

! Characteristics of acute stress reaction are shock, numbness, limitation of consciousness, disorientation, inability to process stimuli, depression, withdrawal or fear, and hyperreactivity in alternating degrees.

A protracted and delayed reaction to trauma defines the long-term sequelae in the sense of posttraumatic stress disorder.

! Typical signs of posttraumatic disorder are repeated experiencing of the trauma in incursive memories, emotional withdrawal, apathy, avoidance, deadening of feelings, or/and dramatic acute eruptions of aggression, rage, fear, or panic.

As an example, this problem of traumatization and the long-term consequences, which has received little attention to date, is discussed in connection with sexual abuse in Chap. 11.

Further Reading

Seikowski K, Gollek S (1999) Belastende Lebensereignisse bei hautkranken Personen. Z Dermatol 185: 56–61

3.3.5 Dissociative Disorders

Dissociative disorders describe the inner turmoil of relational consciousness and the breakdown and displacement of experience content, including the emotional origin of physical symptoms. Charcot (1825 to 1893) demonstrated very early in France the symbolic importance of fainting in hysteria. Freud later coined the historical term conversion hysteria. The outmoded terms hysteria and conversion neurosis have been incorporated into the current definition of the term dissociative disorder.

Definition. Dissociative (or conversion) disorders (ICD-10: F44) are characterized by a partial or complete loss of the normal integration among memories of the past, awareness of identity, immediate sensations, and control of bodily functions.

! In dissociative disorders, there is impairment of integration with partial or complete *decoupling* (dissociation) of *emotional and physical functions.*

Dissociative disorders may play a decisive role in numerous diseases in dermatology.

Dermatoses in Which Dissociative Disorders May Be Present

- Artefacts
- Urticaria
- Acute pruritus
- Anesthetic skin areas (ICD-10: F44.6)
- Pseudoallergic reactions

Patients with dissociative disorders are not aware of the relationship between their skin disease and emotional causes due to the decoupling of skin and psyche. Even a minimal expression of a dissociative disorder can be important if the dermatologist thematizes a connection between an emotional cause and a dermatosis with the patient, who strictly denies it (patient quote: “I'm not crazy”).

This phenomenon can be explained by splitting off as a central defense mechanism of the dissociative disorder. Separation phenomena occur as a protective mechanism, usually in the framework of severe traumatization. The body is emotionally decoupled and numb during abuse in order to achieve overall emotional stabilization, whereby stressful feelings are faded out.

! Dissociative disorders comprise fading out of stressful feelings.

If in certain situations, such as a presumed physical disease, this cleaving mechanism is reactivated as a defense mechanism, the patient cannot recognize the unconscious, psychosomatic relationships of his or her skin disease. Patients often appear to be hardly involved emotionally, or are present with rapidly changing moods.

A classic example of maximum split between body and psyche in dermatology is the group of patients with artefacts. The dissociative amnesia in unconscious, self-caused artefacts is of decisive importance: The patient, because of the separation, often cannot remember the self-manipulation and does not feel pain during the manipulation. A confrontation is usually useless or even contraindicated due to the amnesia.

Conversion disorders may also be signs of a dissociative disorder, whereby unbearable and unresolved conflicts are expressed symbolically by physical symptoms. Conversion is a mechanism by which emotional conflicts are transposed (converted) to physical symptoms. The recordable physical symptoms are usually a brief means of emotional relief and stabilization for the patient. Hysterical fainting, paralysis, or deafness is characteristic of conversion disorders. The symbolic importance of the minimal forms, which are more common today, are not usually taken as lightly as the "arc-de-cercle" (opisthotonus, catatonia). In this connection, it should be discussed whether the somatoform disorders have replaced the classic symptoms noted in the 19th century.

Examples of conversion disorders in dermatology can be found in acute psychogenic-elicited urticaria, genital pruritus, pseudoallergic reactions, and anesthetic skin areas (ICD-10: F44.6; Fig. 3.7). Dissociative sensibility and sensitivity disorders may comprise different losses of various sensory modalities where no neurological disease is present; the anesthetic skin areas correspond to the patient's understanding of body functions.

An experienced dermatologist often has the impression that the skin changes have symbolic meaning as representatives of conflicts, which the patient expresses nonverbally. The symptom unconsciously expresses the patient's fantasy, and the dermatosis takes on a sensual expressive content.

Overall, the initial motivation of patients with a dissociative disorder for psychotherapy is usually very low compared with patients with other disorders. Persuasiveness and a lot of patience, as well as a stable doctor–patient relationship, are prerequisites for motivation for an indicated psychotherapy.

3.3.6 Personality Disorders

Personality disorders may occur as comorbidities with other dermatological diseases. Often, both the emotional disorder and the skin disease are difficult to treat. We refer the reader to appropriate textbooks and classification systems for the detailed diagnostics, differential diagnosis, and treatment of personality disorders (ICD-10).

Borderline disorders (emotionally unstable personality disorders) have been gaining in importance in recent years and are presented here.

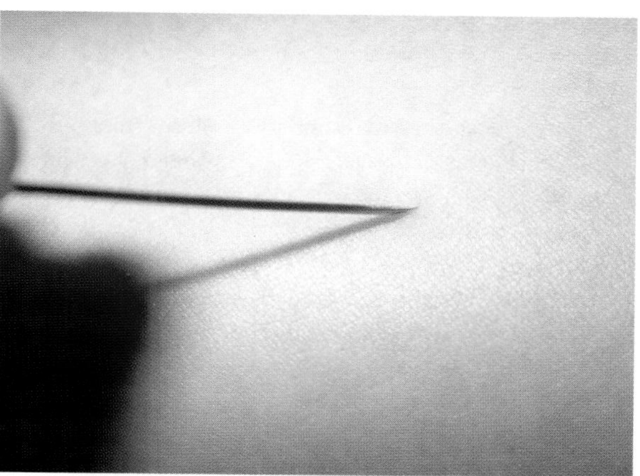

Fig. 3.7 Woman with skin anesthesia in dissociative disorder

Emotionally Unstable Personality Disorders (Borderline Disorders)

A steady increase in the frequency of patients with emotionally unstable personality disorders (ICD-10: F 60.3 borderline disorders) has been determined in recent years.

Occurrence/prevalence. Borderline disorders have a prevalence of 1.6–1.8% of the population. Women are predominantly affected. Patients tend to be city dwellers. The suicide rate is high, and 75% of borderline patients attempt suicide.

Definition. The main presentation of borderline personality disorders is a deep instability in interpersonal relationships and in self-image and affect, often with intensive impulsiveness. The borderline disorder occurs frequently with affective disorders.

Diagnostics. These severe personality disorders are among the greatest diagnostic and therapeutic challenges in psychosomatic dermatology. The skin, as a border organ, plays an important and often symbolic role.

The dermatologist sees patients with borderline disorders because of skin lesions from self-injury or self-manipulation, which are one diagnostic criterion of the disorder.

3

Diagnostic Criteria for Borderline Disorders (DSM-IV)

A pervasive pattern of instability of interpersonal relationships, self-image, and affects, and marked impulsivity beginning by early adulthood and present in a variety of contexts, as indicated by five (or more) of the following:

1. Frantic efforts to avoid real or imagined abandonment. **Note:** Do not include suicidal or self-mutilating behavior covered in criterion 5.
2. A pattern of unstable and intense interpersonal relationships characterized by alternations between extremes of idealization and devaluation
3. Identity disturbance: markedly and persistently unstable self-image or sense of self
4. Impulsivity in at least two areas that are potentially self-damaging (e.g., spending, sex, substance abuse, reckless driving, binge eating). **Note:** Do not include suicidal or self-mutilating behavior covered in criterion 5.
5. Recurrent suicidal behavior, gestures, or threats, or self-mutilating behavior
6. Affective instability due to a marked reactivity of mood (e.g., intense episodic dysphoria, irritability, or anxiety usually lasting a few hours and only rarely more than a few days)
7. Chronic feelings of emptiness
8. Inappropriate, intense anger or difficulty controlling anger (e.g., frequent displays of temper, constant anger, recurrent physical fights)
9. Transient, stress-related paranoid ideation or severe dissociative symptoms

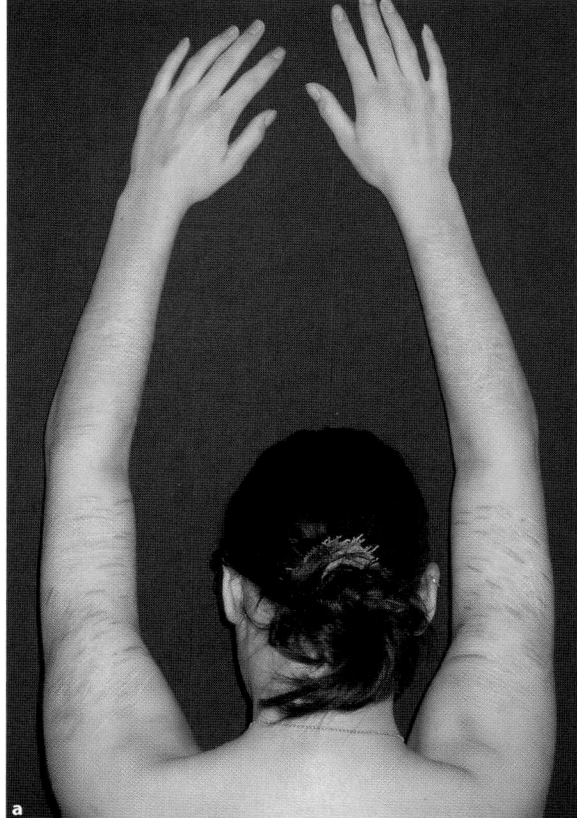

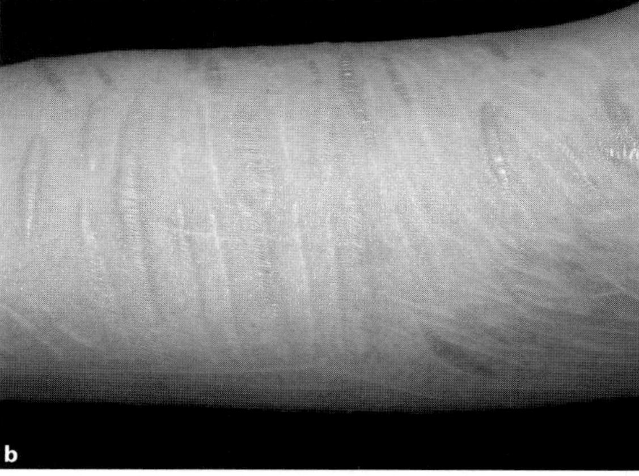

Fig. 3.8a–c Borderline personality disorder. **a** Cutting. **b** Close-up.

Clinical findings. The skin changes are typically artefacts caused by the patient by conscious or unconscious scratching, scouring, or rubbing, or are paraartefacts based on a preexisting dermatosis. Skin artefacts are one of the diagnostic criteria of borderline disorders (Fig. 3.8a–c).

Emotional symptoms. Emotionally, there is a broad and diverse spectrum, with a dominance of restlessness, feelings of being driven, eruptions of rage, impulsiveness, problems on the job, inner emptiness, rage at oneself, and problems in the spousal relationship (Figs. 3.9, 3.10).

Moreover, there are phobias, free-floating fear, compulsive symptoms, conversion symptoms, dissociative reactions, depression, impaired sexuality, loss of impulse control, impaired social behavior, delinquency and suicidal tendency, as well as other psychosomatic or even psychotic symptoms.

Typical splitting phenomena dominate in the defense mechanism spectrum and often include the treatment

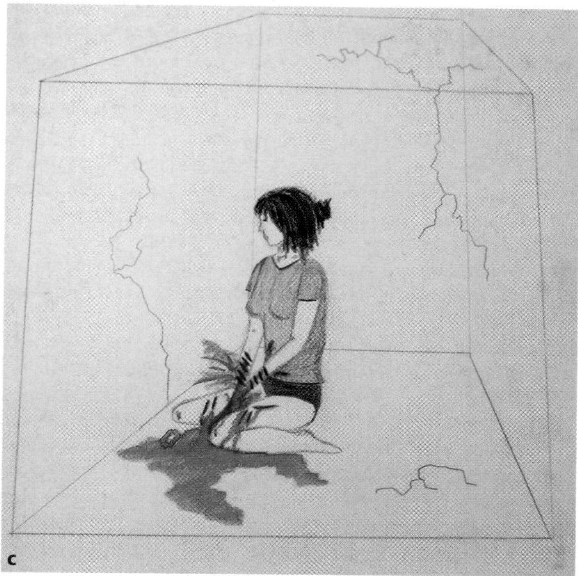

Fig. 3.8a–c *(continued)* **c** Clinical picture of self-inflicted injuries in art therapy

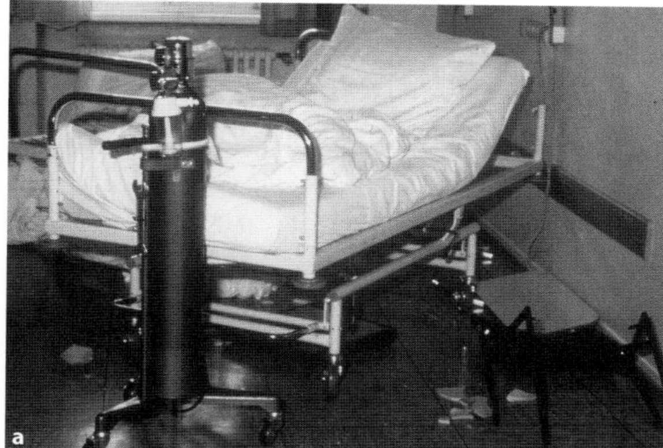

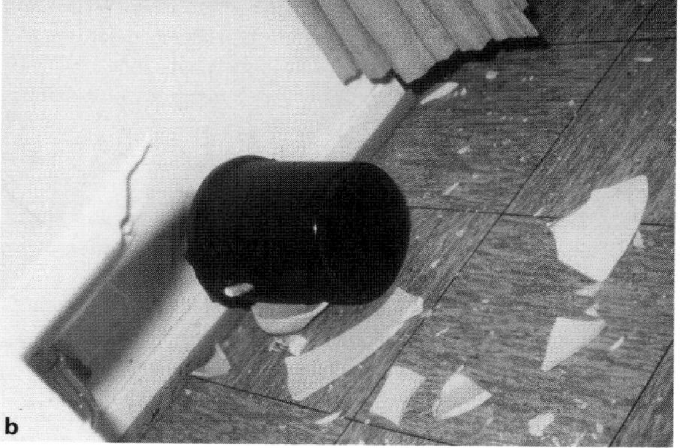

Fig. 3.9a,b Destroyed hospital room of an unstable 36-year-old woman with borderline syndrome; rage episode after emotional mood swing because the ward team set a limit (limited leave)

team. Other characteristic defense mechanisms are a primitive idealization, identification with the aggressor, projective identification, feelings of omnipotence/devaluation, and denial.

Differential diagnosis. Other serious personality disorders and psychiatric diseases, especially paranoid psychoses, must be ruled out in the differential diagnosis of patients with borderline disorders.

Psychotherapy. Due to the severity of the symptoms, hospitalization is needed in 20% of patients with borderline disorders. For the dermatologist, it is important to recognize the disorder, especially in the context of self-injury, and to involve an appropriate specialist as early as possible.

Psychotherapeutic approaches initially comprise a holding function phase depending on the patient's possibilities. In the second phase of external structuring, limits and structures are increasingly set while maintaining the holding function, and integration of "good" and "bad" components is promoted.

In the third phase of beginning inner structuring, there is improved access to the emotions. Accompanying drawing therapy, trauma work, and relaxation procedures have proven useful.

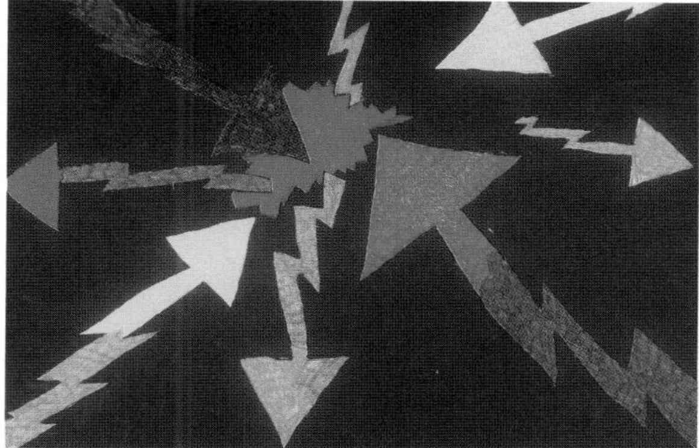

Fig. 3.10 Painting by the same patient as in Fig. 3.9, with emotionally unstable personality disorder and rapid mood swings. Undirected, sometimes colliding bolts of lightning are shown in painting therapy

We refer the reader to pertinent monographs and textbooks on psychiatry and psychotherapy for the special therapeutic concepts.

Psychopharmaceuticals. A combination therapy of psychotherapy with neuroleptics is usually required.

Further Reading

American Psychiatric Association (1994) Diagnostic and statistical manual of mental disorders, 4th edn. American Psychiatric Association, Washington, DC

Bohus M, Limberger M, Ebner U, Glockner FX, Schwarz B, Wernz M, Lieb K (2000) Pain perception during self reported distress and calmness in patients with borderline personality disorders and self mutilating behavior. Psychiatry Res 11: 251–260

Gunderson JG, Kolb JE (1978) Discriminating features of borderline-patients. Am J Psychiatry 135: 792–794

Kernberg O (1967) Borderline personality organization. J Am Psychoanal Assoc 15: 641–685

Harth W, Linse R (2000) Dermatological symptoms and sexual abuse: a review and case reports. J Eur Acad Dermatol Venereol 14: 489–494

Herman JL, Perry JC, Kolk BA van der (1989) Childhood trauma in borderline personality disorder. Am J Psychiatry 146: 490–495

Koblenzer CS (2000) Dermatitis artefacta. Clinical features and approaches to treatment. Am J Clin Dermatol 1: 47–55

Moffaert MM van (2003) The spectrum of dermatological self-mutilation and self destruction including dermatitis artefacta and neurotic excoriations. In: Koo JMY, Lee CS (eds) Psychocutaneus medicine. Dekker, New York, pp 169–189

Rinne T, Kloet ER de, Wouters L, Goekoop JG, Rijk RH de, Brink W van (2003) Fluvoxamine reduces responsiveness of HPA axis in adult female BPD patients with a history of sustained childhood abuse. Neuropsychopharmacology 28: 126–132

Rocca P, Marchiaro L, Cocuzza E, Bogetto F (2002) Treatment of borderline personality disorder with risperidon. J Clin Psychiatry 63: 241–244

Rothenhäusler HB, Kapfhammer HP (1999) Outcome in borderline disorder. A literature review. Fortsch Neurol Psychiatr 67: 200–217

Sass H, Koehler K (1983) Borderline syndromes: borderline area or no-man's land? On the clinico-psychiatric relevance of borderline diagnoses. Nervenarzt 54(5) 221–230

Schindler W (1979) Das Borderline Syndrom – ein Zeichen unserer Zeit. Z Psychosom Med Psychoanal 25(4): 363–375

Zanarini MC, Yong L, Frankenburg FR, Hennen J, Reich DB, Marino MF, Vujanovic AA (2002) Severity of reported childhood sexual abuse and its relationship to severity of borderline psychopathology and psychosocial impairment among borderline inpatients. J Nerv Ment Dis 190: 381–387

Part III

Special Focal Points in Dermatology

In the specialist discipline of dermatology are further subspecialties, some of which have additional recognized titles or organizations within special professional societies and which are associated with characteristic traits from a psychosocial point of view.

Allergology

4

Psychosomatic disorders play an important role in allergology. The practical importance is seen, for example, in patients with pseudoallergies with intolerances to foods, medications, and insect bites, as well as in special forms of urticaria. Moreover, there may be potentiating effects of emotional comorbidities and impairment of coping.

Pathogenesis and differential diagnosis. Differentiation between real allergies and pseudoallergies is one of the central psychosomatic problems (Table 4.1).

Real allergies are characterized by immunological interactions according to the basic definition and classification of Gell and Coombs (1963).

In *pseudoallergies,* no immune-mediated reactions occur, but rather intolerance reactions or somatoform disorders as the cause.

In intolerance reactions, the symptoms are comparable to a real allergy, but there is no proof of a specific IgE-mediated or cellular-mediated reproducible allergic reaction. Predisposing factors may be histamine intolerance or dermographism (urticaria factitia in the European literature).

Table 4.1 Differential diagnostics of allergy

Diagnosis	Cause
Allergy	Immune-mediated
Pseudoallergy	1. Intolerance (multifactorial)
	2. Somatoform disorder (psychogenic)

By contrast, the somatoform disorders are purely emotionally caused disorders, with repeated presentation of physical symptoms despite repeated negative test results and the doctor's assurance that the symptoms cannot be physically explained.

Classification and clinical findings. Due to the various pathogenesis (antibodies, T cells) of allergic diseases, differentiation is possible between immediate reactions and delayed reactions from both a somatic and a psychosomatic point of view (Table 4.2).

Nothing is yet known from a psychosomatic point of view about type VI allergies with specific antigen–antibody reactions in rare autoimmune diseases.

Emotional symptoms (general). Patterns of relationship and interactions with other people have repeatedly been described that are supposedly typical of allergy patients.

Learning-conditioning models. Learning-conditioning models have practical relevance, and detailed studies are available on this. In a basic animal experimental study of classical conditioning, Ader and Cohen (1982) demonstrated that immunological suppression elicited by concurrent cyclophosphamide injection and drinking of saccharin solutions was later elicited also by only drinking saccharin solutions. This remains one of the fundamental experiments on classical (Pavlovian) conditioning of the immune system. Since their seminal study, hundreds of reports have supported these findings, showing that classical conditioning can mediate significant immune suppression.

In 1989, MacQueen et al. achieved a specific increase in mast cell activity by means of classical conditioning.

Table 4.2 Psychosomatic allergology (*AD* atopic dermatitis)

Gell and Coombs classification	Clinical symptoms	Psychosomatic relevance
Type I: IgE-mediated allergic immediate reaction	Pruritus, urticaria, asthma, shock, rhinoconjunctivitis	Anxiety and panic disorder, emotional triggering
Type II: Cytotoxic reaction	Tumor defense, Transplant rejection, thrombopenic purpura	Not confirmed (Gardner–Diamond syndrome in framework of artefacts possible)
Type III: Immune complex reaction	Vasculitis, drug exanthema	Not confirmed, possible in framework of artefacts
Type IV: Cellular allergy, delayed type hypersensitivity	Contact dermatitis, eczematous diseases, AD?	Emotional triggering of eczematous diseases and multifactorial dermatoses: acute episodes of AD, some forms of dyshidrotic eczema
Type V: Granulomatous allergy of delayed type	Granuloma, foreign body reactions	Delayed granulomatous sensitivity reactions that may occur, for example, after artificial injection of foreign body materials

Audiovisual stimuli served as the conditioning stimulus, after which there was significant release of mast cell enzymes.

Russell et al. (1984) showed that histamine can be released as a learned classical conditioning paradigm when associated with odor as a conditioned stimulus.

Scholz (1995) demonstrated that the histamine reaction following a prick test was greater in patients with atopic dermatitis who received dramatizing instructions than that in a control group with soothing instructions.

It thus appears that the allergic reaction can be influenced both by classical conditioning and by eliciting expectation.

Psychodynamic concepts. No typical personality structure has yet been proven in allergic diseases. The controversial but basic allergic object relationship theory defined by Marty (1958) should be mentioned: In the allergic object relationship, the person desires to be symbiotically closer to the person opposite (the "object") in the form of identification or projection than is emotionally healthy, in order to stabilize his or her unstable structure by the constant presence and unity with a partner. This other person may be the doctor. Eczema or allergy occurs, according to Marty, when the object withdraws, does not play along, or holds fast to traits that the subject (patient) cannot accept. In the case of real or symbolic loss of such an object, the subject experiences regression and an outbreak of the disease.

References

Ader R, Cohen N (1982) Behaviorally conditioned immunosuppression and murine systemic lupus erythematodes. Science 215: 1534–1536

Gell PGH, Coombs RRA (1963) The classification of allergic reactions underlying disease. In: Gell PGH, Coombs RRA (eds) Clinical aspects of immunology, 1st edn. Blackwell, Oxford, pp 317–320

MacQueen G, Marshall J, Perdue M, Siegel S, Bienenstock J (1989) Pavlovian conditioning of rat mucosal mast cells to secret rat mast cell protease II. Science 243: 83–85

Marty P (1958) La relation objectale allergique. Rev Fr Psychanal 22: 5–35

Russell M, Dark KA, Cummins RW, Ellmann G, Callaway E, Peeke HVS (1984) Learned histamine release. Science 17: 733–734

Scholz OB (1995) Verhaltensmedizin allergisch bedingter Hauterkrankungen. In: Petermann F (Hrsg) Asthma und Allergie. Hogrefe, Göttingen, S 225–265

Further Reading

Djuric VJ, Bienenstock J (1993) Learned sensitivity. Ann Allergy 71: 5–14

Khansari DN, Murgo AJ, Faith ER (1990) Effects of stress on the immune system. Immunol Today 11: 170–175

Newman ME (1990) Can an immune response be conditioned? J Natl Cancer Inst 82: 1534–1535

Niemeier V, Gieler U, Richter R (2005) Psychosomatische Aspekte bei allergologischen Erkrankungen. In: Saloga J, Klimek L, Buhl R, Mann W, Knop J (Hrsg) Allergologiehandbuch. Schattauer, Stuttgart

Schmidt-Traub S, Bamler KJ, Schaffrath-Rosario A (1995) Vermehrte Angst und andere psychische Auffälligkeiten bei Allergikern? Allergologie 18: 13–19

4.1 Immediate Reactions, Type I Allergy

Type I allergies may present a heterogeneous pattern of clinical symptoms. Among these are generalized pruritus, flush, urticaria, allergic rhinitis, and allergic asthma; the latter is a psychosomatic disease in the classical sense.

Patients with panic disorders and concurrent allergy form a special problem group (Fig. 4.1). Patients with proven allergies have a five times higher risk for the occurrence of panic disorders, and 74% of anxiety patients present with allergies requiring treatment (Schmidt-Traub et al. 1995).

Anxiety disorders are of central importance in allergology.

In psychological test-questionnaire studies in dermatology, patients with anxiety disorders characteristically show a high somatization tendency, which can manifest clinically as pseudoallergic symptoms.

The immune system and controlling neuropeptides appear to play a central key role in pseudoallergic reactions as well. Although little attention has been paid to the connection between anxiety disorders and allergy, this will be a challenge for diagnostics and therapy in psychosomatic dermatology in the future. When evidence is found in allergology of an emotional disorder, a psychotherapist should be consulted.

In allergological emergencies, pseudoallergies may be present that are hard to interpret.
Anxiety disorders with panic attacks may imitate anaphylactoid allergic symptoms or allergic shock equally well.

In emergencies, genuine type I allergies according to Gell and Coombs may often be difficult to differentiate in the initial stages from psychosomatic pseudoallergies, since panic attacks present with symptoms similar to an allergic type I reaction (Table 4.3).

Stage I (German Society for Allergology and Clinical Immunology, DGAI) of the anaphylactoid reaction is characterized by itching, urticaria, or flushing. Starting in stage II, there are gastrointestinal, respiratory, or cardiovascular problems with tachycardia and hypotension, and starting in stage III shock and loss of consciousness occur, up to failure of vital organs in stage IV.

Differentiation of a panic attack from an anaphylactoid reaction or allergic shock reaction may be especially difficult in stage I because no specific cardiovascular symptoms can be proven in this stage. In the differentiation, a hypotensive reaction is more typical of an anaphylactoid shock, while a hypertensive regulation more likely indicates a panic disorder. In addition to psychodynamic concepts, Pavlovian concepts and stress models can be applied especially well with respect to the elicitation and coupling of threatening situations.

As with "real allergies", there is a sensitization phase. Avoidance behavior is characteristic for the anxiety disorder with pseudoallergy, comparable to the stabilization by avoidance and withdrawal of the allergen in allergic reactions.

The treatment of allergic reactions (specific immunotherapy) and panic disorders (behavior therapy) may be performed in both cases by means of "hyposensitization".

Clinical symptoms and presentations in immediate reaction. The following clinical symptomatics are among the important biosocial and psychosocial immediate reactions in dermatology: rhinitis, itching, flush, urticaria, undifferentiated somatoform idiopathic anaphylaxis, the special form of pseudo-sperm allergy, and individual "food allergies".

Urticaria. Urticaria may occur in the framework of a pseudoallergic reaction and is discussed in detail in Chap. 2.

Rhinitis allergica/vasomotor rhinitis. Rhinitis allergica (ICD-10: I30.1–I30.3, F54) is a multifactorially triggerable disease, regarding which only a few biopsychosocial studies are available. As early as 1886 in an article in the *American Journal of the Medical Sciences*, Mackenzie

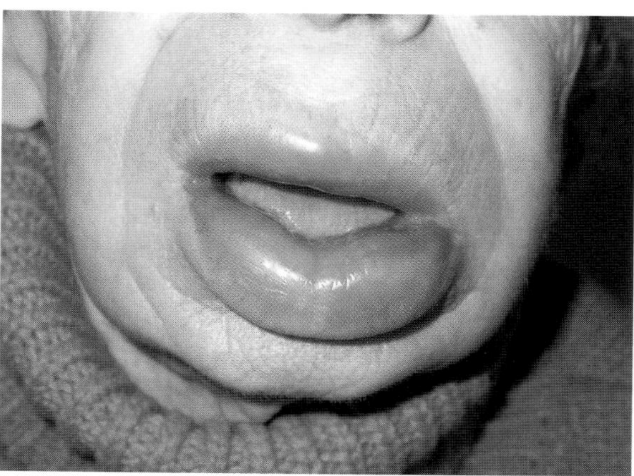

Fig. 4.1 Genuine recurrent angioedema with pronounced anxiety disorder as comorbidity

4

Table 4.3 Comparison of panic and type I allergies

Symptomatics	Panic attacks	Allergic anaphylaxia
Skin	Pruritus, urticaria, flush, sweating	Pruritus, urticaria, flush, sweating
Cardiovascular	Dizziness, tachycardia	Dizziness, tachycardia
Respiratory	Rhinorrhea, dyspnea, chest pain, constriction	Rhinorrhea, dyspnea, chest pain, constriction
Gastrointestinal	Dry mouth, vomiting, defecation	Dry mouth, vomiting, defecation
Emotional	Fear of death	Fear of death
Therapy	Hyposensitization	Hyposensitization

described a pseudoallergic reaction to an artificial rose in the sense of classical conditioning. A woman who was allergic to roses developed hay fever asthma on encountering an artificial rose. In this connection, attention must be paid especially to vasomotor rhinitis, which may often occur due to stress.

More detailed psychological studies reveal increased anxiety and depression scores in rhinoconjunctivitis allergica and vasomotor rhinitis. Vasomotor rhinitis can become symptomatic, for example, due to emotional stress, characteristically during examinations or in public speaking situations.

References

Mackenzie JN (1886) The production of the so-called "rose cold" by means of an artificial rose. Am J Med Sci 91: 45–47

Schmidt-Traub S, Bamler KJ, Schaffrath-Rosario A (1995) Vermehrte Angst und andere psychische Auffälligkeiten bei Allergikern? Allergologie 18: 13–19

Further Reading

Addolorato G, Ancona C, Capristo E, Graziosetto R, Di Rienzo L, Maurizi M, Gasbarrini G (1999) State and trait anxiety in women affected by allergic and vasomotor rhinitis. J Psychosom Res 46: 283–289

Kozel MM, Mekkes JR, Bossuyt PM, Bos JD (1998) The effectiveness of a history-based diagnostic approach in chronic urticaria and angioedema. Arch Dermatol 134(12): 1575–1580

Rueff F, Przybilla B, Fuchs T, Gall H, Rakowski J, Stolz W, Vieluf D (2000) Diagnose und Therapie der Bienen und Wespengiftallergie. Positionspapier der Deutschen Gesellschaft für Allergologie und klinische Immunologie (DGAI). Allergo J 8: 458–472

Russell M, Dark KA, Cummins RW, Ellmann G, Callaway E, Peeke HVS (1984) Learned histamine release. Science 17: 733–734

Scholz OB (1995) Verhaltensmedizin allergisch bedingter Hauterkrankungen. In: Petermann F (Hrsg) Asthma und Allergie. Hogrefe, Göttingen, S 225–265

Undifferentiated Somatoform Idiopathic Anaphylaxis

No cause can be found in one-third of patients with shock symptoms (34%; Kemp et al. 1995), and the diagnosis of idiopathic anaphylaxis is made.

The patients are usually young (30.0±17.3 years) females (68%). Typically, more than two-thirds of the patients have suffered several anaphylactoid episodes. Idiopathic urticaria has also been noted in 58% (Tejedor et al. 2002).

Like genuine anaphylaxis, idiopathic anaphylaxis usually responds well to prednisolone because it can be assumed that this is an allergic reaction although the eliciting allergen could not be identified anamnestically or with the usual diagnostic procedures.

There is also a subgroup of purely emotionally caused anaphylaxis, known as undifferentiated somatoform idiopathic anaphylaxis.

Undifferentiated somatoform idiopathic anaphylaxia is a purely emotionally caused anaphylaxia with no specific antigen–antibody interaction.

The term was coined by Choy et al. (1995). As with genuine anaphylaxia, undifferentiated somatoform idiopathic anaphylaxia in acute presentation is primarily treated as shock by the emergency medical team with H1 blockers, epinephrine, prednisolone, and volume substitution (Lenchner and Grammer 2003).

Characteristically, patients with undifferentiated somatoform idiopathic anaphylaxia do not respond to high-dose therapy with histamine blockers or prednisolone.
Note: **A C1 esterase inhibitor deficiency must be ruled out.**

Antiallergic shock therapy is usually unsuccessful in undifferentiated somatoform idiopathic anaphylaxia. The symptoms usually improve with administration of anxiolytics. The diagnosis of undifferentiated somatoform idiopathic anaphylaxia is then made according to the criteria of somatoform disorders (Sect. 1.3).

Diagnostic Criteria for Undifferentiated Somatoform Idiopathic Anaphylaxia

1. No response to corticosteroids, epinephrine, or antihistamines
2. Presence of a somatoform disorder (ICD-10: F45)

Characteristic of somatoform disorders is the repeated presentation of physical symptoms combined with a stubborn demand for medical examination, despite repeated negative results and assurance from the doctor that the symptoms cannot be physically explained.

When the diagnosis has been confirmed in retrospect, there is denial by the patient and often termination of the doctor–patient relationship.

Motivation for initiating psychotherapy is the exception (Choy et al. 1995). Emergency/medical "doctor hopping" can often be observed.

Therapy. The first priority in therapy is psychoeducation within psychosomatic primary care. Direct confrontation is usually useless. In psychosomatic primary care, special attention should be paid to possible connections between anxiety and allergy.

Most of the available experience in psychosomatic therapy of allergy patients has been gained in allergic asthma and allergies in broad connection with atopic dermatitis patients.

Education (Chap. 18) with the following central components has been found useful:

- Training and providing knowledge about self-management
- Working out of new emotional experiences in dealing with the disease and behavior modification
- Training in relaxation procedures

In allergological diseases (food, medication, and insect allergies, and also urticaria), there is a clear indication for psychotherapy in 8% of the patients (Augustin et al. 1999). The question of when psychotherapy is indicated depends on the comorbidities.

References

Augustin M, Zschocke I, Koch A, Schöpf E, Czech W (1999) Psychisches Befinden und Motivation zu psychosozialen Interventionen bei Patienten mit allergischen Erkrankungen. Hautarzt 50: 422–427

Choy AC, Patterson R, Patterson DR, Grammer LC, Greenberger PA, McGrath KG, Harris KE (1995) Undifferentiated somatoform idiopathic anaphylaxis: nonorganic symptoms mimicking idiopathic anaphylaxis. J Allergy Clin Immunol 96(6 Pt 1): 893–900

Kemp SF, Lockey RF, Wolf BL, Lieberman P (1995) Anaphylaxis. A review of 266 cases. Arch Intern Med 155(16): 1749–1754

Lenchner K, Grammer LC (2003) A current review of idiopathic anaphylaxis. Curr Opin Allergy Clin Immunol 3(4): 305–311

Tejedor A, Sastre DJ, Sanchez-Hernandez JJ, Perez FC, de L (2002) Idiopathic anaphylaxis: a descriptive study of 81 patients in Spain. Ann Allergy Asthma Immunol 88(3): 313–318

Further Reading

Ditto AM, Harris KE, Krasnick J, Miller MA, Patterson R (1996) Idiopathic anaphylaxis: a series of 335 cases. Ann Allergy Asthma Immunol 77: 285–291

Patterson R, Tripathi A, Saltoun C, Harris KE (2000) Idiopathic anaphylaxis: variants as diagnostic and therapeutic problems. Allergy Asthma Proc 21(3): 141–144

Ring J, Darsow U (2002) Idiopathic anaphylaxis. Curr Allergy Asthma Rep 2(1): 40–45

Scholz OB (1995) Verhaltensmedizin allergisch bedingter Hauterkrankungen. In: Petermann F (Hrsg) Asthma und Allergie. Hogrefe, Göttingen, S. 225–265

Pseudo-Sperm Allergy/Sperm Allergy

Psychologization of a Rare Somatic Phenomenon.

Definition. Genuine "sperm allergy" (Specken 1958), a specific sensitization to seminal plasma protein, can be proven, in which contact may lead to reactions ranging from allergic local effects to anaphylactoid systemic reactions.

The symptoms of pseudo-sperm allergy are similar to genuine sperm allergy, but there is no proof of a specific IgE-mediated reproducible allergic reaction. Broad allergological clarification is required because of the similar symptoms.

Occurrence. The women tend to be young and atopic. About 80 genuine cases of "sperm allergy" had been documented as of 2006. Currently no studies are available on pseudo-sperm allergy. A pseudoallergy to sperm or a somatoform disorder is present in five of six patients with suspected sperm allergy.

Pathogenesis. Specific sensitization and IgE-mediated allergic reaction (type I) with histamine release by the mast cells is responsible for genuine sperm allergy.

The sensitization develops to specific components of the seminal plasma. Some results indicate that the allergens originate from the prostate with a molecular weight of 12–40 kDa. No case of sperm allergy is known of in homosexual men, which can be attributed to their own tolerance of prostate antigens.

Clinical findings. Within 20 min after vaginal contact with sperm, patients experience vaginal itching, burning, erythema, mucosal swelling, generalized urticaria, rhinoconjunctival complaints, vomiting, abdominal pain, diarrhea, difficulty swallowing, bronchospasms, angioedema, and cardiovascular dysregulation up to anaphylactic shock. The allergy-related symptoms may also occur after body contact with seminal fluid.

In our experience, the symptoms are usually limited to the genitals in pseudo-sperm allergy, without systemic shock symptoms or panic attacks.

Emotional symptoms. The number of patients presenting for examination with presumed sperm allergy is considerably higher than those in whom genuine sperm allergy can be confirmed. The proof of a specific sensitization (type I) to seminal plasma is the exception. The patients report, "I react allergically to my partner." No publications are available on psychosomatic diagnostics in larger collectives. The patients in whom no specific sensitization can be confirmed show heterogeneous disorders in psychosomatic diagnostics, including compulsive personality structure (with a high need to control), vulvodynia (somatoform disorder), hypochondriacal uprooting depression, psychosexual disorders with somatization disorder, and conversion-neurotic assimilation of a posttraumatic stress disorder in a status following experienced sexual abuse.

No typical emotional disorder or typical personality structure has yet been demonstrated in patients with pseudo- or genuine sperm allergy.

Diagnostics. The examinations listed in the following overview should be performed for somatic clarification.

Diagnosis of Sperm Allergy

- Total IgE
- Specific IgE
  - Specific IgE antibody to latex
- Prick test
  - Latex, house dust, grass pollen
  - Food components and medications that might be found in sperm, e.g., nuts
  - Proteins (albumin)
  - Native sperm
- Intra-cutaneous testing
  - Latex
- Epicutaneous tests
  - Perfumes
  - Soap ingredients
  - Lubricant ingredients
  - Rubber and vulcanization substances
- Other
  - Physical urticaria testing
  - Sexually transmitted disease
  - House allergens (apartment environment)

A sperm allergy is confirmed by proof of specific IgE antibodies and a positive prick test with native sperm of the partner (after ruling out HIV infection and hepatitis serology) in a dilution series beginning at 1:10 (Fig. 4.2).

The prick test in vivo is, however, rejected by some authors because of the danger of infection and for ethical reasons.

Differential diagnoses. A genuine sperm allergy is rare, and proof of a specific sensitization is required. Latex allergy, perfume, lubricant allergy, atopic diathesis with vaginal lubrication impairment, urticaria factitia, and sexually transmitted diseases must be ruled out. A psychosomatic diagnosis should always be made in light of negative allergological findings.

Local allergens in the partner's apartment, such as animal hairs (especially cats) or grass pollen in hay fever or foodstuffs (nuts) and medications (penicillin) that may be present in the partner's sperm must also be considered.

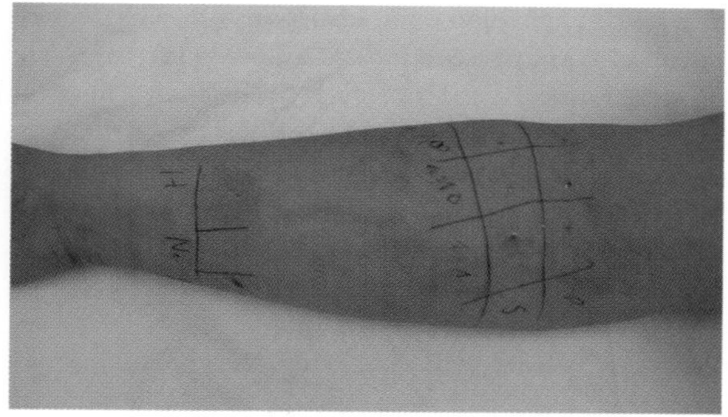

Fig. 4.2 A 26-year-old woman with suspected sperm allergy; positive test reactions in the prick test

Dermatological therapy. Stage-appropriate emergency therapy is indicated in the stage of acute anaphylactoid reaction after sperm contact in a sperm allergy.

After confirmation of a specific sperm allergy, allergen restriction with the use of condoms, availability of an emergency EpiPen set, and an attempt at hyposensitization is necessary. Moreover, active coping that also involves the partner is important.

Taking antihistamines 20 min prior to sexual intercourse leads to sufficient improvement in complaints in some cases. If the desire for a child is unfulfilled because of a sperm allergy, intrauterine insemination with washed spermatozoa can be done.

Changing partners does not help because the allergy is to components of the seminal plasma common to all men.

Psychotherapy. Little is known about psychotherapeutic therapy measures in presumed sperm allergy. In the individual psychosomatic interviews, it is conspicuous that the patients have a high need for control and that often there is no sexual contact because of the so-called sperm allergy. Attention should be paid to masked connections and posttraumatic stress disorders resulting from sexual abuse in childhood.

The pseudo-sperm allergy is a somatoform disorder and should be treated according to the guidelines for therapy of somatoform disorders.

First, a trusting doctor–patient basis should be established and any existing sexual problems discussed. Relaxation techniques may be helpful.

It is important that the suspected diagnosis of sperm allergy not be made too hastily. This could potentiate a misinterpretation by the patient and lead to chronification of an emotional disorder. A broad, open discussion of the phenomenon "sperm allergy" in the media, should also not be held in order to avoid creating or directing hypochondrias and phobias.

If there is a confirmed, genuine sperm allergy, active coping mechanisms should be strengthened in the partnership to also enable anxiety-free sexuality.

Reference

Specken JLH (1958) Een merkwaardig geval van allergie in de gynaecologie. Ned Tjidschr Verloskd Gynaecol 58: 314–318

Further Reading

Bangard C, Rosener I, Merk HF, Baron JM (2004) Typ-I-Sensibilisierung gegenüber Spermaflüssigkeit. Urtikaria und Angioödem. Hautarzt 55(1): 79–81

Bernstein JA, Sugumaran R, Bernstein DI, Bernstein IL (1997) Prevalence of human seminal plasma hypersensitivity among symptomatic women. Ann Allergy Asthma Immunol 78(1): 54–58

Iwahashi K, Miyazaki T, Kuji N, Yoshimura Y (1999) Successful pregnancy in a woman with a human seminal plasma allergy. A case report. J Reprod Med 44(4): 391–393

Kohn FM, Ring J (2000) Sperm intolerance. "My partner has an allergic reaction to me." MMW Fortschr Med 142(37): 34–35

Pevny I, Peter G, Schulze K (1978) Sperm allergy of the anaphylactic type. Hautarzt 29(10): 525–530

Food Intolerances

Definition. Foods may cause symptoms that are similar to allergic reactions but are not based on immunological mechanisms. These are food intolerances, which are also called pseudoallergic food intolerances. Sometimes these are purely somatoform disorders.

Prevalence. The prevalence is estimated at 0.2–2% of the population. By contrast, 33–45% of the general public subjectively attributes various complaints to food allergies (Schafer and Breuer 2003; Raithel et al. 2002; Sampson 1999).

Clinical presentation. In dermatology, chronic recurrent urticaria, the "oral syndrome", or, rarely, even atopic dermatitis is diagnosed as the clinical correlate. Laboratory tests are often interpreted uncritically by patients and sometimes also by physicians. There is often little agreement between skin tests or specific IgE-RAST classes when double-blind provocation testing is performed (Vatn et al. 1995).

Emotional symptoms. Pearson et al. (1983) found fewer emotional anomalies in patients with confirmed food allergies than in patients with *suspected* food allergy that could not be allergologically confirmed. Depressive disorders dominated.

! Patients with suspected food allergies are emotionally more labile than patients with confirmed food allergies.

The comorbidities of depression and social phobia often arise from negative coping. Patients with "food allergies" often have transitions to a somatoform environmental disease or hypochondria (Sect. 1.3).

There are connections between allergies, panic disorders, and agoraphobia (Schmidt-Traub and Bamler 1997). The authors point out that the symptoms of real anaphylactic and anaphylactoid reactions are initially similar to those of panic patients (vasomotor reactions, tachycardia, and hyperventilation) and that knowledge of panic disorders is therefore mandatory for allergologists. Moreover, the uncontrollability of an allergic reaction apparently also contributes to the degree of limitation in quality of life (Augustin et al. 1996).

Moreover, 74% of examined patients with panic attacks reported having had allergic reactions requiring medical treatment in the past (Schmidt-Traub and Bamler 1997).

Summary of Food Intolerance

- No specific personality disorders can be proven.
- Transitions to multiple chemical sensitivity syndrome and polysensitization to multiple environmental allergens have been described.
- Food intolerances may be an expression of anxiety disorders or depression.
- Hypochondriacal disorders may play a decisive role.

Gastrointestinal symptoms are often observed in anxiety (diarrhea) and depression and also belong to the somatic diagnostic criteria of these emotional disorders. Gastrointestinal symptoms in suspected food intolerances may thus be an expression of an anxiety disorder or depression (Rix at al. 1984; Seggev and Eckert 1988).

Intolerances in the transition to multiple chemical sensitivity syndrome and polysensitization to multiple environmental allergens must be clarified under the aspect of an ecosyndrome and in the framework of a somatoform/hypochondriacal disorder. Frequently there is mycophobia or fear of amalgam as a comorbidity.

Therapy. Patients with confirmed, life-threatening allergies or pseudoallergies should receive additional psychosocial care to prevent unfavorable coping. For this, appropriate guidance with sufficient psychosocial consultation is necessary (Carroll et al. 1992). Psychoeducation and training, such as that being used for patients with allergic asthma and atopic dermatitis, may be meaningful. The question of when psychotherapy is indicated depends on the comorbidity of emotional disorders.

References

Augustin M, Zschocke I, Koch A, Dieterle W, Müller J, Schöpf E, Czech W (1996) Lebensqualität und psychosoziale Belastungsfaktoren bei Patienten mit Allergien vom Soforttyp und mit Pseudoallergien. Allergo J 5(1): 13

Carroll P, Caplinger KJ, France GL (1992) Guidelines for counseling parents of young children with food sensitivities. J Am Diet Assoc 92(5): 602–603

Pearson DJ, Rix KJ, Bentley SJ (1983) Food allergy: how much in the mind? A clinical and psychiatric study of suspected food hypersensitivity. Lancet 1(8336): 1259–1261

Raithel M, Hahn EG, Baenkler HW (2002) Klinik und Diagnostik von Nahrungsmittelallergien. Dtsch Ärztebl 99 [Heft 12]: 780–786

Rix KJB, Pearson DJ, Bentley SB (1984) A psychiatric study of patients with a supposed food allergy. Br J Psychiatry 145: 121–126

Sampson HA (1999) Food allergy. Part 1: immunopathogenesis and clinical disorders. J Allergy Clin Immunol 103: 717–728

Schafer T, Breuer K (2003) Epidemiologie von Nahrungsmittelallergien. Hautarzt 54(2): 112–120

Schmidt-Traub S, Bamler KJ (1997) The psychoimmunological association on panic disorder and allergic reaction. Br J Clin Psychol 36: 51–62

Seggev JS, Eckert RC (1988) Psychopathology masquerading as food allergy. J Fam Pract 26(2): 161–164

Vatn MH, Grimstad IA, Thorsen L, Kittang E, Refnin I, Malt U, Lovik A, Langeland T, Naalsund A (1995) Adverse reaction to food, assessment by double-blind placebo-controlled food challenge and clinical, psychosomatic and immunologic analysis. Digestion 56(5): 421–428

Further Reading

Kozel MM, Mekkes JR, Bossuyt PM, Bos JD (1998) The effectiveness of a history-based diagnostic approach in chronic urticaria and angioedema. Arch Dermatol 134(12): 1575–1580

Ring J (1996) Öko-Syndrom (Multiple-Chemical-Sensitivity): Krank durch Umwelt oder krank durch Angst. Allergo J 5: 210

4.2 Late Reactions

Allergic late reactions are cell-mediated type IV hypersensitivity reactions and occur 24–48 h after exposure to an allergen. It is often difficult to identify a direct psychosomatic connection due to the delayed temporal relationship.

Overall, apart from contact dermatitis, individual cases and certain types of dyshidrosiform hand eczema and special forms of food allergies can be classified in the group of late reactions.

Dyshidrosiform Hand Eczema

The so-called dyshidrosiform hand eczema is a special form that is discussed in a separate section (Chap. 2). It may be a variant of contact dermatitis, or it may have other causes (atopic, mycotic, or idiopathic).

Contact Dermatitis

Contact dermatitis (ICD-10: L25.0, F54) is a cell-mediated allergic reaction (type IV) that results in acute dermatitis at the point of contact 24–48 h after exposure to the allergen. Earlier contact with the allergen is a prerequisite for this reaction.

A variety of substances can be considered as allergens. These are usually low-molecular-weight substances that become full antigens in connection with a hapten in the epidermis, or they may be high-molecular substances such as proteins. The most common allergen is nickel (jewelry). Allergies may be acquired at work (occupational dermatoses) or iatrogenically (for example, sensitization to medications or ointments, e.g., in leg ulcers). The localization of the contact dermatitis may be indicative of the possible allergens (jeans-button dermatitis!). A subtle history, taken several times, is often the only way to track down an assumed contact dermatitis.

Clinically, the acute contact dermatitis appears as a more-or-less sharply defined erythema that is usually slightly raised due to cellular infiltrates and edema and shows very small vesicles on close inspection. It is usually accompanied by severe pruritus. Stronger reactions differ especially in their expanse and vesicular components, which appear as bullae and exudative erosions (Fig. 4.3).

Chronic courses lose their exudative character, which becomes visible again only with intensive new contact with the allergen. Otherwise, the presentation of chronic dermatitis may develop with scaly crusts, lichenification, and formation of rhagades.

The epicutaneous or patch test required to confirm the diagnosis shows the above described characteristics of acute contact dermatitis and confirms it in positive cases.

Emotional factors. Allergies may be multifactorial in origin. Allergic and emotional elicitors may mutually supplement effects or even potentiate them. Although there does not appear to be a typical "allergy personality," a greater level of individual emotional phenomena has been demonstrated in allergic patients. For example, elevated aggression scores are often reported. Some authors conclude from this that the allergic symptoms serve to relieve aggressive struggles that would otherwise be directed against oneself (as in depression).

It has also been proven that allergies can be triggered by suggestion and that severe anxiety causes the skin to react more sensitively to potential allergens.

It has been demonstrated in already existing contact eczemas that nonautonomic behavior and ignoring of feelings or inappropriate handling of emotions in conflict and decisional situations have an unfavorable influence on the course of disease (Wirth 1989).

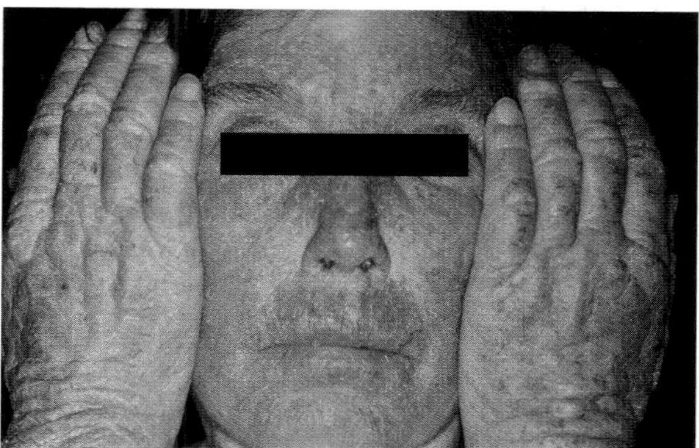

Fig. 4.3 Generalized contact eczema after use of a facial mask with oils

4

Psychotherapy. No detailed controlled studies are available on psychotherapy in late reactions. Initially, therapy should be performed as part of psychosomatic primary care. Strengthening of positive and active coping is especially necessary in chronic-recurrent courses. Coping with contact allergy depends, of course, on the patient's possibility of avoiding the probable allergen – when one has been identified.

Relaxation therapies such as autogenic training and progressive muscle relaxation may be beneficial in reducing stress-dependent attacks.

If depressive or phobic disorders occur, the indication for more intensive psychotherapy should be checked. For phobias that may develop in connection with contact allergy, behavior therapy is indicated with top priority. Psychodynamic psychotherapy may be indicated for patients whose hands are predominantly afflicted and who have dependence and detachment problems.

Psychopharmaceuticals. No detailed experience reports are available. To start, antihistamines according to the stepwise plan (Chap. 15) – nonsedating or sedating such as hydroxyzine – or doxepin are recommended.

Reference

Wirth K (1989) Psychosomatik des Kontaktekzems. Psychomed 1: 43–46

Further Reading

Hansen O, Küchler T, Lotz G, Richter R, Wilckens A (1981) Es juckt mich an den Fingern, aber mir sind die Hände gebunden. Z Psychosom Med Psychoanal 27: 275–290

Khansari DN, Murgo AJ, Faith ER (1990) Effects of stress on the immune system. Immunol Today 11: 170–175

Roudebush RE, Bryant HU (1991) Conditioned immunosuppression of a murine delayed type hypersensitivity response: dissociation from corticosterone elevation. Brain Behav Immun 5: 308–317

Russell M, Dark KA, Cummins RW, Ellmann G, Callaway E, Peeke HVS (1984) Learned histamine release. Science 17: 733–734

Schmidt-Traub S, Bamler KJ, Schaffrath-Rosario A (1995) Vermehrte Angst und andere psychische Auffälligkeiten bei Allergikern? Allergologie 18: 13–19

Stangier U, Gieler U (2000) Hauterkrankungen. In: Senft W, Broda M (Hrsg) Praxis der Psychotherapie, 2. Aufl. Thieme, Stuttgart, S 566–581

Zachariae R, Bjerring P (1993) Increase and decrease of delayed cutaneous reactions obtained by hypnotic suggestions during sensitization. Studies on dinitrochlorobenzene and diphenylcyclopropenone. Allergy 48: 6–11

Andrology

5

In Germany and other parts of Europe, andrology is seen as a subspecialty of dermatology, urology, and endocrinology. A survey in doctors' practices revealed that about 29% of the women and 25% of the men (disregarding age differences) suffered from a functional sexual disorder (Buddeberg 1983).

In an andrological practice, potency impairments are reported by 57.7% of the men (mean age 44.8 years), followed by an additional 14.6% who also report loss of libido (Seikowski and Starke 2002). The focal points in andrological practice are erectile dysfunction; loss of libido, also in connection with the "aging man" symptom complex; and impaired orgasm, such as ejaculatio praecox in young men. Erection problems are a characteristic multifactorial model example of biopsychosocial diseases and require biopsychosocial clarification and interdisciplinary cooperation.

Classification and clinical symptoms. The ICD-10 provides a systematized classification of psychosocial sexual disorders after exclusion of organic causes (Table 5.1).

Sexual Aversion and Lack of Sexual Enjoyment

In sexual aversion (ICD-10: F52.10), the thought of a sexual partner relationship is coupled strongly with negative feelings and causes so much fear and anxiety that sexual acts are avoided. A lack of sexual enjoyment (ICD-10: F52.11) is related, in which sexual reactions may proceed normally, but orgasm is experienced without the corresponding feelings of lust.

Excessive Sexual Drive

Augmented sexual desire (ICD-10: F52.7) denotes the presence of an excessively increased sex drive. In this connection, the definition of "augmented" is difficult due to the increasing liberalization in society. Women with excessive sex drive (sex mania) are generally termed nymphomaniacs. For men, the terms are Don Juan complex or satyriasis. The patients often have incorrect fantasies, incomplete knowledge, or even somatoform disorders, including body dysmorphic disorders.

Dyspareunia

Purely psychogenic pain during coitus (ICD-10: F52.6) is rare among men. Usually there is a nonspecific persistent anogenital pain syndrome (Sect. 1.3.4). Chronic prostatitis must be considered first in painful ejaculation. Thorough urological diagnostics should be performed for differential-diagnostic clarification.

Table 5.1 Classification of nonorganic sexual dysfunction (ICD-10: F52)

ICD-10	Nonorganic sexual dysfunction
F52.0	Lack or loss of sexual desire
F52.1	Sexual aversion and lack of sexual enjoyment
F52.2	Erectile dysfunction: failure of genital response
F52.3	Orgasmic dysfunction
F52.4	Premature ejaculation
F52.5	Nonorganic vaginismus
F52.6	Nonorganic dyspareunia: pain during sexual intercourse
F52.7	Excessive sexual drive

Impaired Orgasm

Characteristically, in impaired orgasm (ICD-10: F52.3) there is a lack of or blocked orgasm despite maintained rigidity, whereby this may occur after a delay. Emotionally caused anorgasm in men is an absolute rarity in andrological practice.

Impaired orgasms are also a characteristic side effect of the use of psychopharmaceuticals, including selective serotonin reuptake inhibitors (SSRIs), and may make a change of medication necessary.

Premature Ejaculation

Definition. Ejaculatio praecox (ICD-10: F52.4) is the inability to control ejaculation, which occurs prior to immissio (ejaculatio ante introitus vaginae) or shortly thereafter. Coitus is thus unsatisfying for both partners.

Classification. To better understand the emotional symptoms, two forms of premature ejaculation are differentiated: primary ejaculatio praecox and secondary ejaculatio praecox.

Primary ejaculatio praecox manifests at the beginning of sexual experience, that is, usually in youth or early adulthood, and the course persists. In secondary ejaculatio praecox, by contrast, normal ejaculation is initially possible, and the sexual disorder occurs at a later time in life.

Pathogenesis. Ejaculatio praecox is almost exclusively due to a psychosomatic disorder. A purely somatic hypothesis is hypersensitivity of the glans penis with excessive stimulation of spinal ejaculation centers (St. Lawrence and Madakasira 1992).

Emotional symptoms. Ejaculatio praecox often becomes manifest in connection with a new partnership, partnership conflicts, or other erectile dysfunctions and adjustment disorders (Fig. 5.1).

Concepts of learning theory are an important basis for understanding negative conditioning of the ejaculation reflex, from which the following central behavior therapy treatment concepts were directly developed (Masters and Johnson 1970).

Differential diagnosis. In prolonged stimulation time and rapid ejaculation, an apparent ejaculatio praecox, attributable in fact to an erectile dysfunction, must be clarified.

Psychotherapy. Premature ejaculation is relatively normal in young men, especially in early sexual experiences. Many men learn to have more or less good control over the ejaculation reflex over time.

Psychotherapeutic interventions are indicated in cases of persistent problematic ejaculatio praecox. Basic behavior therapy concepts and training programs have been developed especially for this (Masters and Johnson 1970).

Pharmacological therapy. Good effectiveness has been achieved with beta-receptor blockers (propanolol 120 mg/day), and SSRIs, especially sertraline as well as paroxetine and fluoxetine, led to clear improvement in the symptoms in studies (Salonia et al. 2002). The therapy of choice is sertraline (100 mg/day).

Hypersensitivity can also be reduced by the use of condoms.

Lack of Desire

Lack of sexual desire (ICD-10: F52.0) means primarily that sexual activities are initiated less often. Loss of libido is also a diagnostic part-symptom and somatic criterion for definition of a depression (somatic syndrome).

Lack of Desire

- Specific symptomatics
  - Decrease in libido
  - Lack of sexual desire
  - Erections and orgasm impairment/reduced potency
  - Decrease in the number of morning erections
- General complaints (aging-male syndrome has not been scientifically confirmed)
  - Depressive mood
  - Deterioration of general well-being
  - Joint and muscle complaints
  - Heavy sweating
  - Insomnia
  - Increased need to sleep; often tired
  - Irritability
  - Nervousness
  - Anxiety
  - Physical exhaustion/reduced energy
  - Decreased muscular strength
  - Feeling of having passed one's prime
  - Feelings of discouragement; "the doldrums"
  - Reduced beard growth

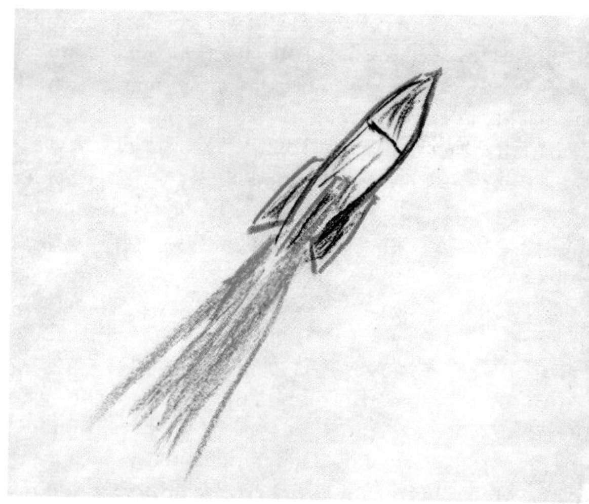

Fig. 5.1 Ejaculatio praecox in art therapy

Biopsychosocial Aspects of Impotence

- Somatic
  - Age
  - Physical diseases (Metabolic syndrome)
  - Hormones
  - Medications
- Emotional
  - Stress
  - Fear (of failure)
  - Emotional disorders and conflicts
  - Sexually deviant tendencies
  - Impaired self-image
  - Projection from partner
  - Identification with partner
  - Somatopsychic adjustment disorder
- Social
  - Sex-typical role behavior
  - Sexual norms
  - Media reports

In "aging male syndrome," which has been in the focus in recent years, an age-dependent testosterone deficiency (late-onset hypogonadism) is considered responsible for the loss of libido. The discussion of whether all of the general symptoms listed can be attributed to advancing age or particularly to a decrease in testosterone levels has not yet been concluded. Clearly, libido impairments can be in a causal relationship with lower testosterone levels. The use of testosterone gels as lifestyle medications against the midlife crisis, including their use for depression, listlessness, and fatigue, has not, however, been scientifically confirmed and should be rejected.

Libido impairments are often found in combination with erectile dysfunction.

Failure of Genitale Response

Definition. Erectile dysfunction (ICD-10: F52.2) or impotentia coeundi describes a chronic presentation lasting at least 6 months in which at least 70% of the attempts to consummate coitus are unsuccessful.

Pathogenesis. The causality of erection disorders is multifactorial (Hartmann 1998; Morelli et al. 2000).

Emotional symptomatics. The most common comorbidity of erectile disorders is depression or anxiety disorder (Hartmann 1998).

Depressive disorder. A manifest erectile dysfunction frequently occurs within the framework of depression or/and leads secondarily to a depressive mood state, especially if it is not adequately treated early on and has possibly resulted in serious partnership conflicts and estrangement at the physical level.

Anxiety disorder. Even prior to sexual contact, the fear of failure and the fear of a possible erectile dysfunction may be so dominant that no erection occurs. Moreover, after successful immissio, the fear of not being able to maintain the erection long enough may result in anxiety and loss of erection during coitus.

If the patient has experienced this several times, the anxiety problems intensify, in which the fear of failure is in the foreground.

Fear of failure leads to failure.
Failure leads to anticipatory fear and avoidance.

If the patient is aware of his fear of failure, there are additional anticipatory fears that lead to a vicious cycle, and the fear of failure may lead to avoidance of any sexual contact and resignation.

A broad spectrum of other cofactors may potentiate erectile dysfunction, such as situations of physical tension or fear of discovery (children, parents), or other factors such as those presented below may play a role and prevent relaxed spontaneous sexuality.

Anxiety Disorders and Erectile Dysfunction

- Specific disorders
  - Fear of failure
  - Sexual performance anxiety
  - Fear of discovery
  - Fear of pregnancy
  - Sexual boredom
  - Unclear sexual orientation
  - Religious reasons
  - Emancipation problems, idealized image of women
  - Male self-conception
  - Body dysmorphic disorders
  - Feelings of inferiority
- General
  - Generalized anxiety disorders
  - Mixed patterns with depressive disorders
  - Adjustment disorders
  - Compulsive thinking
  - Situations of tension, "daily hassles", schedule pressure
  - Private family or professional problems
  - Partnership conflicts
  - Dissatisfaction
  - Rage

Other fears up to compulsive thinking that result in sexual disorders include the worry of not being able to satisfy the woman long enough or intensively enough (Masters and Johnson 1970). A central role here is played by false information, including that from the media, or body dysmorphic disorders, and feelings of inferiority, which may inhibit sexuality. This may also be seen with relationship changes between the genders, whereby strong and emancipated women can elicit conflicts in the male self-conception, which may then be expressed as erection problems.

On the other hand, erection disorders can be induced by projections of the woman's sexual disorders to the man and lead to complete withdrawal from sexual life, with the causal feminine disorder remaining hidden. Caring for the impaired and needy male but impotent partner can, in turn, stabilize the relationship.

Moreover, sexual abuse in the woman's history must be taken into account in this connection, since coitus is experienced as a danger and a threat and may reactivate the historical abuse or lead to splitting phenomena and dissociative disorders.

Psychotherapy. Psychotherapeutic interventions are indicated especially in clear emotional disorders, partnership problems, and the fear of failure. One central question is the couple's motivation for shared partnership programs (Master and Johnson 1970) and whether these are offered or can be realized locally.

An interdisciplinary combination therapy with drug therapy of the erectile dysfunction (e.g., phosphodiesterase inhibitors) for relief and concurrent performance of psychosomatic primary care or psychotherapy has proven beneficial.

Stress and Fertility

The unfulfilled wish for a child remains a relevant medical problem. Overall, according to statistical projections, more than a million German couples are involuntarily childless. A connection between stress, stress hormones, and a tendential limitation of fertility could be demonstrated in some studies that took psychosomatic aspects into account (Fig. 5.2). Prolactin and neopterin are stress-responder markers. Subgroups of stress responders with an unfulfilled wish for a child have significantly higher levels of the stress parameters prolactin, cortisol, follicle-stimulating hormone, and the immunological marker neopterin. At the same time, there is subfertility as noted by limited motility, the hypoosmotic swell test, and penetration capacity.

The neuroendocrinological and neuroimmunological differences are associated in the psychological test questionnaires of stress responders with a significantly higher reaction control. This means that nonstress responders may possibly have a fertility advantage. Here again, the central question of primary or secondary genesis arises. Does increased need for reaction control lead to increased stress, or does elevated stress lead to greater need for reaction control and thus possibly to a detriment to fertility?

Sterile marriages. Partners in sterile marriages are a heterogeneous group, without any specific personality anomalies that can be claimed as characteristic of all patients.

When the wish for a child is not spontaneously achieved, serious doubts arise about the person's own perfection, first by the woman because, traditionally, the man's fertility is presumed to be self-evident as long as intercourse and ejaculation function (Seikowski and Starke 2002).

This is followed by self-accusation, accusations, and feelings of guilt toward the partner up to instability of the partner relationship, marital crisis, and even separation. Lack of libido and withdrawal of love are often the consequence of a frustrated wish for children.

Psychogenic sterility. Purely psychogenic sterility in marriage is extremely rare, but it is occasionally encountered in andrological practice and is then usually a surprise finding.

! Sterility is clearly psychogenic when, despite medical clarification, the couple with an unfulfilled wish for children do the following:
- **Continue self-damaging behavior (drug or alcohol abuse, eating disorders, and the like)**
- **Have sex only on infertile days or not at all**
- **Agree to necessary measures of fertility treatment but do not take them**

References

Buddeberg C (1987) Sexualberatung, 2. Aufl. Enke, Stuttgart

Hartmann U (1998) Psychological stress factors in erectile dysfunctions. Causal models and empirical results. Urologe A 37(5): 487–494

Masters W, Johnson V (1970) Human sexual inadequacy. Little, Brown, Boston (Dt. Ausgabe: Master W, Johnson V, 1987, Liebe und Sexualität. Ullstein, Frankfurt am Main)

Morelli G, De Gennaro L, Ferrara M, Dondero F, Lenzi A, Lombardo F, Gandini L (2000) Psychosocial factors and male seminal parameters. Biol Psychol 53(1): 1–11

Salonia A, Maga T, Colombo R, Scattoni V, Briganti A, Cestari A, Guazzoni G, Rigatti P, Montorsi F (2002) A prospective study comparing paroxetine alone versus paroxetine plus sildenafil in patients with premature ejaculation. J Urol 168(6): 2486–2489

Seikowski K, Starke K (2002) Sexualität des Mannes. Pabst, Lengerich Berlin

St Lawrence JS, Madakasira S. (1992) Evaluation and treatment of premature ejaculation: a critical review. Int J Psychiatry Med 22(1): 77–97

Further Reading

Bernstein J, Mattox JH, Keller R (1988) Psychological status of previously infertile couples after a successful pregnancy. J Obstet Gynecol Neonatal Nurs 17: 404–408

Domar AD, Clapp D, Slawsby EA, Dusek J, Kessel B, Freizinger M (2000) Impact of group psychological interventions on pregnancy rates in infertile women. Fertil Steril 73: 805–811

Harth W, Linse R (2000) Psychosomatic andrology: how to test stress. J Psychosom Res 48: 229

Harth W, Linse R (2004) Male fertility: endocrine stress-parameters and coping. Dermatol Psychosom 5: 22–29

Seikowski K (1997) Psychological aspects of erectile dysfunction. Wien Med Wochenschr 147(4–5): 105–108

Special Case: Somatoform Disorders in Andrology

The Koro syndrome (ICD-10: F48.8) is an epidemic and culture-dependent syndrome that occurs suddenly in Asia, in which sociocultural factors predominate as elicitors.

Definition. In Koro syndrome, there is an episode of sudden and intensive fear that the penis could be drawn back into the body and possibly cause death (Fig. 5.3). This fear often occurs as a mass phenomenon, in which many men hold onto their penis or try to prevent the presumed event by placing wooden tongs on their penis. The classical Koro epidemics occur regularly in Southeast Asia and China (Tseng et al. 1992), and confirmed reports of up to 300 attacks within a few days have been published. Retrospective studies show that the lower socioeconomic class is especially affected, representing 61.3% of cases. In psychological test studies, the symptom checklist SCL-90 revealed significant differences for somatization, anxiety/depression, and compulsiveness.

Classification Recommendation for Koro

- Primary (culture-dependent)
  - Sporadic
  - Epidemic
- Secondary (Koro-like syndrome)
  - Central nervous system disorder: tumor, epilepsy, cerebrovascular impairment
  - Drug induction
  - Primary emotional disorder: schizophrenia, affective disorder, anxiety disorder, hypochondria, personality disorder, sexual disorder
  - Infectious diseases: HIV/AIDS, syphilis
  - In combination with other culture-dependent syndromes: Amok, Dhat, Shen-k'uei

Individual cases that may occur as a comorbidity in other diseases are differentiated. Isolated cases of this

5

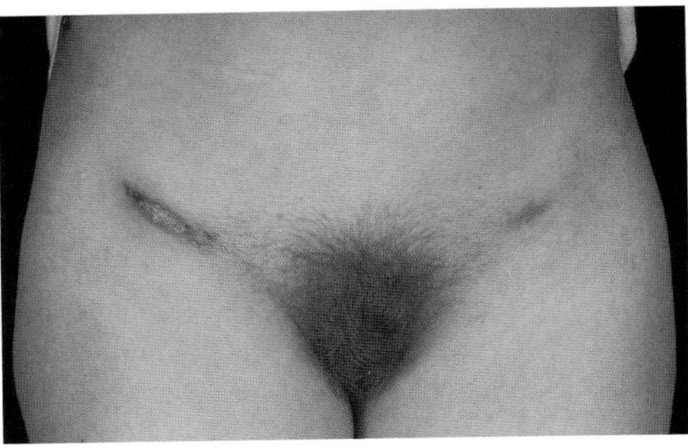

Fig. 5.2 Artefacts in the actual sense: 27-year-old woman with unfulfilled desire for a child and artefacts in the lower abdomen

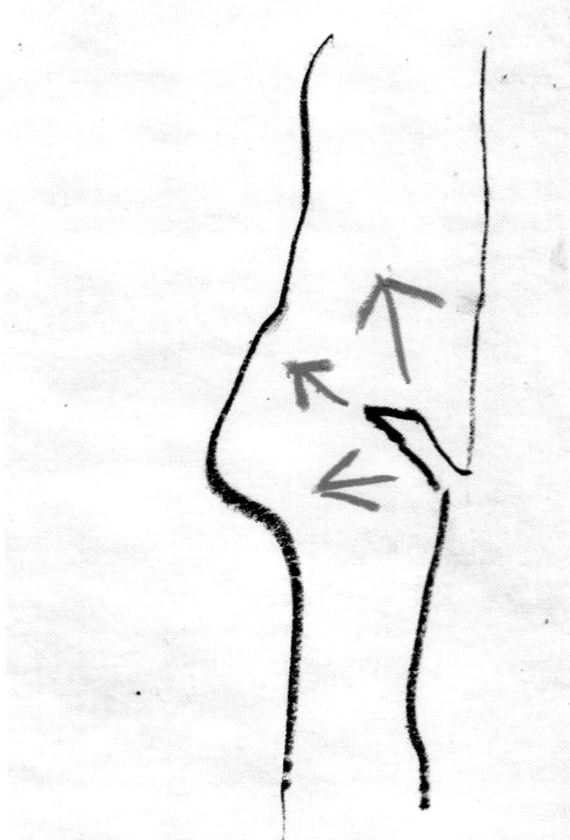

Fig. 5.3 Caucasian with Koro-like syndrome. The patient's drawing illustrates the assumption that the glans penis will be drawn into the body and the fear of dying from that. No objective findings could be noted in physical examination

Koro-like syndrome outside the original cultural circle have been described in Europe as a complex psychosomatic-andrological disorder. The presence of a somatoform disorder must be discussed.

The differential diagnosis includes the frequent Dhat syndrome, which is characterized by the fear of detriment to health and debility due to loss of semen.

Reference

Tseng WS, Mo KM, Li LS, Chen GQ, Ou LQ, Zheng HB (1992) Koro epidemics in Guangdong, China. A questionnaire survey. J Nerv Ment Dis 180(2): 117–123

Further Reading

Adeniran RA, Jones JR (1994) Koro: culture-bound disorder or universal symptom? Br J Psychiatry 164(4): 559–561

Bernstein RL, Gaw AC (1990) Koro: proposed classification for DSM-IV. Am J Psychiatry 147(12): 1670–1674

Chowdhury AN (1996) The definition and classification of Koro. Cult Med Psychiatry 20(1): 41–65

Fishbain DA, Barsky S, Goldberg M (1989) "Koro" (genital retraction syndrome): psychotherapeutic interventions. Am J Psychother 43(1): 87–91

Harth W, Linse R (2001) Koro und kulturabhängige Syndrome in der psychosomatischen Dermatologie. Z Hautkr 76 (Suppl 1): 35

Jilek W, Jilek-Aall L (1977) Mass-hysteria with Koro-symptoms in Thailand. Schweiz Arch Neurol Neurochir Psychiatr 120(2): 257–259

Keshavan MS (1983) Epidemic psychoses, or epidemic koro? Br J Psychiatry 142: 100–101

Kranzler HR, Shah PJ (1988) Atypical koro. Br J Psychiatry 152: 579–580

Malinick C, Flaherty JA, Jobe T (1985) Koro: how culturally specific? Int J Soc Psychiatry 31(1): 67–73

Chong TM (1968) Epidemic koro in Singapore. Br Med J 1(592): 640–641

Sachdev PS, Shukla A (1982) Epidemic koro syndrome in India. Lancet 2(8308): 1161

Scher M (1987) Koro in a native born citizen of the U.S. Int J Soc Psychiatry 33(1): 42–45

Venereology

A drastic increase in sexually transmitted viral infections appears to be one of the outstanding cultural-psychosocial challenges in the coming years (Stanberry et al. 1999). The increasing prevalence of primarily sexually transmitted viral diseases, such as herpes simplex virus (HSV), human papilloma virus (HPV), and human immunodeficiency virus (HIV), is resulting in a "new venereology" compared with the classical venereal diseases that had to be reported (Adler and Meheust 2000; Wutzler et al. 2000).

In the new federal German states, the lowest number of reportable venereal diseases was reached in 1967 (Elste and Krell 1973), but thereafter, there was another increase after years of decreasing numbers. Improved therapeutic possibilities alone were not sufficient to achieve a decrease in incidence, which was reversed again to a negative trend due to changes in lifestyle and habits. Increasing promiscuity; increasing homosexuality; intensification of sexual behavior with an increase in premarital and extramarital sexual intercourse; increasing migration, immigration of foreign workers, and tourism; prostitution; and a reduction in individual precautions due to taking ovulation inhibitors are discussed as the causes (Haustein and Pfeil 1991).

In 2002, there was a reincrease in syphilis in all of Germany (Fig 5.4).

All sexually transmitted diseases are directly dependent on the risk behavior (Jäger 1992). A low educational level, joblessness, and poverty are associated with especially high-risk sexual behavior. The underlying influence of sociocultural developments and aspects of society on the diagnosis spectrum and the resultant further spread of diseases was described very differentially very early on the basis of venereal diseases. The disclosure of a high-risk sociocultural lifestyle is decisive for mobilizing health potentials in dermatology and for working out concepts of prevention.

References

Adler MW, Meheust AZ (2000) Epidemiology of sexually transmitted infections and human immunodeficiency virus in Europe. J Eur Acad Dermatol Venereol 14(5): 370–377

Elste G, Krell L (1973) Zur Epidemiologie des Morbus Neisser. Dtsch Gesundheitsw 28(3): 139–144

Jäger H (1992) Sexuell übertragbare Erkrankungen und öffentlicher Gesundheitsdienst – Vorschläge zur Neugestaltung von Beratungsstellen bei sexuell übertragbaren Erkrankungen. Gesundheitswesen 54: 211–218

Haustein UF, Pfeil B (1991) Drastischer Anstieg der Syphilis Inzidenz in Westsachsen. Hautarzt 42: 269–270

Stanberry L, Cunningham A, Mertz G, Mindel A, Peters B, Reitano M, Sacks S, Wald A, Wassilew S, Woolley P (1999) New developments in the epidermiology, natural history and management of genital herpes. Antiviral Res 42(1): 1–14

Wutzler P, Doerr HW, Färber I, Eichhorn U, Helbig B, Sauerbrei A, Brandstadt A, Rabenau HF (2000) Seroprevalence of herpes simplex virus type 1 and type 2 in selected German populations – relevance for the incidence of genital herpes. J Med Virol 61: 201–207

Skin Diseases and Sexuality

Chronic-recurrent skin diseases such as psoriasis vulgaris, AD, severe acne, and venereal diseases have a negative influence on sexual behavior (Fig. 5.5).

Acne and psoriasis patients fear rejection and react to the environment with emotional inhibition. Disfiguring skin diseases are associated with avoidance of body contact and less exchange of caresses compared with people with healthy skin (Niemeier et al. 1997). Psoriasis patients present with a greater deficit than atopic dermitis patients with respect to caressing and increased inhibition. Patients with atopic dermitis suffer more than psoriasis patients and have greater emotional stress, but the psoriasis patients feel considerably more stigmatized. It is conspicuous that there is no dif-

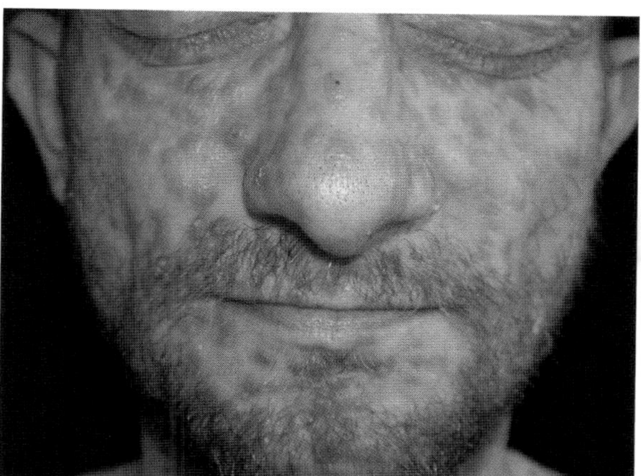

Fig. 5.4 Secondary syphilis (lues II)

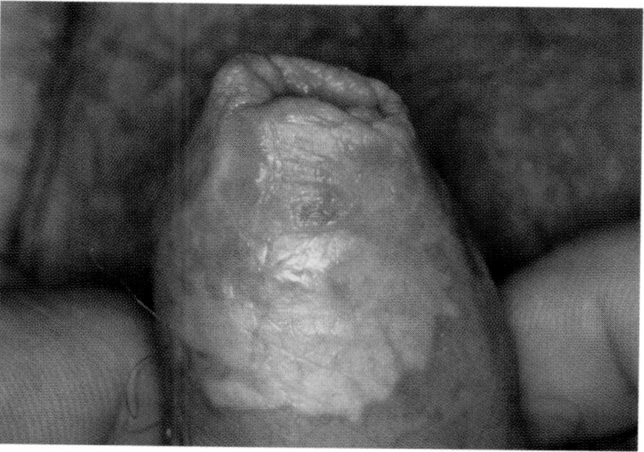

Fig. 5.5 Patient with lichen sclerosus et atrophicus on the penis and massive fear of rejection in a sexual relationship

5

ference between the groups examined with respect to coitus frequency.

The negative assessment of skin diseases is also expressed in the attitude of people with healthy skin. Disgust is a frequent association with skin diseases. Hornstein et al. (1973) determined that two-thirds of the people with healthy skin questioned were reluctant to visit a dermatology clinic. Often, they saw a parallel between skin diseases and venereal diseases and said that the cause of skin diseases was "lack of hygiene" and "frequent change of sex partner." The danger of contamination by shaking hands alone was considered high by half of those questioned.

References

Hornstein OP, Brückner GW, Graf U (1973) Social evaluation of skin diseases in the population. Methods and results of an informing inquiry. Hautarzt 24(6): 230–235

Niemeier V, Winckelsesser T, Gieler U (1997) Skin disease and sexuality. An empirical study of sex behavior or patients with psoriasis vulgaris and neurodermatitis in comparison with skin-healthy probands. Hautarzt 48(9): 629–633

Further Reading

Dorssen IE van, Boom BW, Hengeveld MW (1992) Experience of sexuality in patients with psoriasis and constitutional eczema. Ned Tijdschr Geneeskd 136(44): 2175–2178

Musaph H (1977) Skin, touch and sex. In: Money J, Musaph H (eds) Handbook of sexology. Elsevier, Amsterdam, pp 1157–1165

Niemeier V, Gieler U (2003) Skin and sexuality. In: Koo J, Lee CS (eds) Psychocutaneous medicine. Dekker, New York, pp 375–382

Pasini W (1984) Sexologic problems in dermatology. Clin Dermatol 2: 59–65

Spector JP, Carrey MP (1990) Incidence and prevalence of the sexual dysfunctions: a critical review of the empirical literature. Arch Sex Behav 19: 389–408

6 Cosmetic Medicine

The overall state of health has significantly improved, especially in the economically privileged middle and upper classes (World Health Organization 2001). Simultaneously, the public's expectations of medicine and the demand for beauty and rejuvenation have markedly increased in the Western industrialized nations (Wijsbek 2000). The economic situation in industrialized nations allows ever increasing numbers of individuals to fulfill their wishes for medical aesthetic procedures. This has been accompanied in recent years by advertising campaigns and repeated reports in private print media and on television and the Internet, producing ever changing fashion and beauty ideals.

The current ideals in Western industrialized nations are leading in dermatology to an increasingly broad and also lucrative subspecialization in cosmetic dermatology (Fig. 6.1). The dermatologist is consulted because of the central desire for youth and beauty.

Botox and filler injections, laser therapy, microdermabrasion, and chemical peels accounted for 6,635,250 aesthetic cosmetic procedures performed in the year 2005, as reported by the American Society for Aesthetic Plastic Surgery (Table 6.1).

Moreover, the technical and pharmaceutical industries are undertaking an increasing number of research projects to develop new lasers and lifestyle medications. Their popularity is then spread by advertising campaigns and lifestyle media as the fashion-related ideals of beauty change.

The people involved often have an exact idea of the procedures they wish to obtain from the dermatologist, such as filler application, skin resurfacing, dermablation, chemical peels, and botulinum-A therapy. The doctor–patient contact is often established with the clear intention of obtaining a defined desired therapy.

Questions about side effects of the methods applied are asked in relatively few cases, and risk is accepted here more than in any other area of medicine. Among the risks reported are complications after liposuction or laser therapy, abusive use of tanning salons, allergic contact dermatitis after procedures such as tattooing, and foreign-body granulomas and infections after piercing

Table 6.1 Aesthetic cosmetic procedures in 2005; data from the American Society for Aesthetic Plastic Surgery

Type of procedure	Number
Wrinkle treatment by laser surgery	271,000
Wrinkle treatment with Botox	3,800,000
Liposuction	324,000
Hyaluronic acid injections	778,000
Sclerotherapy	590,000
Lid correction	231,000
Breast enlargement	291,000
Nose correction	298,000
Chemical peels	1,000,000
Breast reduction	114,000
Face-lift	109,000
Laser hair removal	783,000
Microdermabrasion	838,000

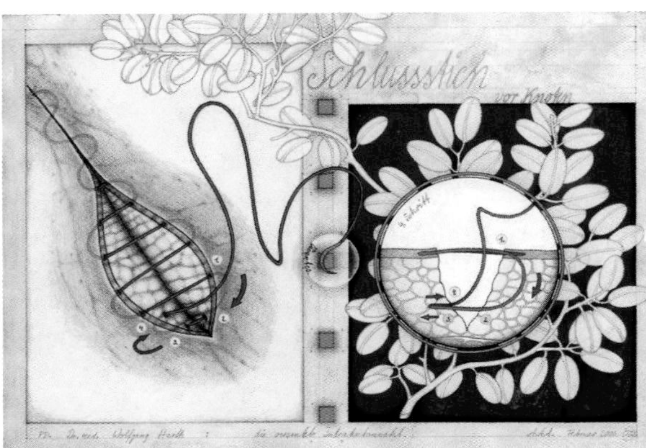

Fig. 6.1 Aesthetic medicine

(Fig. 6.2). However, this group of patients is also characterized by a considerable proportion of primary or secondary emotional disorders that should be recognized by the health care provider and adequately addressed. Often there are somatoform disorders, or the procedure may be done to please a third party. Frequently, the underlying emotional disorder is not readily recognized, so several repeated interviews prior to invasive cosmetic procedures may be needed, with more detailed care initiated in a special liaison consultation if an emotional disorder is suspected. In dermatological cosmetology, particular attention must be paid to body dysmorphic disorder (Sect. 1.3.2), which must be ruled out.

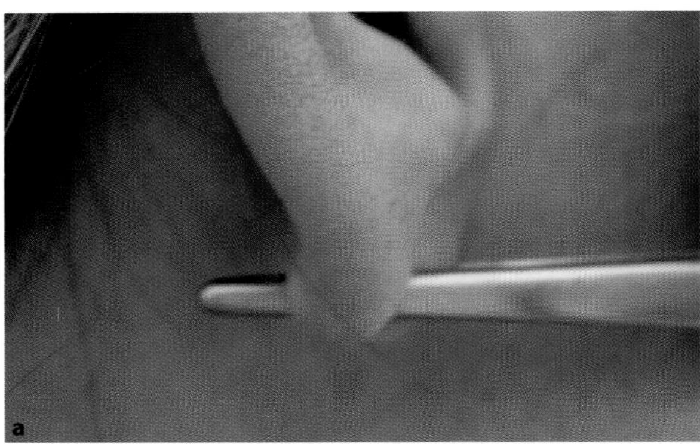

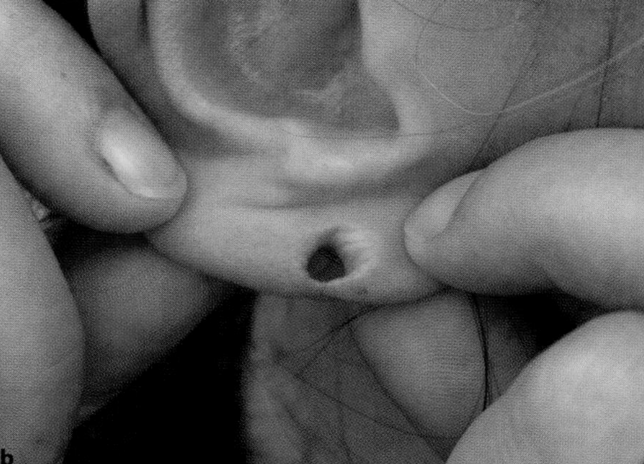

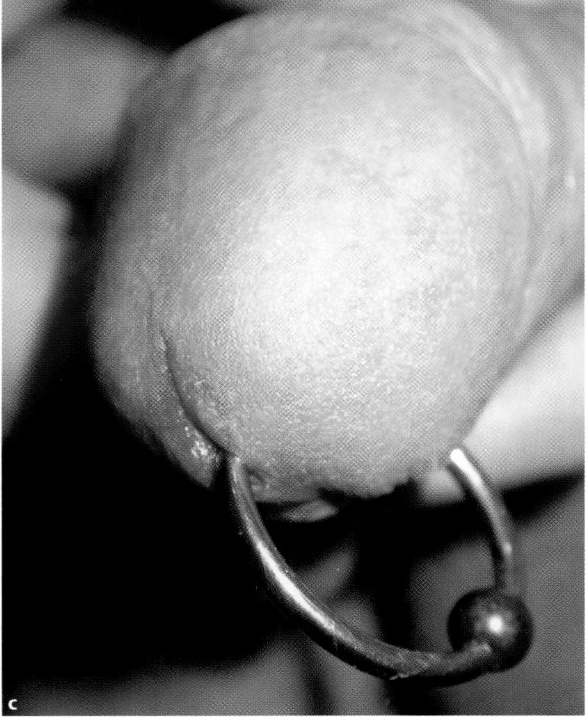

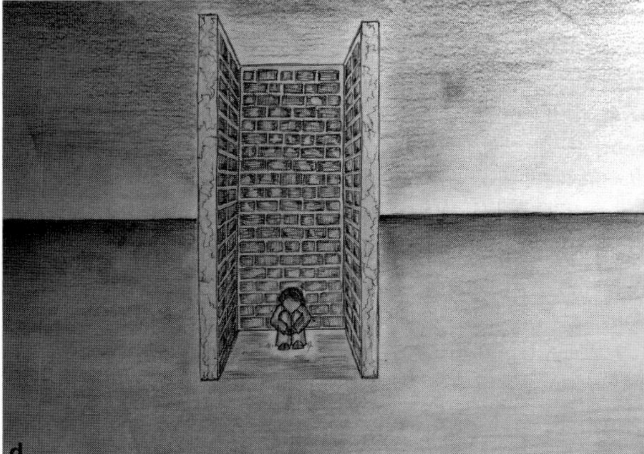

Fig. 6.2 a,b Views of skin lesion as a sequela of traumatization by costume jewelry. **c** Genital piercing. **d** Body dysmorphic disorder: hidden lonely place depicted in art therapy

Need and Indication: the Doctor in a Jam

In body dysmorphic disorder, the desire for therapy with lifestyle medications or operations is an attempt to stabilize emotional equilibrium with the help of a drug or the scalpel (Bishop 1983; Cash 1992) and to achieve a pseudosolution at the organic level. These individuals interpret mild, brief symptoms or even physiological body functions (sweating, hair cycle, heartbeat) as illnesses.

> **Misinterpretations by Healthy People in Medicine**
>
> - Risks become illnesses: cholesterol, bone calcium loss
> - Mild or brief symptoms become illnesses: pain, flatulence, erection disorders
> - Physiological body functions become diseases: sweating, hair cycle, heartbeat
> - Psychosomatic problems are taken for purely somatic diseases: body dysmorphic disorders, somatoform disorders, compulsive disorders, somatization disorders

"Medicalization" of physiological life is then expected to solve psychosocial problems. The demand by healthy people for therapy, but especially in cases in which an emotional disorder cannot be completely ruled out, puts emotional pressure on the doctor in the ambivalence between insistence and lack of indication. This is medication abuse in a broad sense. Central and important is the early and adequate determination of indication (Brin 1997), and the doctor should refuse to provide the desired treatment if in doubt.

Two main areas of cosmetic medicine can be differentiated: cosmetic surgery procedures (both invasive and noninvasive) and lifestyle drugs.

Psychosomatic Disturbances and Cosmetic Surgery

In no other field of medicine does the decision for surgery depend on biopsychosocial aspects as it does in establishing the indication for elective aesthetic surgery. Reich showed that in a group of 750 patients seeking correction of their outward appearance, 62% were emotionally unstable and 2% had unrealistic expectations (Reich 1982). Fashion-dependent lifestyle factors and trends in our Western culture play a major role. Ohlsen et al. found in 1979 that 81% of women considering breast augmentation got the idea from from the media. Requesting surgery can be a substitute solution for mental problems, with underlying psychosocial conflicts being suppressed.

In elective cosmetic treatment, even more attention must be paid to contraindications and complications than in medically indicated surgery, and this must be included in the detailed preoperative patient information. For example, the typical risks of liposuction include permanent asymmetry, skin dimpling, altered skin pigmentation, sensory disturbances, infections, seromas, scars, and bleeding. Serious complications such as pulmonary embolism, hematogenic shock, sepsis, or death occur in 0.1–0.2% of cases (Lehnhardt et al. 2003).

The question of operating or not operating in aesthetic surgery is, as in no other field of medicine, dependent on the patient's conscious and unconscious emotional motivations, and thus the psychosocial background must also be considered. Several studies have shown an incidence of emotional disturbances in connection with aesthetic surgical procedures of up to 47.7% in Japan (Ishigooka et al. 1998). In a French study (Meningaud et al. 2001), up to 50% of patients had previously used psychopharmacologic agents, especially antidepressants (27%). Studies in women undergoing breast augmentation reveal a two- to threefold higher rate of suicide compared with the normal population (McLaughlin et al. 2003). The spectrum of emotional disturbances in aesthetic surgery is quite heterogeneous and can range from mild adjustment disorders to severe psychiatric diseases. The most important disorders reported in the literature are outlined in Table 6.2. They can be classified into primary and secondary disturbances.

Possible Psychosomatic/Mental Disorders

Reactive Disorders and Adjustment Disorders

In cases of objective disfigurement such as congenital defects, scars, keloids, or neoplasia, secondary reactive mental disturbances as well as subjective suffering, and reduced quality of life often occur (Crisp 1981). Reactive disorders can appear as acute stress reactions or in a delayed manner as posttraumatic stress disorder. Among burn patients, depression was found in up to 23% and posttraumatic stress disorder in 45% (Van Loey and Van Son 2003).

If prior emotional vulnerability exists, an adjustment disorder is possible. Adjustment disorders are heterogeneous and can be characterized by desperation, depressive reaction, anxiety, and, finally, social withdrawal.

Table 6.2 Mental disorders associated with aesthetic surgery

Primary mental disorders
Psychiatric disorders • Affective/bipolar disorder (F30–F39) • Factitious disorders/Münchhausen syndrome (F68.1) • Schizophrenia/body dysmorphic delusion (F20–F29) • Intentional self-harm (suicide) (X60–X84)
Social phobia (anxiety disorders F40)
Somatoform disorders (F45) • Hypochondriasis (F45.2) • Body dysmorphic disorder (F45.2) • Somatization disorder (multiple complaints of physical illness) (F45.0)
Personality disorder (F60) • Emotionally unstable personality disorder (borderline disorder) (F60.3) • Narcissistic personality disorder (F60.8) • Obsessive-compulsive personality disorder (F60.5)
Secondary mental disorders and comorbidities
Reactions to severe stress (F43) • Acute stress reaction (F43.0) • Posttraumatic stress disorder (F43.1) • Adjustment disorder (F43.2)
Comorbidities • Anxiety disorder/social phobia (F40)
Depressive disorder (F30–39)

A clear indication usually exists for reconstructive plastic surgery on the basis of physical findings.

With concomitant reactive emotional disturbances, aesthetic surgery can lead to cure or improvement of associated signs and symptoms (Honigman et al. 2004). Surgery that fulfills the patient's expectations can lead to higher self-esteem, improved quality of life, and self-assurance at work as well as self-assurance in a partnership. Women with breast reduction surgery showed the greatest improvement in postoperative quality of life of all aesthetic surgical procedures (Freire et al. 2004).

When the emotional disturbance stands in the forefront, even successful surgery can lead to destabilization of the psychological status.

This can occur when emotional problems are blamed on a physical defect, which then becomes an excuse for the psychological problem.

Comorbidity

A coexisting emotional problem can have a great influence on the motivation for and outcome of elective surgery for a definite physical problem. Because mental disturbances such as affective disorders (6.3%), anxiety disorders (9%), and somatoform disorders (7.5%) have a high prevalence in the German population, as in other countries, they have to be considered as comorbidities alongside the physical defects. In numerous international studies, groups undergoing elective surgical treatment display significantly higher rates of coexisting mental disease (Ishigooka et al. 1998).

Depressive Disorders

In elective surgical treatment, affective disorders are particularly prominent, at 20% (Meningaud et al. 2001). The main symptoms of affective disorders are depressed mood, loss of interest or happiness, lack of motivation, and rapid fatigue. The spectrum of depression ranges from mild, temporary disturbances to severe psychotic disorders with suicidal ideation. Additional symptoms of depression, according to ICD-10, are reduced self-esteem or self-confidence, feelings of guilt or uselessness, a negative or pessimistic outlook on the future, reduced vigilance, and ideation of or attempted suicide.

In aesthetic medicine, special attention must be paid to additional symptoms and disturbed body image with reduced self-esteem, as these draw the motivation for elective aesthetic surgical treatment into question.

Anxiety Disorders

Anxiety before surgery is a common phenomenon. Patients undergoing elective aesthetic surgery have higher anxiety scores in comparison to patients undergoing plastic reconstructive surgery (Sonmez et al. 2005). Preoperative panic disorders (ICD-10:F41.0) can occur with clearly demarcated episodes of intensive anxiety or uneasiness, palpitations, rapid pulse, sweating, trembling, shortness of breath or respiratory distress, fear of death, paresthesia, numbness, hot flushes, or chills.

Nonspecific diffuse or generalized anxiety disorder (ICD-10:F41.1) is differentiated from acute panic disorders. It is characterized by excessive chronic anxiety, fearful expectations, motor tension, and vegetative irritability.

Social Phobias

A special form of anxiety that can play a role in disfigurement and elective cosmetic surgery is social phobia (ICD-10:F40.1). Here, the anxiety reaction focuses on the fear of judgmental observation by individuals or groups. Furthermore, certain social situations are avoided with resulting psychosocial isolation and chronic disturbance of relationships.

Primarily pure social phobias without physical defects are usually associated with low self-esteem and fear of criticism and can be the prime motive for requesting aesthetic surgical treatment.

A body dysmorphic disorder could be diagnosed in 11% of patients with social phobia (Hollander and Aronowitz 1999).

When a mental disorder is projected onto a presumptive physical defect, a "corrective" procedure is contraindicated.

The surgery should be refused, as it is likely to worsen the primarily mental symptoms.

Obsessive-Compulsive Disorders

In connection with cosmetic surgery, patients often report continual preoccupation with their outward appearance. In obsessive-compulsive disorders, either obsessive thoughts (ICD-10:F42.0), compulsive behavior (ICD-10:F42.1), or mixed symptoms (ICD-10:F42.2) exist. Obsessive thoughts can be defined as repeated and continual thoughts, impulses, and imaginations regarding aesthetic factors that are perceived as obtrusive and inappropriate and cause much anxiety and great discomfort.

Compulsive behavior includes repeated aesthetic procedures, including requested elective surgery, highly repetitive skin care, or control of outward appearance.

Hour-long care, such as combing of hair, compulsive control of hair in front of the mirror, and touching, is performed. When no objective defect is present, a somatoform disorder must be excluded.

Somatoform Disorders

By definition, the characteristic of somatoform disorders (ICD-10:F45) is the repeated presentation of physical symptoms in connection with the persistent demand for medical diagnosis (therapy) despite repeated negative results and assurance by the physician that symptoms have no organic basis. Among patients that requested cosmetic surgery, the subgroups of somatization disorder (F45.0) and dysmorphophobia (F45.2; body dysmorphic disorder) as a special hypochondriac disorder are important. Divergent opinions on the question "to operate or not to operate?" may exist here, leading to conflicts in the physician–patient relationship.

Somatization Disorder (Multiple Complaints of Physical Illness)

Somatization disorders encompass a pattern of recurrent, multiple physical complaints that lead to medical treatment or surgery. Often one finds a combination of pain and various gastrointestinal, sexual, and pseudoneurological symptoms.

Hypochondriasis/Body Dysmorphic Disorder

Hypochondriasis (ICD-10:F45.2) denotes continual preoccupation with the fear or conviction of having one or multiple severe or progressive bodily diseases. In a study of 415 patients in Japan seeking cosmetic surgery, every 10th patient exhibited a hypochondriacal disorder (Ishigooka et al. 1998). In aesthetic medicine, physiological processes (sweating, hair growth cycle) are often interpreted by healthy patients as disease, and the aging process is denied or misinterpreted.

In hypochondriacal preoccupation with outward appearance, a body dysmorphic disorder might be present.

Body Dysmorphic Disorder (Dysmorphophobia)

Some patients requesting cosmetic procedures may present with nonobjective symptoms and have a body dysmorphic disorder. Despite no objective physical defect, a subjective perception of disfigurement exists. The definition of body dysmorphic disorder includes as a central criterion the preoccupation with a defect or disfigurement of outward appearance. This defect is either nonexistent or minimal.

In the field of aesthetic medicine, patients with body dysmorphic disorder constitute the most frequent and important problem.

The prevalence of body dysmorphic disorder in the entire American population is estimated at 1% and in American and German study collectives up to 4% (Bohne et al. 2002), and among patients seeking cosmetic surgery it is estimated to be up to 15% (Glaser and Kaminer 2005).

The spectrum of presumed defects is highly variable and includes the quality and quantity of skin and skin appendages as well as asymmetry and disproportionality. Patients often complain of presumed hair loss or hypertrichosis, pigmentation disorders, pore size, vascular images, paleness, erythema, or sweating as abnormalities.

Patients with body dysmorphic disorder often request elective treatment. In a study of 289 patients with body dysmorphic disorder (DSM-N), 45.2% of adults had already undergone dermatologic and 23.7% surgical intervention without improvement of symptoms (Phillips et al. 2001). Because subjective judgment is crucial in aesthetic medicine, a patient with a body dysmorphic syndrome might, due to the different appearance postoperatively, find the results unusual and disturbing and view a good surgical outcome as a failure.

For these reasons, body dysmorphic disorders are an absolute contraindication for elective aesthetic treatment (Fig. 6.2d).

Personality Disorders

In some individuals seeking elective cosmetic surgery, a personality disorder may be present and influence the surgical outcome. In histrionic personality disorder, a consistent pattern with excessive emotion and desire for attention exists. The main feature of obsessive-compulsive personality disorder is thorough perfectionism and inflexibility. Narcissistic personality disorder is characterized by fantasized greatness with concomitant sensitivity to the judgment of others. Other personality disorders include dependent, anxious-reluctant, paranoid, and schizoid forms. Particular attention must be paid to the recently more often reported emotionally unstable personality disorder (borderline disorder).

Emotionally unstable personality disorder is one of the most difficult mental diseases confronted in elective surgery. The main feature of borderline personality disorder is severe instability in interpersonal relationships, in self-image and in emotions, often with intense impulsiveness. In dermatology one often sees factitial disease in such patients with self-injury, or the patient may attempt to involve the physician in the manipulations by demanding surgery. Characteristically, the phenomenon of splitting occurs, with belief in "good" and "bad" parts of the own body. The "bad" is to be removed by the surgeon so that only the "good" remains.

All mental and physical problems are attributed to the negative part of the body.

Polysurgical Addiction and Münchhausen Syndrome

In contrast to the anxiety many patients have before surgery, some patients seem to welcome surgery. Often a liking of or frenzy for surgery exists [formerly termed "mania operativa" (Küchenhoff 1993)] and can particularly be observed in elective cosmetic surgery. Patients enjoy the dramatic event of surgery because of the attention they receive from the surgical team or from friends and family. The diagnosis of the wish for nonindicated surgery can be presumed when there is a history of multiple previous surgeries with unclear explanations (Table 6.3).

Münchhausen syndrome (ICD10:F68.1) is characterized by the triad of wandering from hospital to hospital, pseudologia phantastica, and self-inflicted injury (Oostendorp and Rakoski 1993). In Münchhausen syndrome the physician can be misused as the executor of the manipulation.

The surgeon becomes the tool of a psychopathological attempt at a solution. After initially being idealized by the patient, the doctor can become the object of much anger as soon as he or she refuses to provide the requested treatment.

Regardless of whether surgery is performed or refused by the surgeon, in the further course a conflict can be actively staged ("expert-killer" behavior) so that the patient

Table 6.3 Alarm signals in aesthetic surgery

- Aggression, lack of insight, hostility, impulsivity, self-manipulation
- Idealization of the surgeon
- Life crisis, suicidal tendencies
- Pessimism, affective disorder, anxiety disorders
- Regression and childlike behavior
- Attribution of guilt or charges (toward other therapists)
- Secondary gain due to disease (especially attention by others)
- Somatization of mental problems (multiple complaints of illness)
- Carelessness (side effects), denial of reality
- Disturbed compliance, lack of independence
- Disturbed coping with the disease
- Treatment for the sake of another person
- Deep disturbance of self-valuing/self-image, self-valuing problems
- Overattribution: exaggeration of the physical defect
- Overidentification with the defect
- Unclear motivation
- Unclear previous surgeries
- Expectations of treatment that are too high

can free himself or herself from the role of the putative passive sufferer (Beck 1977). The pressure for surgery can unconsciously be based on the desire for self-mutilation, self-punishment, or partial suicide.

Primarily Psychiatric Disorders and Special Forms

Severe psychiatric disorders such as schizophrenia can exist in patients seeking surgery and are often evident and easy to recognize due to bizarre delusions or hallucinations (Lee and Koo 2003). Body dysmorphic delusion deserves special attention. Paranoid-hallucinatory, hebephrenic, and catatonic schizophrenia are differentiated, with each displaying various symptoms such as delusion, hallucinations, formal disorder of thoughts, disordered ego, affective disorders, and psychomotor disorders. Severe affective disorders can manifest as unipolar depression (major depression), bipolar disorder or mania, or long-term affective disorder. Mixed forms with schizophrenia and depression or mania appearing in rapid succession or together occur in so-called schizoaffective disorders.

! A high risk of suicide with mortal danger must be expected in depressed patients.

Suicidal tendencies must be asked about and excluded when establishing the indication for surgery. When appropriate signs of ideations of suicide or attempted suicide with acute suicidal tendencies exist, surgery is absolutely contraindicated, and immediate psychiatric treatment is necessary. In cases with chronic or reactive suicidal tendencies due to disfigurement or when there is a history of attempted suicide, the situation is more difficult, and the indication for cosmetic surgery should be made in an interdisciplinary manner in cooperation with a psychiatrist.

Indication for Cosmetic Surgery and Psychosomatic Disturbances

Considering psychosomatic components in the treatment concept before planned surgery will help surgical dermatologists or surgeons minimize dissatisfaction and litigation by the patient. If, despite this, the patient is operated on, the surgery cannot alleviate the (primary) mental disorder. Further destabilization and acute exacerbation of mental symptoms can occur. The patient is dissatisfied and complains excessively, up to the point of damaging the surgeon's reputation. Especially with the background of rising malpractice suits by patients following requested, often not indicated, surgery, dermatologists performing surgery may find themselves in unpleasant situations.

It is therefore advisable for those in the surgical disciplines to adequately consider psychosomatic aspects. Here in particular, preoperative idealization of the surgeon may convert to furious disappointment and pure hatred followed by litigation. Before performing elective surgery, the physician must check the indications (Table 6.4) very carefully and protect everyone concerned from false expectations. The patient must receive comprehensive information and counseling. At this point it should again be stressed how important it is to precisely document the information that the patient is given on the possibilities and risks of surgery. Photodocumentation can be of great benefit.

Research (Honigman et al. 2004) shows that risk factors for a poor treatment result include youth, male gender, only minimal deformity, previous unsatisfactory cosmetic surgery, unrealistic expectation of surgery, motivation for operation for the sake of another person, anxiety disorder, depressive disorder, and personality disorder (Tables 6.1–6.4). It is all the more important to exclude mental disorders from the outset.

Body dysmorphic disorder, in particular, is characterized by the discrepancy between the investigator's assessment and the patient's perception of the defect (objective and subjective). Diagnosis and follow-up of body dysmorphic disorder can be simplified by a visual analog scale (VAS) without much sacrifice of time ("2-min diagnosis"; Gieler 2003; Fig. 6.3).

The results of the VAS should be verified in a discussion with the patient. The first structured interview modules for screening for body dysmorphic disorder were developed in the United States and Germany in 1993 (Dufresne et al. 2001: Stangier et al. 2003; Table 6.5). If the answer to the first five questions is "yes", it is highly likely that the patient has body dysmorphic disorder, and elective aesthetic surgery should not be performed. An absolute contraindication exists if the additional questions are answered "yes." One should be particularly careful if professional failure or problems in social relations are attributed to outward appearance. The use of the VAS and a structured questionnaire can aid surgeons in diagnosing body dysmorphic disorder in clinical practice. In all cases, a mental disorder should be excluded, and if one is found, a psychotherapist should be consulted.

Table 6.4 Pros and cons: aids in decision making regarding requested surgery

Surgery: yes **Possible indications**	**Surgery: no** **Contraindications**
• No mental disease	• Mental disturbance
• High degree of torment	
• Objective physical defect	• No objective physical defect
	• Body dysmorphic disorder
	• Suicidal tendencies
• Realistic expectations	• Unrealistic expectations
• Feasibility of surgery	• Multiple unsuccessful corrective surgeries
• Acceptable risk	• Unacceptable surgical risk
• Improvement	• Impending deterioration

Table 6.5 Screening for body dysmorphic disorder

Key questions:

1. Do you believe that a part of your body is abnormal?
2. Have you ever been very concerned about your appearance?
3. Do you often and carefully view yourself in the mirror? How much time do you spend doing so?
4. Do you attempt to hide your defect with your hands, cosmetics, or clothes?
5. What effects does your preoccupation with appearance have on your life in the areas of your profession, social contacts, and partnerships? Have you neglected normal activities because of the defect?

Additional questions:

6. Do you expect a radical change in your life as the result of surgery?
7. Are you sometimes so desperate that you wish you were dead or want to harm yourself?

Brief diagnostics of body dysmorphic disorder

How strongly are your feelings about yourself affected by your appearance?

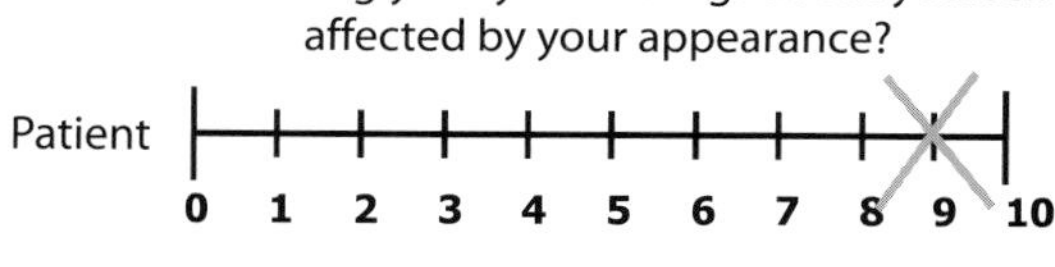

How strongly is the patient affected by his or her appearance?

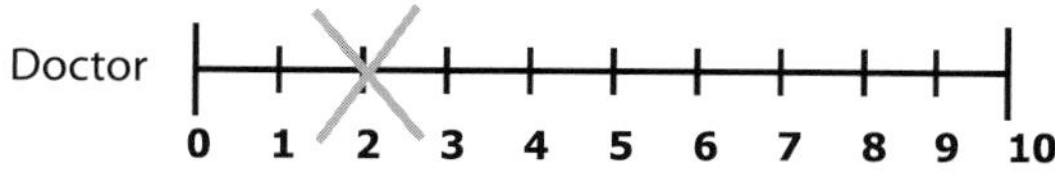

Body dysmorphic disorder likely

Fig. 6.3 Visual analog scale (VAS) for body dysmorphic disorder. The doctor and patient independently rate disfigurement and record severity on the optical VAS using values between 0 and 10 (with 0 meaning "no disfigurement" and 10 meaning "most severe disfigurement"). When a discrepancy of more than 4 points on the VAS occurs, body dysmorphic disorder is highly suspicious

Management of Psychosomatic Patients Requesting Cosmetic Surgery

When aesthetic surgery is sought, treatment of a mental disorder instead of surgery may be indicated, and the motivation to undergo psychotherapy may be the main treatment concept. Patients with a somatoform disorder present a particular challenge, as psychosocial factors connected with the patient's complaints are usually strictly denied. Successful referral to a psychotherapist is possible only in rare cases. In an optimized treatment plan, these patients might be treated in the office in a liaison consultation with a psychotherapist. If this is not possible, a psychosomatic approach through thematization of the psychosocial situation, consequences of the putative defect, coping with the disease, past experience with disease, severe stress situations, or provocative situations might be possible. The direction of the conversation is away from symptoms and in the direction of psychosocial aspects. Building a supportive relationship by taking the patient seriously and showing understanding of the complaints is fundamental in basic psychosomatic care.

In building a durable physician–patient relationship with broad biopsychosocial aspects in mind, structural psychoeducation with the aim of a working alliance with problematic patients has been successful. The basis of psychoeducation is imparting information through a biopsychosocial disease model. The question of when psychotherapy is indicated depends on coexisting diseases and existing conflicts as well as on the patient's motivation.

The efficacy of behavioral therapy with cognitive reconstruction in body dysmorphic disorder has been reported. The success of behavioral programs has been demonstrated in some studies with 2-year follow-up (McKay 1999; Wilhelm et al. 1999).

The indication for psychopharmacologic therapy depends on the mental disorder in the forefront and thus the primary symptoms to be addressed. A randomized, placebo-controlled trial has shown the efficacy of fluoxetine, a selective serotonin reuptake inhibitor (SSRI), for treating body dysmorphic disorder (Phillips et al. 2002).

! Requested cosmetic surgery can be successful only if biopsychosocial aspects governing motivation are taken into consideration. Mental disturbances must be excluded before performing aesthetic surgery.

References

Beck D (1977) Das Koryphäen-Killer-Syndrom. Dtsch Med Wschr 102: 303–307

Bishop ER (1983) Monosymptomatic hypochondriacal syndromes in dermatology. J Am Acad Dermatol 9(1): 152–158

Bohne A, Keuthen NJ, Wilhelm S, Deckersbach T, Jenike MA (2002) Prevalence of symptoms of body dysmorphic disorder and its correlates: a cross-cultural comparison. Psychosomatics 43: 486–490

Brin FM (1997) Botulinum toxin: new and expanded indications. Eur J Neurol 4:59–63

Cash TF (1992) The psychological effects of androgenetic alopecia in men. J Am Acad Dermatol 26(6): 926–931

Crisp AH (1981) Dysmorphophobia and the search for cosmetic surgery. Br Med J (Clin Res Ed) 282 (6270): 1099–1100

Dufresne RG, Phillips KA, Vittorio CC, Wilkel CS (2001) A screening questionnaire for body dysmorphic disorder in a cosmetic dermatologic surgery practice. Dermatol Surg 27: 457–462

Freire M, Neto MS, Garcia EB, Quaresma MR, Ferreira LM (2004) Quality of life after reduction mammaplasty. Scand J Plast Reconstr Surg Hand Surg 38 (6): 335–339

Gieler U (2003) Psychodynamische Diagnostik und Therapie der körperdysmorphen Störung. In: Stirn A, Decker O, Brähler E (Hrsg) Körperkunst und Körpermodifikationen. Psychosozial 26(4): 58

Glaser DA, Kaminer MS (2005) Body dysmorphic disorder and the liposuction patient. Dermatol Surg 31 (5): 559–561

Hollander E, Aronowitz, BR (1999) Comorbid social anxiety and body dysmorphic disorder: managing the complicated patient. J Clin Psychiatry 60 (suppl 9): 27–31

Honigman RJ, Phillips KA, Castle DJ (2004) A review of psychosocial outcomes for patients seeking cosmetic surgery. Plast Reconstr Surg 2004; 113 (4): 1229–1237.

Ishigooka J, Iwao M, Suzuki M, Fukuyama Y, Murasaki M, Miura S (1998) Demographic features of patients seeking cosmetic surgery. Psychiatry Clin Neurosci 52 (3): 283–287

Küchenhoff J (1993) Der psychogen motivierte Operationswunsch. Chirurg 64: 382–386

Lee E, Koo M (2003) Psychiatric issues in cutaneous surgery. In: Koo JMY, Lee CS (eds) Psychocutaneus medicine. Dekker, New York, pp 383–410

Lehnhardt M, Homann HH, Druecke D, Steinstraesser L, Steinau HU (2003) Liposuktion – Kein Problem? Chirurg 74 (9): 808–814

McKay D (1999) Two-year follow-up of behavioral treatment and maintenance for body dysmorphic disorder. Behav Modif 23: 620–629

McLaughlin JK, Lipworth L, Tarone RE (2003) Suicide among women with cosmetic breast implants: a review of the epidemiologic evidence. J Long Term Eff Med Implants 13 (6): 445–450.

Meningaud JP, Benadiba L, Servant JM, Herve C, Bertrand JC, Pelicie Y (2001) Depression, anxiety and quality of life among scheduled cosmetic surgery patients: multicentre prospective study. J Craniomaxillofac Surg 9 (3): 177–180

Ohlsen L, Ponten B, Hambert G (1979) Augmentation mammaplasty: a surgical and psychiatric evaluation of the results. Mammoplastik – the surgical and psychiatric evaluation of the results. Ann Plast Surg 2(1): 42–52

Oostendorp I, Rakoski J (1993) Münchausen syndrome. Artefacts in dermatology. Hautarzt 44 (2): 86–90

Phillips KA, Grant J, Siniscalchi J, Albertini RS (2001) Surgical and nonpsychiatric medical treatment of patients with body dysmorphic disorder. Psychosomatics 42 (6): 504–510

Phillips KA, Albertini RS, Rasmussen SA (2002) A randomized placebo-controlled trial of fluoxetine in body dysmorphic disorder. Arch Gen Psychiatry 59: 381–388

Reich J (1982) The interface of plastic surgery and psychiatry. Clin Plast Surg 9 (3): 367–377

Sonmez A, Biskin N, Bayramicli M, Numanoglu A (2005) Comparison of preoperative anxiety in reconstructive and cosmetic surgery patients. Ann Plast Surg 54 (2): 172–175

Stangier U, Janich C, Adam-Schwebe S, Berger P, Wolter M (2003) Screening for body dysmorphic disorder in dermatological outpatients. Dermatol Psychosom *4: 66–71*

Van Loey NE, Van Son MJ (2003) Psychopathology and psychological problems in patients with burn scars: epidemiology and management. Am J Clin Dermatol 4(4): 245–272

Wijsbek H (2000) The pursuit of beauty: the enforcement of aesthetics or a freely adopted lifestyle? J Med Ethics 26: 454–458

Wilhelm S, Otto MW, Lohr B, Deckersbach T (1999) Cognitive behavior group therapy for body dysmorphic disorder: a case series. Behav Res Ther 37: 71–75

World Health Organization (2001) World health report 2000, www.who.int/whr

Lifestyle Medicine in Dermatology

Lifestyle drugs have become more and more a part of our daily lives because of their widespread presence on the Internet, commercials, and television, and because of medical demands. They have become an important new group of medications that are taken to increase the individual's well-being and quality of life.

These drugs have also been labeled smart drugs, life-enhancement drugs, vanity drugs, and quality-of-life drugs and are influenced by fashion trends and private lifestyles.

6

In dermatology, the current focus of lifestyle medications is on skin rejuvenation, including antiwrinkle therapy, and on hair loss, as well as treatment for sweating. The additionally reimbursable services have caused a shift in the activity spectrum of many dermatologists to cosmetic medicine. Lifestyle interventions are an apparently harmless, noninvasive minimal therapy, but they may be detrimental in the presence of emotional disorders or if side effects occur (Table 6.6).

With the increase in press coverage related to lifestyle drugs in lifestyle magazines and television programs and the availability of information on the Internet, requests to obtain such treatments for well-being are rapidly on the rise (Lexchin 2001).

The increasing availability of drugs that can be used to alter appearance, physical and mental capabilities, or even character is changing the social fabric of our culture and poses a difficult challenge to our healthcare systems. It is also revolutionizing the traditional doctor–patient relationship.

A generally accepted definition of lifestyle drugs is not available in the current literature. Therefore, we propose the following (Harth et al. 2003):

Lifestyle drugs are those medications taken solely to increase personal life quality and to attain a current psychosocial beauty ideal, without a medical need for treatment.

Based on this definition, a pharmaceutical substance, such as a nootropic or SSRI, that has been approved to treat a specific medical disease could also be improperly used or abused without indication as a lifestyle drug to enhance well-being. Accordingly, a drug could be a lifestyle drug or not, depending on its use. Two types of lifestyle drugs may be differentiated:

1. Drugs approved for a specific lifestyle indication (e.g., baldness that is not a disease)
2. Drugs approved for specific indications but used for other purposes

Phosphodiesterase inhibitors, for example, are indicated for erectile dysfunction but are also used by young healthy subjects to increase sexual performance. Sometimes the male population has been driven by the unreal fantasy of a 100% controllable erection. As a consequence, somatizations of psychosocial causes of erectile dysfunction are observed, and otherwise "normal" occasional failures become a widespread disease. In this particular case, the drug becomes a lifestyle drug depending on where one draws a line to represent normal.

The use of lifestyle drugs in Germany was shown in one representative nationwide survey study (n=2,455) to be as follows (Hinz et al. 2006): psychotropic drugs, 7.3% (12.4% women 45–54 years); weight reduction, 5.3% (13.6% women 25–34 years); and hair growth, 2.4% (8.0% men 45–54 years).

In the United States, 3–10% of students take stimulating drugs during their final exams (Kadison 2005).

Among 1,802 visitors to 113 fitness centers in Germany, 13.5% confessed to having used anabolic substances at some point in time (Striegel et al. 2006). Besides health-threatening cardiovascular, hepatotoxic, and psychiatric long-term side effects, acne occurs in about 50% as an important clinical indicator of anabolic substance abuse (Fig. 6.4).

The users consciously accept known and frequent side effects such as possible cardiovascular complications of sildenafil. In recent years, additional rare side effects of phosphodiesterase inhibitors have been seen, including nonarteritic anterior ischemic optic neuropathy (50 cases) in the treatment of erectile dysfunction (Bella et al. 2006).

Increasingly, physicians are contacted with the request for a specific lifestyle drug. The ones most frequently asked for are lifestyle drugs for erectile dysfunction, increased sexual potency, or improvement of hair growth, and drugs for weight loss or appetite inhibitors for the regulation of body weight. Sildenafil was discussed in 0.5% (68 of 13,394) of consultations in general practice in London and orlistat in 0.3% (42 of 13,394). Nearly 20% of general practitioners thought such prescriptions were inappropriate (Ashworth et al. 2002).

The main drugs involved – all requiring a prescription from the physician – are discussed in the following section.

Lifestyle Drugs in General

Nowadays, lifestyle drugs are mostly represented by nootropics, psychopharmaceuticals, hormones, and "ecodrugs" (Hesselink 1999; see Table 6.6).

- Overweight is a central problem of our society. Orlistat and sibutramine are used to treat obese patients, but they are also used as lifestyle drugs in subjects with normal body weight. They function as inhibitors of gastrointestinal lipid-metabolizing enzymes. Possible side effects are pigment disorders, flatulence, bowel incontinence, and rectal pains (Halford and Blundell 2000).
- Antidiabetics such as metformin and lipid-lowering drugs (simvastatin, rosuvastatin, and cerivastatin) are popular substances that are also abused as life-

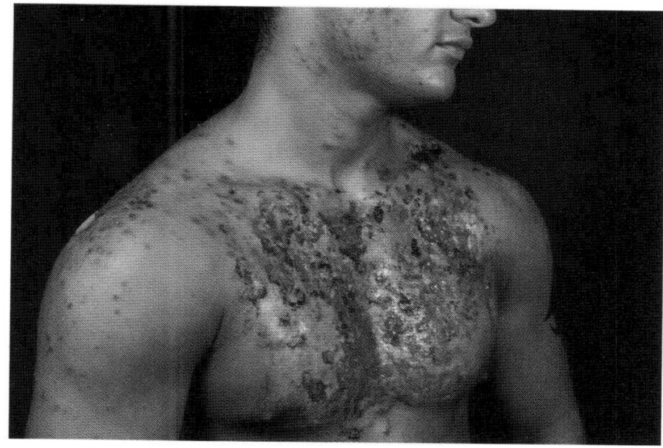

Fig. 6.4 Body-builder acne after taking anabolic hormones (Illustration provided by H.-C. Schuppe, from Assmann et al. 1999)

Table 6.6 Available lifestyle drugs (modified from Hesselink 1999)

Nootropics	Psychopharmaceuticals	Hormones	"Ecodrugs"	Others
Dimethylaminoethanol (DMAE)	Gamma hydroxybutyrate (GHB)	Dehydroepiandrosterone (DHEA)	Absinth	Dextromethorphan (DXM)
Hydergine	Ketamine	Pregnenolone	Echinacea	Metformin
Piracetam	Fluoxetine	Melatonin	Kava-kava	Propranolol
Pramiracetam	Selegilin	Desmopressin (DDAVP)	Herbal ecstasy	Coenzyme Q
Acetyl-L-carnitine	S-adenosyl-methionine (SAM)	Norethisterone	Ritual spirit	Orlistat
Oxiracetam	Methylphenidate	Contraception drugs	Guarana	Nimodipin
Aniracetam	Adrafinil/modafinil	Growth hormone	Chinese herbs	Centrophenoxin
Vinpocetine	Sibutramine	Anabolic steroids	Rose of Sharon	Clenbuterol
Idebenone	L-tryptophan		Vitamins	NADH
Vincamin	Serotonin		Minerals	Phenytoin
Cyprodenat	Dexfenfluramine		Amino acids	Deprenyl
Yohimbin	Ecstasy (MDMA)		Ginkgo biloba	Bupropion
	Ondansetron			
	Parlodel			

style drugs for weight reduction or to counterbalance high-fat meals ("the pill after the fat"). Lulled by the alleged safety of these medications, people indulge in uncontrolled binging, accepting imbalanced metabolism and unnecessary drug side effects.

- Psychopharmaceuticals, especially SSRIs such as fluoxetine (Prozac), are also taken as lifestyle drugs by persons in search of increased psychological drive or to facilitate social contacts or lose weight or obtain delayed ejaculation. Ritalin and atomoxetine (Strattera), indicated to treat attention deficiency syndromes, are improperly used as stimulants to increase alertness and improve intellectual performance (Teter et al. 2005). Benzodiazepines are also being widely used without proper indication.
- Modafinil (Vigil), a medication for the treatment of narcolepsy, is improperly taken as a lifestyle drug to prolong waking periods and alertness (Kruszewski 2006). In Germany, the prescription and use of this substance are regulated by the laws concerning narcotics.
- Donepezil (Aricept) is used for the treatment of Alzheimer's disease; currently, students take it as a lifestyle drug to increase cognition and improve learning, global function, and memory. But its real efficacy is questionable, and side effects are problematic.
- In Germany, andrology is a subdiscipline of dermatology. Hardly any other medication has raised worldwide such a broad and public discussion of private sexual behavior as has sildenafil (Viagra). A phosphodiesterase inhibitor for therapy of erectile dysfunction, it was introduced to the market in 1998. Meanwhile, in addition to sildenafil, new drugs including tadalafil and vardenafil with longer-lasting effects ("weekend pill") are available.
  The possible side effects of sildenafil must be considered, especially possible cardiovascular complications that may even lead to death. Some physicians have already admitted to using sildenafil in women, as sildenafil has demonstrated a dose-dependent effect in female sexual arousal disorder (Claret et al. 2006).
- Testosterone patches, transdermal systems, and injections have been used for substitution in deficiency syndromes. In the actual discussion of the "aging male syndrome," a decrease in testosterone is held responsible for a decline or loss of libido and for other complaints such as impaired general well-being, less muscle power, sleeping disorders, depression, and nervousness. However, scientific correlation of these symptoms to testosterone serum levels has not yet been proven. The new testosterone formulation (testosterone undecanoate) possesses long-term kinetics for application only four times a year, mimicking eugonadal testosterone serum levels without supraphysiological or subphysiological serum concentrations. The gel application, which has been available since 2003, is especially abused as a lifestyle medication without proof of pathologically reduced testosterone levels.
- In a randomized double-blind placebo-controlled study, the testosterone patch Intrinsa improved sexual function and decreased distress in surgically menopausal women, but it was not approved by the U.S. Food and Drug Administration (Simon et al. 2005).
- Bremelanotide (PT-141 nasal spray) is a hormone-like synthetic peptide melanocortin analog of alpha-melanocyte-stimulating hormone that is an agonist at melanocortin receptors. Its effect on female and male libido is currently being investigated. The preliminary evaluation suggests a positive effect on desire and arousal in women with sexual arousal disorder (Diamond et al. 2006). The erectogenic potential and its ability to cause significant erections in patients who do not have an adequate response to a PDE5 inhibitor suggest that bremelanotide may provide an alternative treatment for erectile dysfunction. It was safe and well tolerated in two studies, but the drug is still not available on the market.
- Growth hormones including somatotropin are available at low cost. The abuse of somatotropin by sportsmen is based on belief in its potent anabolic effects. Furthermore, it is considered a "fountain of youth" that will make those who take it younger and thinner (Van der Lely 2003). As a lifestyle drug, this hormone is currently broadly used to strengthen muscles, reduce body fat, decrease wrinkles, increase energy, and improve sexual life. Severe side effects, especially induction of diabetes mellitus and malignant neoplasms and facilitation of the progression of already existing lesions, cannot be ruled out.

Special Lifestyle Drugs in Dermatology

In dermatology, the current focus of controlled (prescription only) lifestyle drugs is on skin rejuvenation, including antiwrinkle therapy, hair loss, and sweating, and lifestyle drugs are requested to influence cosmetic findings, which usually are simply a result of the natural aging process of the skin or normal variants such as hyperhidrosis (Table 6.7). These patients believe that skin and hair should reveal youth and beauty at first sight.

In dermatology, lifestyle drugs are probably generally rather harmless and noninvasive, but they may be noxious if side effects occur.

- Vitamins, nutrient supplements, minerals, and skin creams have been aggressively promoted as being able to delay aging and prolong life. Vitamins A, E, and C are used in prophylaxis and therapy of skin aging. In vitro investigations suggest positive effects of the vitamins A, C, and E as potent antioxidants and partial stimulants of collagen synthesis. On the contrary, increased mortality was observed in people who consumed very high amounts of vitamin E (more than 1,000 IU per day; Schmidt 2000).
- Low-dose isotretinoin medication is used to overcome a physiological seborrhea and prevent a shining face. The side effects, especially teratogenicity and metabolic impairments, are disproportional to the desired effect as a lifestyle medication (Geissler et al. 2003).
- Finasteride (Propecia) as a typical lifestyle drug is used to treat androgenetic alopecia, which is not a disease in the proper sense. Finasteride is a 4-azasteroid, which inhibits the human type II of 5-alpha-reductase in the hair follicles and blocks the peripheral conversion of testosterone to androgen dihydrotestosterone. Reported side effects include reduced libido, a reduction in ejaculation volume, erectile dysfunction, and an increase in breast size (Libecco and Bergfeld 2004). Numerous new market launches can be anticipated in this area (Dutasterid: 5-alpha-reductase types I and II, latanoprost).
- Botulinum toxin is the neurotoxin of the anaerobic bacterium *Clostridium botulinum* and is used broadly in cosmetic medicine for wrinkles and sweating. It binds to presynaptic cholinergic nerve terminals and blocks the quantal exocytosis of acetylcholine at the motor and vegetative nerve ends (Harth 2001a). Botulinum toxin is responsible for the clinical signs and symptoms of botulism, a type of food poisoning. The use of botulinum toxin in aesthetic dermatology is a lifestyle medication "par excellence".

Psychosomatic Patients Requesting Lifestyle Drugs

The skin, as a visible organ, represents a special focus for the observation of physical symptoms. People consulting a dermatologist often have an exact idea of the desired procedure. Massive affects including anger and rage may arise in the doctor–patient relationship when healthy people aggressively demand a lifestyle drug of a prescription-only group and the doctor refuses because of contraindications or side effects. Initially the patient idealizes the physician, but as soon as the expectations are not met, the patient instigates a conflict, with the physician becoming an object of anger ("expert-killer" behavior).

Table 6.7 Lifestyle drugs in dermatology

Medication	Indication	Lifestyle abuse
Isotretinoin/tretinoin	Acne vulgaris	Dorian Gray syndrome (dream of eternal youth), inhibition of normal seborrhea
Minoxidil, finasteride	Androgenetic alopecia	Body dysmorphic disorder with unremarkable findings
Botulinum toxin, methanthelinium bromide	Hyperhidrosis	Suppression of normal exercise-dependent sweating, body dysmorphic disorder, sociophobia, shame disorder
Sildenafil, tadalafil, phentolamine, apomorphine	Erectile dysfunction	Eternal potency and 100% controllable erection
Testosterone	Testosterone deficiency	Midlife crisis
Somatotropin	Hypophyseal dwarfism	Maintenance of youthfulness, doping
Metformin, Crestor, simvastatin, orlistat, sibutramine	Adiposity, diabetes, hypercholesterinemia	Anorexia nervosa, Sisi syndrome

Additionally, however, the group of lifestyle drug users in medicine is characterized by a considerable proportion of emotional disorders. The question of using or not using a lifestyle drug without medical need is, as in no other field of medicine, dependent on the patient's conscious or unconscious emotional motivations; therefore, the patient's psychosocial background must also be considered.

Hair loss, especially the common androgenetic alopecia in men, is a frequent reason for consulting a dermatologist. With the introduction of the new lifestyle drug finasteride (Propecia) in January 1999, there has been a simultaneous increase in consultations of patients with somatoform disorders (body dysmorphic disorder) and regular scalp hair or with the wish of a preventive prescription for this lifestyle drug (Harth 2001b).

Patients with body dysmorphic disorder (preoccupation with an imagined defect in appearance) also seek costly treatment with botulinum toxin. The term "botulinophilia" was inaugurated as a new diagnosis to designate a body dysmorphic disorder of patients with subjectively experienced hyperhidrosis that objectively cannot be verified. In dermatology, patients with body dysmorphic disorder often request elective cosmetic treatment. In a study of 289 patients with such a disorder, 45.2% of adults had already undergone dermatologic treatment without improvement of their body dysmorphic disorder symptoms (Phillips 2002). Hence, lifestyle problems in medicine are partly characterized by somatoform disorders, the somatization of normal variants, and the desire for somatic therapy of psychosomatic disorders.

The relevant somatoform disorders in dermatology can be differentiated as hypochondriacal disorders, somatization disorders, somatoform autonomous disorders, and persistent somatoform pain disorders. These patients complain of numerous symptoms that cannot be medically objectified. A precise differential diagnostic division is necessary in order to initiate adequate therapy strategies.

Additionally, the concept of illness may be inappropriate. Physical variants, mild or brief symptoms (erection disorders), and even physiological body functions (sweating, hair cycle, heartbeat) may be interpreted as illnesses, or psychosomatic problems are taken to be purely somatic diseases.

This group of skin patients is often labeled with diagnoses such as "dermatological nondisease" (Cotterill 1996).

Usually, depressive disorders, anxiety disorders, and additionally compulsive disorders, sociophobic tendencies, or shame are predominant.

For example, patients with hair loss have lower self-confidence, higher depression scores, greater introversion, higher neuroticism, and feelings of being unattractive (Cash 1992). Patients with objectively normal hair often report an amount of hair loss that they subjectively deem disfiguring, and they suffer greatly from their assumed disease. The excessive preoccupation with an imagined deficit with objectively normal telogenic effluvium is called psychogenic effluvium in the sense of a body dysmorphic disorder.

Men with muscle dysmorphia among males with body dysmorphic disorder were significantly more likely to have abused anabolic-androgenic steroids (21.4%) (Pope et al. 2005). In one study, 48.9% of individuals with body dysmorphic disorder (n=86/176) had a lifetime substance use disorder (Grant 2005). Body-image pathology is associated with illicit use of anabolic-androgenic steroids.

A special form of body dysmorphic disorder is the wish of patients to stay young forever, termed Dorian Gray syndrome (Brosig et al. 2001). The name was taken from an 1891 novel by Oscar Wilde. Dorian Gray syndrome is associated with narcissistic regression, sociophobia, and the strong desire to maintain youth. Lifestyle medicaments are often used with the intention to stop or reverse the natural aging process.

The physician should consider the possibility of facing a patient suffering from a psychosocial disorder if the patient requests prescription of a lifestyle drug. In these cases, generous prescriptions of lifestyle drugs may lead to chronification of unrecognized emotional disorders. Patients with somatoform disorders will usually strictly deny a psychosocial relationship to the complaints reported.

Great resistance to psychosomatic models of explanation is generally accompanied by the expectation of a purely somatic treatment. Thus, the desire for therapy with lifestyle drugs is often an attempt to achieve an emotional balance with the help of a drug, thus attaining a pseudosolution of an unconscious emotional conflict at the organic level. Medicalization of physiological life is expected to solve psychosocial problems. But such treatment is doomed to fail if the causally significant emotional disorder behind the symptoms is ignored. Frequently, the underlying emotional disorder is not even recognized by the person affected and sometimes also not recognized by the consulted physician. When confronted with the diagnosis of an emotional disorder, the patient refuses to face reality, and the referral to a psychological or psychiatric outpatient service is very difficult.

The psychosomatic approach can be achieved by thematization of the overall current psychosocial situation, coping with the disease, earlier experience with disease, and possible serious eliciting situations. The question of when psychotherapy is indicated depends on coexisting diseases and conflicts as well as on the patient's motivation.

Lifestyle drugs need a precise indication, and the dermatologist must pay attention to possible abuse, long-term risks, complications, and side effects. Patients with psychological disturbances sometimes push aside possible risks and complications or deny side effects. Psychosomatic disorders must be excluded in the entire area of lifestyle medicine in any patient. Because patients with somatoform disorders often have strong expectations from somatic treatment, they consult the physician (dermatologist) first, and it is up to the doctor to make the early diagnosis of an emotional disorder to avoid chronification of psychosocial disturbances.
The use of lifestyle medications in an uncritical manner is contraindicated. Psychotherapy or psychopharmacological treatment comes first.

References

Ashworth M, Clement S, Wright M (2002) Demand, appropriateness and prescribing of "lifestyle drugs": a consultation survey in general practice. Fam Pract 19: 236–241

Assmann T, Arens A, Becker-Wegerich P, Schuppe HC, Lehmann P (1999) Acne fulminans mit sternoklavikulären Knochenläsionen und Azoospermie nach Abusus anaboler Steroide. Z Hautkr 74: 570–572

Bella AJ, Brant WO, Lue TF, Brock GB (2006) Non-arteritic anterior ischemic optic neuropathy (NAION) and phosphodiesterase type-5 inhibitors. Can J Urol. 13: 3233–3238

Brosig B, Kupfer J, Niemeier V, Gieler U (2001) The Dorian Gray syndrome: psychodynamic need for hair growth restorers and other fountains of youth. Int J Clin Pharmacol Ther 39: 279–283

Cash TF (1992) The psychological effects of androgenetic alopecia in men. J Am Acad Dermatol 26: 926–931

Claret L, Cox EH, McFadyen L, Pidgen A, Johnson PJ, Haughie S, Boolell M, Bruno R (2006) Modeling and simulation of sexual activity daily diary data of patients with female sexual arousal disorder treated with sildenafil citrate (Viagra). Pharm Res 23: 1756–1764

Cotterill JA (1996) Body dysmorphic disorder. Dermatol Clin 14: 457-463

Diamond LE, Earle DC, Heiman JR, Rosen RC, Perelman MA, Harning R (2006) An effect on the subjective sexual response in premenopausal women with sexual arousal disorder by bremelanotide (PT-141), a melanocortin receptor agonist. J Sex Med 3: 628–638

Geissler SE, Michelsen S, Plewig G (2003) Very low dose isotretinoin is effective in controlling seborrhea. J Dtsch Dermatol Ges 1: 952–958

Grant JE, Menard W, Pagano ME, Fay C, Phillips KA (2005) Substance use disorders in individuals with body dysmorphic disorder. J Clin Psychiatry 66(3): 309–316

Halford JC, Blundell JE (2000) Pharmacology of appetite suppression. Prog Drug Res 54: 25–58

Harth W, Linse R (2001a) Botulinophilia: contraindication for therapy with botulinum toxin. Int J Clin Pharmacol Ther 39(10): 460–463

Harth W, Linse R (2001b) Body dysmorphic disorder and life-style drugs. Overview and case report with finasteride. Int J Clin Pharmacol Ther 39: 284–287

Harth W, Wendler M, Linse R (2003) Lifestyle-Medikamente Definitionen und Kontraindikationen bei körperdysmorphe Störungen. Psychosozial 26, 4(94): 37–43

Hesselink JM (1999) Surfen mit Nebenwirkungen: Probleme rund um die Smartdrugs. Dtsch Med Wochenschr 124(22): 707–710

Hinz A, Brähler E, Brosig B, Stirn A (2006) Verbreitung von Körperschmuck und Inanspruchnahme von Lifestyle-Medizin in Deutschland. BZgA Forum Sexualaufklärung und Familienplanung 1: 7–11

Kadison R (2005) Getting an edge – use of stimulants and antidepressants in college. N Engl J Med 353: 1089–1091

Kruszewski SP (2006) Euphorigenic and abusive properties of modafinil. Am J Psychiatry 163: 549

Lexchin J (2001) Lifestyle drugs: issues for debate. CMAJ 15: 1449–1451

Libecco JF, Bergfeld WF (2004) Finasteride in the treatment of alopecia. Expert Opin Pharmacother 5: 933–940

Phillips KA, Albertini RS, Rasmussen SA (2002) A randomized placebo-controlled trial of fluoxetine in body dysmorphic disorder. Arch Gen Psychiatry 59: 381–388

Pope CG, Pope HG, Menard W, Fay C, Olivardia R, Phillips KA (2005) Clinical features of muscle dysmorphia among males with body dysmorphic disorder. Body Image 2: 395–400

Schmidt JB (2000) Neue Aspekte der Prophylaxe und Therapie des Hautalterns. In: Plettenberg A, Meigel WN, Moll I (Hrsg) Dermatologie an der Schwelle zum neuen Jahrtausend. Aktueller Stand von Klinik und Forschung. Springer, Heidelberg

Simon J, Braunstein G, Nachtigall L, Utian W, Katz M, Miller S, Waldbaum A, Bouchard C, Derzko C, Buch A, Rodenberg C, Lucas J, Davis S (2005) Testosterone patch increases sexual activity and desire in surgically menopausal women with hypoactive sexual desire disorder. J Clin Endocrinol Metab 90: 5226–5233

Striegel H, Simon P, Frisch S, Roecker K, Dietz K, Dickhuth HH, Ulrich R (2006) Anabolic ergogenic substance users in fitness-sports: a distinct group supported by the health care system. Drug Alcohol Depend 81: 11–19

Teter CJ, McCabe SE, Cranford JA, Boyd CJ, Guthrie SK (2005) Prevalence and motives for illicit use of prescription stimulants in an undergraduate student sample. J Am Coll Health 53: 253–262

Van der Lely AJ (2003) Hormone use and abuse: what is the difference between hormones as fountain of youth and doping in sports? J Endocrinol Invest 26: 932–936

7 Psychosomatic Dermatology in Emergency Medicine

Only a few isolated studies are available so far on psychosocial disorders in emergency centers. It is certain that, in addition to purely somatic diseases, somatopsychic (reactive) aspects may often play a decisive role – for example, fear of death during asthma crises or myocardial infarctions.

Overall, individual reports confirm that 50% of all patients in the emergency department present with emotional disorders or comorbidities (Klussmann 1999; Byrne et al. 2003). Purely emotional disorders with a predominant psychiatric disorder are present in 10–15% of the patients (Bolk and Wegener 1984).

Dermatological emergencies are generally rare. A single study has revealed that the proportion of psychosomatic disorders in dermatological emergency services is 13.5%, whereby a purely emotional genesis of the dermatosis was present in 4.5% (Harth and Linse 2003). Individual cases of purely emotional disorders, affect artificial disorders, and parasitic delusions as skin-related delusional disorder are rare. Usually, the emotional disorder occurs as a comorbidity in urticaria or atopic dermatitis. Anxiety disorders are in the foreground of emotional problems in more than 40% of the cases.

Thus, there is sometimes a great discrepancy in dermatological emergency care between the subjective symptoms and the objective somatic findings. Anxiety disorders are particularly common in allergological emergency services. An anaphylactoid reaction may be imitated by a panic attack and be psychogenically conditioned (Chap. 4). There may be pseudoallergies, as in undifferentiated somatoform idiopathic anaphylaxis, in which the anaphylaxis is purely emotionally caused without specific antigen–antibody interaction and with no response to corticosteroids.

Based on available data, a psychosocial causality, especially anxiety disorder, should be taken into account in the case of allergological emergencies that are difficult to classify, and psychosocial aspects should be considered to a greater degree in diagnostics and therapy. This is a long-term goal, since patients with psychosocial problems call rescue units several times each year. A biopsychosocial treatment strategy could be developed in cooperation with those providing dermatological emergency care.

References

Byrne M, Murphy AW, Plunkett PK, McGee HM, Murray A, Bury G (2003) Frequent attenders to an emergency department: a study of primary health care use, medical profile, and psychosocial characteristics. Ann Emerg Med 41(3): 309–318

Bolk R, Wegener B (1984) Emergency center patients from the psychiatric and psychosomatic viewpoint. Psychiatr Prax 11: 74–80

Harth W, Linse R (2003) Der psychosomatische Notfall in der Dermatologie. JDDG 1(Suppl 1): 163

Klussmann R (1999) Ongoing conflict situations and physical disease. Wien Med Wochenschr 149(11): 318–322

Further Reading

Moran P, Jenkins R, Tylee A, Blizard R, Mann A (2000) The prevalence of personality disorder among UK primary care attenders. Acta Psychiatr Scand 102(1): 52–57

Pajonk FG, Grunberg KA, Paschen HR, Moecke H (2001) Psychiatric emergencies in the physician-based system of a German city. Fortschr Neurol Psychiatr 69: 170–174

Windemuth D, Stücker M, Hoffmann K, Altmeyer P (1999) Prävalenz psychischer Auffälligkeiten bei dermatologischen Patienten in einer Akutklinik. Hautarzt 50: 338–343

Zdanowicz N, Janne P, Gillet JB, Reynaert C, Vause M (1996) Overuse of emergency care in psychiatry. Eur J Emerg Med 3(1): 48–51

8 Surgical and Oncological Dermatology

Cutaneous surgery has shifted into the focus of psychosomatic dermatology in recent years, particularly because of the increase in aesthetic surgical procedures. The recently established diagnostic criteria for body dysmorphic disorder have simplified the definition of indication in the field of aesthetic surgery.

Special Foci in Psychosomatic Surgery and Oncology

- Cutaneous surgery
  - Body dysmorphic disorder
  - Indication in aesthetic dermatology
  - Fear of operation
  - Polysurgical addiction
  - Münchhausen syndrome
  - Wound healing
  - Premedication
- Oncology
  - Fear in metastasizing tumor disease
  - Quality of life in metastasizing tumor disease
  - Interferon therapy: development of depression (comorbidity)

Cutaneous Surgery

The surgeon's presurgical activity in obtaining the patient's history is critical for defining the indication, operation, and restitution measures.

The definition of indication is the first step and is important in advance, including psychosomatic aspects, particularly if the indication is aesthetic, non-life-threatening, or urgently required and if there are relative indications for surgery that can be planned. Three main groups can be differentiated (Hontschik and Uexküll 1999):

- 1st-order relative indication: Health problems exist that could become threatening.
- 2nd-order relative indication: The disorder of emotional, physical, or social well-being does not definitely outweigh the risks of the operation.
- 3rd-order relative indication: The doctor and patient disagree about the procedure; if the procedure is to be forced, the surgeon must "pull the emergency brake."

Moreover, an increasingly litigation-prone society has led to more medicolegal consequences in the whole field of surgery. These include not only valid operative errors but, for example, disfiguring scars resulting from lifesaving procedures that can often be the cause of malpractice actions.

The definition of indication as well as patient information are central to preparation, particularly in cosmetic procedures with possible complications that could also be the topic of a subsequent lawsuit. From a psychosomatic point of view, this is especially relevant in the case of problem patients who aim to achieve apparent solution of their emotional disorder by means of the scalpel. If there is no somatic finding, a body dysmorphic disorder must generally be ruled out prior to the surgical procedure, especially in aesthetic medicine.

Body Dysmorphic Disorders

In body dysmorphic disorders, the individual is excessively preoccupied with a slight deficiency or a nonexistent disfiguration of his or her physical appearance (Sect. 1.3.2), and an emotional and social disorder predominates in the symptoms of the complaint.

If the patient desires an operation due to imagined disfiguration, surgery should be refused under psychosomatic aspects in body dysmorphic disorder. Therapy for the emotional disorder takes predominance in an adequate treatment concept.

Indication in Aesthetic Dermatology

The indication for surgery must generally be strictly defined in aesthetic dermatology. Compared with required operations, more intensive information about the surgery, focusing on possible complications and worsening of the findings, is needed in cosmetic procedures, and exaggerated expectations must be corrected, as done in the field of reproductive medicine. There are often repeated interviews prior to surgery.

! In aesthetic medicine, a very strict definition of indication and intensive information about the operation and possible complications are required.

This is furthermore necessary because aesthetics are subject to subjective judgment to a particularly high degree, and the patient may experience his or her altered postoperative appearance as unaccustomed and disruptive. Emotional disorders or comorbidities must be given special attention in this respect.

The following findings may hint at a primary emotional disorder in the field of aesthetic surgery:

Alarm Signals in Psychosomatic Surgery

- Exaggeration of the physical defect
- Impairment of self-image
- Body dysmorphic disorder
- Unclear motivation or "expecting too much" of therapy
- Affective disorder and anxiety disorder
- Somatization disorders (multiple other complaints)
- Acute psychosis
- Serious narcissistic personality disorders/borderline disorder
- Operation being done to please a third party

In treatment-on-demand, enormous pressure is often exerted on the physician. If the patient's wish for the operation arises from an emotional disorder, covert or open reproachful behavior must often be expected. If no concession is made by the doctor because of contraindications, enormous rage may sometimes arise, especially in the case of invasive aesthetic procedures.

But beware of performing operations as a favor. Emotionally disturbed patients in particular tend to exhibit derogatory postoperative behavior, to the detriment of the surgeon. Practical experience has shown that such problem patients – even with good surgical results – often remain very unsatisfied (see the section on expert killers in Chap. 17). Even if only for this reason, the indication for surgery in aesthetic medicine should be carefully examined with respect to the possible presence of an emotional disorder.

The operation is then expected to stabilize the patient's emotional instability. This false belief means that an unconscious attempt is made to achieve an apparent solution at the organ level that cannot succeed from a surgical procedure. If a body dysmorphic or other emotional disorder is suspected, the primary indication is for initiation of psychopharmacological and psychotherapy, depending on the underlying condition.

However, aesthetic operations may also lead to emotional healing in patients suffering from severely disfiguring dermatoses with serious adjustment disorder or sociophobia (Crisp 1981).

Fear of Operation

Anxiety disorder is one of the central emotional disorders in the framework of operations. The patient may have anticipatory anxiety or fear of death or fear of surgical complications, including fear of possible disfiguration. In addition, there may be anxieties about separation from the family due to hospitalization, financial losses, and adjustment disorders.

Regression and reactivation of earlier childhood fears may occur in patients who were hospitalized during childhood. Even slight trauma in the vulnerable childhood years often leads to emotional scars. But postoperative emotional disorders are also frequent, such as depressions and even transition syndromes, delirium, and acute psychoses.

Polysurgical Addiction

In contrast to fear of invasive procedures, some patients appear to look forward to operations. Whereas it used to be necessary to combat avoidance of surgery, the battle now is against the tendency or desire for surgery: "mania operativa."

The willingness to undergo surgery and body manipulations may occur in any combination, and artificial wound-healing disorders can result in alternating operations (Hontschik and Uexküll 1999). Patients with polysurgical addition are at risk of iatrogenic damage on the one hand and reinforcement and chronification of the emotional disorder on the other.

Emotional findings. Large studies on procedures are available from the field of abdominal surgery, which is most often confronted with these problematics. In women between 13 and 25 years of age, a histologically controlled misdiagnosis has been found in 44% of all appendectomies (Hontschik and Uexküll 1999). In these situations, the mothers played a decisive role in the emergency admissions, with openly aggressive insistence on surgery. Experience has shown abdominal pain to be the most widespread female form of physical expression of a life crisis. Such life crises occur especially on weekends, so appendectomies peak on Monday. After a new wait-and-see concept was introduced, the number of appendectomies with histologically verified misdiagnoses was reduced to less than 20%.

Polysurgical addiction and insistence on a surgical procedure may unconsciously express a desire for self-mutilation or self-punishment, similar to that found in patients with artificial disorders and Münchhausen syndrome. Deep-psychologically, sadomasochistic and suicidal tendencies are described in the patients (Menninger 1934), or narcissistic organ neuroses are discussed (Siebenmann et al. 1984). Splitting phenomena often occur, whereby the patient has a fantasy of a good and an evil area in his or her own body. The patient believes that the evil organ should be removed by the surgeon so that only the good remains (Figs. 8.1, 8.2). All emotional and physical damage to the body is attributed to the negative, passive part of the body. Such dissociative splitting phenomena (Sect. 3.3.5) occur especially in patients who have earlier experienced violence, which made the splitting necessary for self-defense.

Added to this is the desire for attention and care based on a lack of supportive emotional relational experiences on the one hand and self-punishment desires due to unconscious feelings of guilt on the other.

Patients can enjoy the dramatic event of an operation because of the attention they receive from the treatment team or family and environment. Even with the planning alone, the fantasy of an operation often has a relieving effect for the patient. Characteristic is the selection of the agitation field. Thus, surgeons are particularly selected because they are associated, in the fantasy of the emotionally disturbed patient, with the character traits of omnipotence for the surgery-addicted person.

The surgeon thus becomes a tool for the patient's psychopathological and false attempt at solution. The presumed cure by a surgical intervention is, however, doomed to failure and may strengthen chronic organ

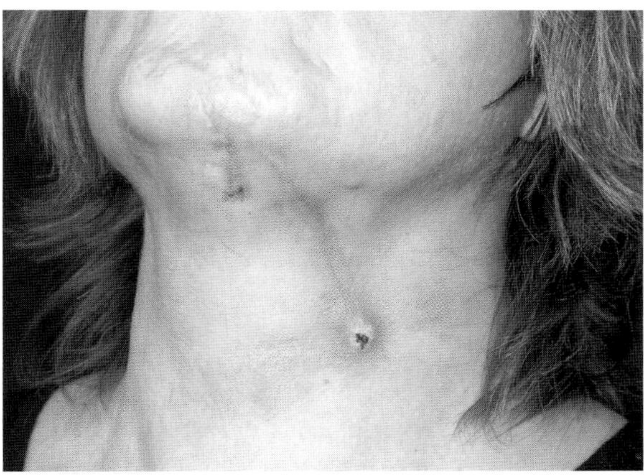

Fig. 8.1 Polysurgical addiction in a woman, with factitial scar caused by self-manipulation in borderline disorder. A 44-year-old woman requested removal of the lesion and scar correction. She had a history of eight previous surgeries in various hospitals in Germany and had contacted 11 university dermatology departments

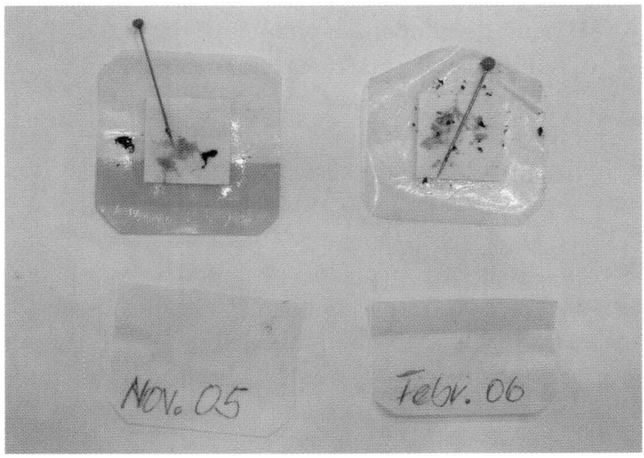

Fig. 8.2 Instruments to eliminate the "bad things" in self operations. These needles were used by the patient to manipulate her wound shown in Fig. 8.1. Staphylococci were cultured from both the needles and the wound

neuroses and reactive injuries or the experience of helplessness, even if the patient cannot recognize this in his or her current situation. The physician runs the risk of the patient's developing enormous rage after initial idealization, especially if the doctor refuses to be abused for delegated pathological self-punishment. Both when an operation is performed and when an operation is refused, there may be active staging of expert-killer behavior later (see Chap. 17), with which the patient attempts to free himself or herself from the role of the passive sufferer.

Diagnostics. The diagnosis of a desire for nonindicated surgery may be suggested in a history of multiple, unclearly necessitated operations and frequent hospitalizations. The record reported in the literature for this is a 52-year-old man with 423 hospital admissions (Küchenhoff 1993).

! Definition of the indication under biopsychosocial aspects is of central importance in preparation for surgery.

Dramatic and yet vague descriptions of symptoms by the patient are characteristic. In these cases, time is well spent in having the complaints described in detail in order to discover inconsistencies and incompatibilities with somatic evidence. Surgeons should be suspicious of dramatizing but vague descriptions of symptoms. A feeling of rage in the reporting is often an alarm signal and hints at an emotional disorder.

! Alarm Signals in Surgery

- **Dramatization**
- **Vague descriptions of symptoms**
- **A feeling of rage (in reporting to the doctor)**

The feeling that "something's not quite right here" may point the way for the physician to recheck the indication or bring it up for discussion with a team of experts.

Therapy. Refusing to do the operation and initiating broad psychosocial treatment strategies is the therapy of choice for the desire for nonindicated surgery. Initiation of psychotherapeutic interventions heads the list, but it is seldom possible because such patients usually lack the motivation.

! If the indication is relative or unclear, the physician should not be forced into surgery. He or she should provide the patient with written information several times and, if possible, wait and see what happens.

To provide psychosomatic primary care, it may be meaningful to make several appointments with the patient, for example at 14-day intervals, and to obtain a second opinion in advance from a psychotherapist. This procedure within liaison consultancy has proven beneficial. More detailed psychotherapy depends on the existing comorbidities.

According to available data and studies, the number of operations in pathological polysurgical addiction and body manipulation can be reduced after introduction of a biopsychosocial indication concept.

Münchhausen syndrome. The Münchhausen syndrome (Sect. 1.1.4) is characterized by the triad of hospital roving, pseudologia phantastica, and self-inflicted injury.

The patient's urge for self-manipulative destructive acts on his own body is expressed in the concept of expanded artefacts and additionally as a willingness to undergo surgery. The manipulation with the scalpel is delegated to the surgeon. A number of hospitalizations and surgical procedures, sometimes with visible multiple scars, is characteristic. Often there is an underlying borderline disorder.

Wound healing. Wound healing is also subject to numerous multifactorial influence factors. Among these are a genetic disposition (wound-healing impairments), self-damaging behavior (nicotine abuse, artefacts), or stress-induced negative influence on the immune system, which is decisive for wound healing. In one of the few studies available, stress showed a clearly negative delaying influence on wound healing in an animal experiment (Tausk and Nousari 2001). Hypnosis has been found to enable improved wound healing (Ginandes et al. 2003).

Thus, numerous different biopsychosocial factors are decisive for good wound healing. Coping with the disease is another factor. The patients logically feel hindered in their activities and worry more about their health. The secondary gain from disease that arises in many patients is especially problematic. Several studies confirm that improved training in independent wound care can improve the patient's quality of life (Augustin and Maier 2003). Attention must be paid to artificial wound-healing impairment in patients with unclear, persistent, and atypical impaired wound healing (see Sect. 1.1).

Premedication. Premedication in surgery can now be considered a routine measure prior to any procedure and is established as a standard to reduce anxiety, especially in the in-hospital setting. Short-acting benzodiazepines and nonbenzodiazepines, some with an amnestic effect, have proven beneficial (Chap. 15).

References

Augustin M, Maier K (2003) Psychosomatic aspects of chronic wounds. Dermatol Psychosom 4: 5–13

Crisp AH (1981) Dysmorphophobia and the search for cosmetic surgery. Br Med J (Clin Res Ed) 282(6270): 1099–1100

Ginandes C, Brooks P, Sando W, Jones C, Aker J (2003) Can medical hypnosis accelerate post-surgical wound healing? Results of a clinical trial. Am J Clin Hypn 45(4): 333–351

Hontschik B, Uexküll T von (1999) Psychosomatik in der Chirurgie. Schattauer, Stuttgart

Küchenhoff J (1993) Der psychogen motivierte Operationswunsch. Chirurg 64: 382–386

Menninger KA (1934) Polysurgery and polysurgical addiction. Psychoanal Q 3: 173–199

Siebenmann R, Biedermann K, Maire R, Oelz O, Largiader F (1984) Mania operativa. Schweiz Rundschau Med Prax 73: 1215–1221

Tausk FA, Nousari H (2001) Stress and the skin. Arch Dermatol 137: 78–82

Further Reading

Krause U, Eigler FW (1990) Artifizielle Krankheiten in der Chirurgie. Das Problem der selbstinduzierten Wundheilungsstörung Dtsch Med Wochenschr 115: 1379–1385

Oncology

Dermatological oncology comprises diagnostics and therapy of skin neoplasias, with which acute or chronic courses of emotional disorders may occur.

Emotional Problem Areas in Oncology

- Being informed of a negative diagnosis
- Coping with the disease
- Reactive adjustment disorders
- Manifestation of a premorbid emotional disorder
- Crisis intervention/suicidal tendency
- Care of and attendance on the dying
- Brain organic psychosyndrome
- Medication side effects
- Quality of life

The proportion of indications for emotional care in oncology is up to 50%, depending on the method of diagnosis (Strittmatter 2004; Sollner et al. 1998). It is certain that informing a patient of a malignant disease is an exceptional situation. A procedure taking biopsychosocial aspects into account in indispensable both in the acute situation and in long-term care, especially in serious metastasizing diseases. Several extensive main foci and shifting problem areas can be delineated here.

Informing a Patient of the Diagnosis

When informing a patient of a serious diagnosis, it is necessary to allow plenty of time, apart from situations of time pressure or stress. It is important to select language that the patient can understand. Sometimes a careful dosing of information, consequences, and prognosis must be made in order to not overwhelm the patient and to allow him or her to understand the full scope of the information. The doctor should ask questions about the patient's expectations, fears, and any unclear items and offer to involve persons close to the patient early on (Augustin et al. 1996).

Coping with Disease/Quality of Life

On being told of the diagnosis, the patient usually reacts with acute "shock" to some degree, which is then followed by beginning to cope with the disease (refer to the section on coping in Chap. 12). The following phases concern various degrees of coping with disease: shock, denial, intrusion, working out, and completion.

The treating physician should promote active coping in each of these phases, during which time a supportive holding function as part of psychosomatic primary care is usually necessary, taking the patient's personal coping style into account (Augustin et al. 1997). This often means that patients question all areas of their lives after learning the diagnosis and also reconsider their current life situations (job, spouse, themselves). Subsequently, a constructive new orientation is worked out. In individual cases the patient may experience an acute crisis with decompensation of an emotional disorder, or there may also be a resignation phase, especially in stressful long-term courses, that may even lead to accomplished suicide.

Increased attention has been paid to quality of life in recent studies of adjuvant therapy/chemotherapy of malignant melanoma in dermatological oncology. The polychemotherapies performed up to a few years ago have largely been abandoned, in part because of long-term poor compliance and marked limitations in quality of life with a lack of prognostic advantages.

Reactive Adjustment Disorders and Comorbidities

Within the framework of oncological diseases, adjustment disorders may occur that affect the problem areas of emotional symptoms, vegetative disorders (sleep disorders, loss of libido and appetite, pain), and work disorders. Acute stress disorders occur, as do posttraumatic stress disorders, so psychosomatic aspects must receive special attention in oncology in general. Pronounced fear of tumor, fear of metastasis and progression, and fear of death may occur, especially in an advanced long-term course of oncological care (tumor dispensaries; Trask and Griffith 2004; Zschocke et al. 1996). Representative of the central importance of fear is the following patient quotation: "Fear of what's coming is the greatest torment."

In addition is the fear of diagnostic and therapeutic interventions. Accordingly, premedication (anxiolytics), pain therapy, or adjusted tumor therapy is conducted. General personality disorders and affective disorders are also codeterminants. Premorbid depressive symptomatics or anxiety disorders may become manifest for the first time as complicating comorbidities in the framework of the tumor disease.

Interferon/Organic Psychosyndrome

Brain-organic psychosyndromes are another problem area, for example, as part of central nervous system metastasis or as side effects of chemotherapy. Serious neuropsychiatric side effects may occur in therapy with interferon alpha, usually with depressive or paranoid disorders that may even include suicidal thoughts and may require therapy adjustment if the side effects are pronounced. Citalopram (Cipramin, Sepram) as well as paroxetine have proven beneficial.

Care of the Dying

Care of the dying patient, pronouncement of death of a patient, and the subsequent discussion with family members is a great burden for the patient, the family, and also for the doctor. Emotional attention is required of the doctor, who is supposed to offer consolation and must continuously signal his or her willingness to provide this, often during the night hours. Physicians themselves can be brought to the end of their strength if, for example, despair, sadness, or discouragement are affectively discharged when they are overtired. One should not foster any false hopes. Just the doctor's presence may be a relief for the dying patient and provide him or her with a sense of security, usually when the family is involved. The family members also need to have an opportunity to take leave after the patient has died; this includes support and consolation from the doctor.

References

Augustin M, Zschocke I, Dieterle W, Schöpf E, Muthny FA (1997) Bedarf und Motivation zu psychosozialen Interventionen bei Patienten mit malignen Hauttumoren. Z Hautkr 5(72): 333–338

Augustin M, Zschocke I, Stein B, Muthny FA (1996) Der Betreuungsbedarf von Melanompatienten in verschiedenen Erkrankungsphasen – Formulierung eines psychosozialen Betreuungskonzeptes. In: Brähler E, Schumacher J (Hrsg) Psychologie und Soziologie in der Medizin. Psychosozial-Verlag, Gießen, S 7–8

Sollner W, Zingg-Schir M, Rumpold G, Mairinger G, Fritsch P (1998) Need for supportive counselling – the professionals' versus the patients' perspective. A survey in a representative sample of 236 melanoma patients. Psychother Psychosom 67(2): 94–104

Strittmatter G (2004) Psychosocial counseling of skin cancer patients in these times of diagnosis related groups (DRG). Hautarzt 55(8): 735–745

Trask PC, Griffith KA (2004) The identification of empirically derived cancer patient subgroups using psychosocial variables. J Psychosom Res 57(3): 287–295

Zschocke I, Augustin M, Stein B, Deußen-Wernicke T, Muthny FA (1996) Vergleichende Betrachtung psychosozialer Belastungsfaktoren bei stationären Patienten mit verschiedenen Hauttumoren. In: Brähler E, Schumacher J (Hrsg) Psychologie und Soziologie in der Medizin. Psychosozial-Verlag, Gießen, S 213

Photodermatology

9

UV Exposition

In recent decades, no lifestyle change has had such significant influence in dermatology as behavior modification regarding exposure to ultraviolet (UV) light.

Malignant melanoma has a variable morbidity worldwide, which can be attributed to geographic, climatic, socioeconomic, and ethnic factors, as well as migration and individual behavior (UV exposition; Dubin et al. 1986; Deutsche Dermatologische Gesellschaft 1987).

In our modern society (MacKie et al. 1997) the incidence of malignant melanoma has increased over the past 40 years (Osterlind and Moller Jensen 1986) as a result of altered vacation habits, such as frequent trips to tropic regions and increased exposure to the sun even in childhood (Sahl et al. 1995). In Germany there is strong evidence for a further increased incidence, highlighted by the findings of the Cancer Registry of the Saarland, which showed that as of 1995 (Statistisches Landesamt Saarland 1998) there had been an increase of 5% in men and 3,3% in women every year.

In part, this problem is due to the lifestyle ideals propagated by society (tanned skin equals success and/or beauty). On the other hand, adverse events occur due to sunlight, such as melasma, which may sometimes be co-caused by the presence of hormone dysregulation or exogenous light sensitizers in cosmetics (Fig. 9.1).

In addition, a number of photodermatoses involve marked limitations in quality of life and may lead to pronounced psychosomatic disorders.

"Light Allergy"

In addition to the so-called persistent light reactions and chronic actinic dermatitis, in which the skin reacts sensitively to sunlight and even artificial light, patients increasingly report so-called light allergies, which are associated with sociophobia and avoidance of public places and which make life a torment, cause the patient to despair, and may lead to suicide.

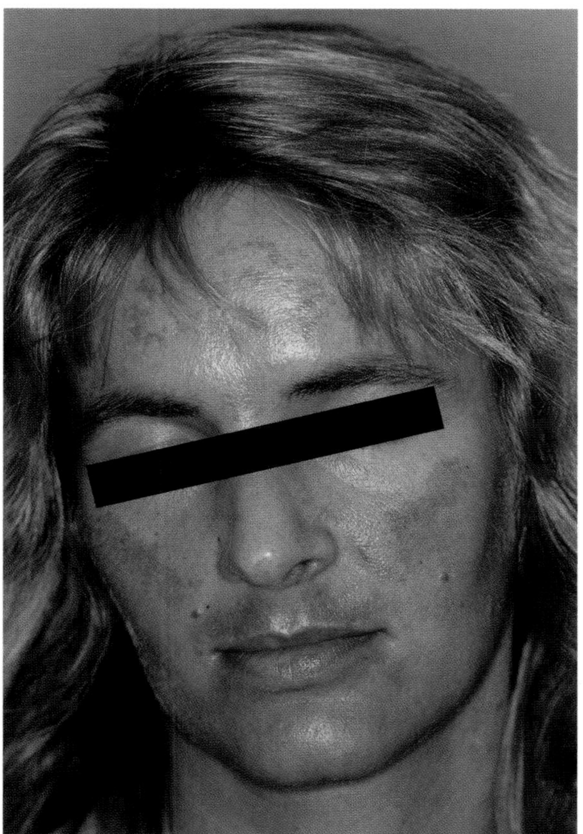

Fig. 9.1 Melasma patient with pronounced sociophobia and adjustment disorder due to light-induced brownish maculae on the face

A broad discussion of „light allergy" [synonym: Hannelore Kohl (wife of the former German federal chancellor) syndrome] was held in the public media after Hannelore Kohl committed suicide. According to the story in the media, her depression was the result of a light allergy that could not be treated by physicians. The members of the professional societies published several reports contending against the incorrect statement that light dermatoses cannot be treated.

In particular, the literature contains no reports of known suicidal tendencies in rare light reactions, such as patients with xeroderma pigmentosum or hydroa vacciniforme. These patients, whose disease is also known as moonlight disease because of the necessity of avoiding sun exposure, cannot lead normal lives; however, there is still no evidence that they regularly commit suicide.

Therefore, there must have been a comorbidity in Mrs. Kohl's case that led to her fatal despair.

The following diagnostic criteria belong to the biopsychosocial phenomenon of so-called light allergy:

1. **Presumed "light allergy"**
2. **Avoidance of public places (sociophobia)**
3. **Depressive disorder**
4. **Suicidal tendencies**

Depression or sociophobia may be present as comorbidities that arise secondarily through poor and negative coping. Patients with "light allergies" often have a somatoform environmental disease or hypochondria (Sect. 1.3), which hides serious depression and sociophobia from the environment under the mask of a light allergy (Fig. 9.2).

The body appears to act psychologically in a logical manner by sending the signal "no light exposure – no more public places"!

By means of cognitive processes, an initially physically existing light reaction can be taken unconsciously as a reason to react to every light.

Medicine has been experiencing an increasing number of patients in recent times who apparently react physically to the "hostile" environment, in this case light and the public. This phenomenon can be recognized in psychosomatic medicine when emotional conflicts and injuries can no longer be compensated. In this situation, the patient "somatizes"; he or she suffers from a disease that can neither be medically explained nor apparently treated.

Furthermore, the patient represses the underlying emotional conflicts that have led to the disease; thus, they are not revealed and made understandable and changeable for the person afflicted.

Treatment of the somatoform disorder and manualized programs to improve coping are in the foreground of psychotherapy.

Tanorexia

Indoor tanning is a common risk behavior with well-known health risks. Motives for UV exposure have been shown to be related to specific attitudes toward the tan

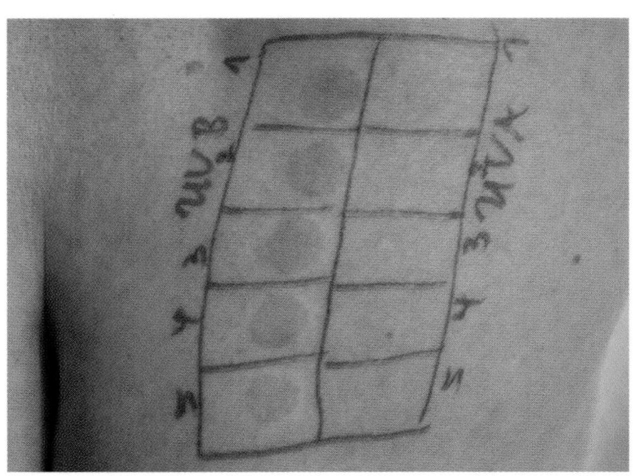

Fig. 9.2 Woman with presumed light allergy in depression. After testing and confirmed hypersensitivity using the UVB test, the patient unnecessarily no longer left the house because of her "light allergy," despite contrary advice from her doctor

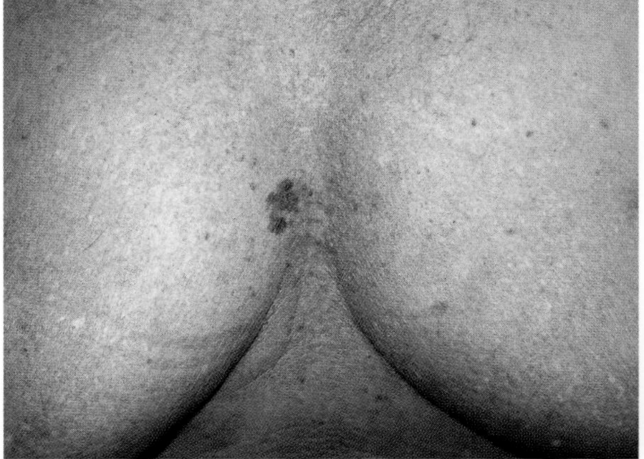

Fig. 9.3 Tanorexia with melanoma and severe light damage of the skin in a 48-year-old female hairdresser with many years of sunbathing and indoor light exposure (tanning booth in the hair salon)

appearance. In a study of college female tanners, six important factors were found: general attractiveness, media influence, influence of family and friends, physical fitness appearance, acne reasons, and skin-aging concerns (Cafri et al. 2006). Individuals who chronically and repetitively expose themselves to UV light in order to tan may have a novel type of UV light substance-related disorder. In one study, a significant proportion of college students demonstrated evidence of UV light substance-related disorder (Poorsattar et al. 2007; Fig. 9.3).

Furthermore, tanning is a relatively frequent behavior that is related to body dysmorphic disorder (Phillips et al. 2006). Among tanners, the skin was the most common body area of concern (84.0%). All tanners experienced functional impairment due to body dysmorphic disorder, and 26% had attempted suicide. Tanners were more likely than nontanners to compulsively pick their skin.

References

Cafri G, Thompson JK, Roehrig M, van den Berg P, Jacobsen PB, Stark S (2006) An investigation of appearance motives for tanning: the development and evaluation of the Physical Appearance Reasons For Tanning Scale (PARTS) and its relation to sunbathing and indoor tanning intentions. Body Image 3(3): 199–209

Deutsche Dermatologische Gesellschaft und Deutsche Krebshilfe (1987) Der entscheidende Punkt, Hautkrebs früh erkennen. Hamburg

Dubin N, Moseson M, Pasternack BS (1986) Epidemiology of malignant melanoma: pigmentary traits, ultraviolet radiation, and the identification of high-risk populations. Recent Results Cancer Res 102: 56–75

MacKie R, Hole D, Hunter JA et al (1997) Cutaneous malignant melanoma in Scotland: incidence, survival, and mortality, 1979–94. The Scottish Melanoma Group. Br Med J 315(7116): 1117–1121

Phillips KA, Conroy M, Dufresne RG, Menard W, Didie ER, Hunter-Yates J, Fay C, Pagano M (2006) Tanning in body dysmorphic disorder. Psychiatr Q 77(2): 129–138

Poorsattar SP, Hornung RL (2007) UV light abuse and high-risk tanning behavior among undergraduate college students. J Am Acad Dermatol 56(3): 375–359

Osterlind A, Moller Jensen O (1986) Trends in incidence of malignant melanoma of the skin in Denmark 1943–1982. Recent Results Cancer Res 102: 8–17

Sahl WJ, Glore S, Garrison P, Oakleaf K, Johnson SD (1995) Basal cell carcinoma and lifestyle characteristics. Int J Dermatol 34(6): 398–402

Statistisches Landesamt Saarland (1998) Morbidität und Mortalität an bösartigen Neubildungen im Saarland 1994 und 1995. Sonderheft 1998, Statistisches Landesamt Saarland, Saarbrücken

Further Reading

Thune P (1991) Life style sun-bathing and tanning – what about UV-A solariums? Tidsskr Nor Laegeforen 111(17): 2085–2087

Suicide in Dermatology

10

In addition to emotional diseases, distress, isolation, and life events, physical diseases are among the risk factors for suicidal tendency. Attention must be paid to the possible danger of suicide in dermatology. Suicidal individuals usually give warning in a presuicidal syndrome with narrowing of thoughts, autoaggression, and suicidal fantasies that may include a consummating plan. In dermatology, men with severe acne conglobata and patients with metastasizing tumor diseases, such as malignant melanoma, are most at risk.

Further risk groups are patients with body dysmorphic disorder, severe progressive systemic scleroderma, and patients with artefact syndrome or borderline disorders (Fig. 10.1).

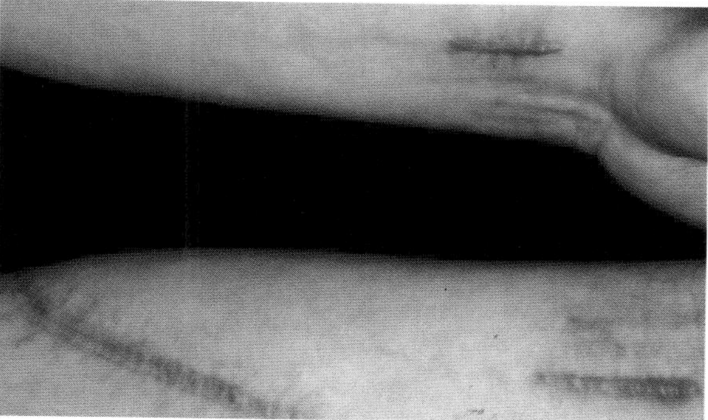

Fig.10.1 Operative care after attempted suicide by slashing the wrists

Risk Groups for Suicide in Dermatology

1. Dermatoses with risk of suicide
   - Acne conglobata (especially men)
   - Metastasizing malignant melanoma
   - Patients with dermatitis artefacta syndrome
   - Progressive systemic scleroderma
   - Body dysmorphic disorder
2. Emotional comorbidities with risk of suicide
   - Depressive disorder
   - Borderline personality disorders
   - Schizophrenia

The incidence of suicide in depressive disorders is estimated at about 4%. Persons who have already attempted suicide once will repeat the act within 2 years with a probability of between 15% and 35%. About half of all suicides are committed by people who were clearly suffering a depressive illness.

Early recognition and estimation of the risk of suicide is one of the most urgent tasks in dermatology. Attempted suicides and suicidal tendencies are usually based on negative subjective, but also often transient, life situations that are correctable.

Of primary importance at first is a supportive holding function and gaining of time. But when necessary, psychiatric therapy should be strictly initiated – by court order if need be – if the patient is a danger to himself or herself. Once a stable relationship has been established, the development of alternative solutions to the problems of the current situation and a plan for the future can be undertaken.

Further Reading

Bronisch T (2002) Psychotherapie der Suizidalität. Thieme, Stuttgart

Cotteril JA, Cunliffe WJ (1997) Suicide in dermatological patients. Br J Dermatol 137: 246–250

Gupta MA, Gupta AK (1998) Depression and suicidal ideation in dermatology patients with acne, alopecia areata, atopic dermatitis and psoriasis. Br J Dermatol 139: 846–850

Traumatization: Sexual Abuse

11

Severe traumatizations or their long-term consequences in medicine and dermatology are caused primarily by forms of sexual abuse, as well as by physical or emotional deprivation or physical abuse in individual cases. The Münchhausen-by-proxy syndrome is presented as a special form in Sect. 1.1.4.

The spectrum of sexual abuse is presented in detail in the following chapter.

Definition. Sexual abuse denotes sexual acts that violate the sexual self-determination of a person who has not reached adulthood, is in a particular relationship to the abuser, or is not able to defend himself or herself physically or emotionally (Egle et al. 1997).

Incidence. Retrospective studies shows that a high percentage of the population has been subject of some sort of sexual abuse.

In Germany (82.5 million inhabitants), 52,321 criminal acts violating sexual self-determination were recorded in 2006, of which the absolute numbers were 8,118 cases of rape and 12,765 cases of sexual abuse of children (Polizeiliche Kriminalstatisti 2007).

Results of a national telephone survey conducted in 2001–2003 indicate that one in 59 U.S. adults (2.7 million women and 978,000 men) experienced unwanted sexual activity in the 12 months preceding the survey and that one in 15 U.S. adults (11.7 million women and 2.1 million men) has been forced to have sex during his or her lifetime (Basile et al. 2007). Findings suggest that victimization rates have remained consistent since the 1990s.

Sociological studies assume, however, that the number of unreported cases is vastly greater. The prevalence figures (Feldman et al. 1991; Lowy 1992; Satin et al. 1992; Spencer and Dunklee 1986) of sexual abuse show a broad scattering with estimates of 9–38% for women and 9–16% for men. Comparison is possible only to a limited extent due to the varying observation periods of the individual studies and the nonuniform definition of sexual abuse.

It is certain, though, that based on the consistently high prevalence of sexual abuse, every dermatologist will be consciously or unconsciously confronted with this problem area and thus with the particular demands of venereal diseases as well as the diagnostics and therapy of psychosomatic disorders.

Classification. Dermatological queries about sexual abuse differ widely and always present a special situation and challenge, in which the procedures must be structured and calm. Practical experience has shown that in addition to the acute effects of the abuse, the latent long-term consequences and the consequences of unnecessary examinations in unconfirmed suspected diagnoses require careful attention. Three focal groups can be particularly differentiated in dermatology:

Sexual Abuse in Dermatology (Harth 2000)

1. Acute direct consequences of sexual abuse
   - Injuries
   - Sexually transmitted diseases
   - Pregnancy
   - Emotional symptoms
2. Long-term sequelae of sexual abuse
   - Physical functioning impairments
   - Psychosomatic/psychiatric diseases
3. Imitations and misdiagnoses
   - Specific dermatoses mimicking sexual abuse
   - Iatrogenically induced, reactive emotional symptoms

Clinical findings. As an acute consequence, there are injuries in the genital area and even more often to the body directly after abuse. Due to the variability of clinical findings and the broad spectrum of normal variants, the diagnostics for sexual abuse of children are difficult, and gynecological findings are very different and ambiguous.

Guiding physical symptoms are injuries to atypical locations (buttocks, back, genitals, groin) and a conspicuous pattern of injury. After the corresponding incubation period, the entire spectrum of sexually transmitted diseases (STDs) can be found. Data especially for gonorrhea, herpes genitalis, condylomata acuminata, chlamydia, pediculosis pubis, scabies, and human immunodeficiency virus (HIV) are available in the literature. Attention must be paid to the different sexual and nonsexual transmission possibilities.

Sexual abuse must also be considered in the case of pregnancy in a very young girl.

As another problem area, specific dermatoses with easily confused morphology may mimic sexual abuse. The differential diagnosis must be undertaken with special tact in this situation, which is out of the ordinary for everyone involved, in order to avoid iatrogenically traumatizing procedures.

The localization of a dermatosis in the genital area alone, as well as an atypical morphology, false-positive laboratory tests, or false history in the framework of neurotic-psychotic illnesses may lead to an incorrectly presumed suspicion of sexual abuse. Imitations require thorough but cautious procedures leading to the diagnosis (Table 11.1).

Scars or functional impairment occur only in the rarest cases as long-term consequences of sexual abuse. More often, dermatoses – as comorbidities in psychosomatic disorders – occur as long-term sequelae, sometimes only decades after sexual abuse.

Table 11.1 Imitations and misdiagnoses: differential diagnoses in sexual abuse (Harth 2000)

Dermatoses in the genital area	Allergic-toxic contact eczema (phytodermatitis)
	Atopic vulva eczema
	Diaper rash
	Hemorrhagias, vasculitis
	Blistering dermatoses
	Lichen sclerosus atrophicans (hemorrhagic after minimal trauma with toilet paper)
	Lichen planus
	Psoriasis
Infections	Bacterial (streptococci)
	Mycoses (candidiasis)
	Viruses (varicellae, herpes simplex, condylomata acuminata)
	Parasites
Neoplasias	Papillomas
	Carcinomas
	Sarcomas
Congenital deformities	Vascular deformity (hemangiomas)
	Epispadia
	Syndrome (Klippel–Trenaunay)
Trauma	Irritations
	Accident (automobile)
	Cultural (circumcision)
Systemic diseases	Crohn's disease
	Megacolon
	Fistulae

! Consideration should be given to psychosomatic long-term sequelae of sexual abuse in the history of patients with dermatitis artefacta syndrome (DAS), self-injuries to the lower arms, borderline disorders, or anorexia nervosa.

The best-confirmed emotional genesis and thus causal association (Gupta and Gupta 1993; van Moffaert 1991) as a sequela of sexual abuse is found in patients with DAS and those with borderline disorders with self-injury, which is often inflicted in the lower arm. Eating disorders may also develop as long-term consequences of sexual abuse (Sect.1.3.2).

In individual cases, possible comorbidity can be proven with urticaria (Borsig et al. 2000), dyshidrosis and hyperhidrosis, alopecia areata, perioral dermatitis, vulvar eczema, vulvodynia, and body dysmorphic disorders. The treatment of the skin lesions is usually successful only when the emotional disorder resulting from the traumatization is taken into account.

Psychopathological symptoms. Acute consequences of sexual abuse vary widely. They depend mainly on the age of the person affected, the severity of the abuse, the relationship to the abuser, and, especially in children, the frequency and duration of the traumatization. Directly after sexual abuse, the most frequently reported changes in emotional behavior among children include disrupted development; learning difficulties; excessive sexualization, including masturbation or touching the genitals of other children; running away; truancy; enuresis; self-injury; insomnia; eating disorders; and suicidal tendencies. Many abused children show characteristic traits in interaction, such as the so-called frozen smile or frozen alertness. Frequently a disruption in proximity–distance regulation is conspicuous. In addition, fears are evident in situations that are reminiscent of the abuse context, such as bathing, showering, or physical examinations.

In abused adults, the acute consequence is often depression and reduction of self-esteem, acute stress disorder, anxiety, shame, or feelings of guilt.

The long-term sequelae, which usually occur only years or even decades later, must be differentiated here. Sexual abuse in the developing years of childhood affects the person's entire later life. As coping or defense mechanisms against the traumatizing situation, patients develop posttraumatic stress disorders, splitting phenomena, and long-term dissociative disorders, up to and including borderline personality disorders and psychoses. The long-term consequences of sexual abuse are often only nonspecific depressive symptoms (83%) or sleep disorders, headache, chronic gastritis, somatoform pain disorders, phobia, eating disorders, addictions, suicidal thoughts, self-injury, frequent consultation with doctors, increased divorce rates, or sexual disorder, including promiscuity or prostitution (Bachmann et al. 1988).

The third problem area is emotional disorder that is iatrogenically induced by an initially suspected but finally rejected diagnosis of sexual abuse.

In general, clinicians are warned against voicing a suspected diagnosis too quickly and thereby disrupting the family ties, which may even lead to divorce. The suspicion alone and the corresponding diagnostic measures to rule out sexual abuse may lead to a lack of trust and feelings of insult on the part of the person affected, the partner, or the family, and may elicit reactive emotional disorders.

Moreover, negative statements about the child's abuser should be avoided because the child may have an ambivalent relationship to this person, especially when it is a relative. Accusations of guilt, aggressive confrontations, or criticisms of the parents are contraindicated.

The doctor should be particularly aware of unconscious reactivation of previous traumatization during diagnostic physical examinations and gynecological examinations of children, including smears and introduction of the speculum.

Diagnostics. Proof of sexual abuse is very difficult and is possible only by means of time-consuming history taking, physical examination, medical tests, and thorough psychological examination. This is normally performed in special regional centers, usually in cooperation with the investigative authorities and specialized clinics or gynecological centers. Occasionally, abuse is simulated, so this must be ruled out.

Sexually transmitted infections and characteristic injuries in the genital and anal areas are important guiding symptoms for confirming sexual abuse.

Quick recording of gynecological findings is required in suspected sexual abuse when there is a possibility of obtaining sperm traces shortly after the fact, or if acute injury must be treated. The dermatologist is usually consulted to rule out any STD according to the guidelines.

In general, venereal disease is rarely found in children. Therefore, if one of the classic venereal diseases is diagnosed in a child or if there are specific gynecological findings, there is a high probability that these are attributable to sexual abuse.

In this context, STDs pose particular difficulties. In principle, transmission of genital papilloma virus infections or herpes infections can occur by contact, but the question of sexual abuse must also be ruled out. Studies of large numbers of patients have concluded that sexual abuse cannot be directly proven in the majority of children with condylomata acuminata and that other causes are possible (Gross 1992).

Atypical dermatoses or protracted courses of treatment in emotionally conspicuous comorbidities often cannot be initially interpreted as late sequelae of sexual abuse, either because the abuse and its consequences can be neither voiced nor thematized by the patient for a long time or because the connection is unconscious. Patients who were abused often show great resistance to revealing this information. The patient often cannot remember the repressed abuse, and this memory becomes accessible only during long-term psychotherapy. Deep-psychological diagnostics regarding sexual abuse in the early development years should be considered in skin patients, especially in the presence of DAS, posttraumatic stress disorders, dissociative disorders, or borderline personality disorders.

There is no specific test or behavior to rule out or confirm sexual abuse at the physical or emotional level. Calmness and patience are important in the acute crisis, avoiding accusations of guilt or aggressive confrontations with the parents. Involving the police is a decision with serious consequences and should not be taken lightly; it should be a team decision whenever possible.

Therapy. Sexual-medical queries, especially in connection with possible sexual abuse, always require psychosomatic primary care or more intensive psychotherapeutic measures.

Protection of the patient has first priority. Treatment aims first at creating security, protection, and trust. Thus, the dermatologist must on the one hand initiate and carry out the necessary exclusion diagnostics cautiously and with reserve in the case of imitations, but on the other hand impartially and thoroughly reveal and treat the acute inflicted abuse, involving the juvenile court if necessary in the case of children. STDs must be treated according to guidelines.

11

Attention must be paid in long-term consequences to repressed, unconscious connections, and shyness must be overcome in initiating combined psychosomatic procedures as standard therapy (Fig. 11.1). Overpsychologizing must be avoided. Not every burden must be relevant or thoroughly worked out. Many patients have erected a stable defense against the traumatization, and forced discussion or reminders of the traumatization may lead to flooding with negative affects and emotional destabilization of the patient. If a patient has an emotional disorder and if sexual abuse is found in his or her history during the course of treatment, focused reduction or assumption of a monocausal origin cannot simply be assumed, and other emotional aspects or personality disorders must be given attention.

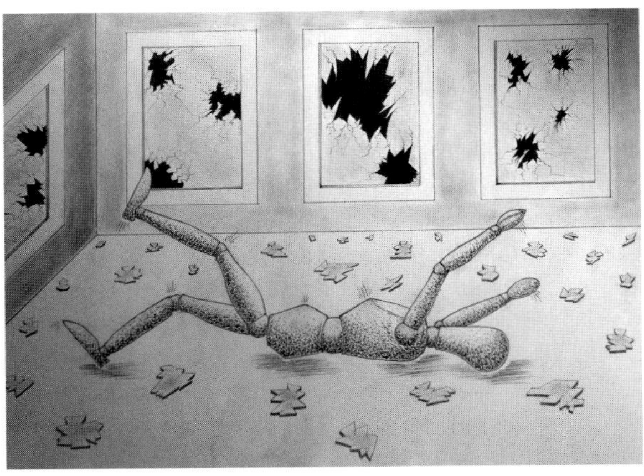

Fig. 11.1 Art therapy by patient with posttraumatic stress disorder

Psychopharmaceuticals. Therapy with psychopharmaceuticals does not take priority in the treatment concept. If an acute stress disorder is present, anxiolytics and sedatives may be necessary. In the case of long-term sequelae, therapy with antidepressants or neuroleptics is indicated depending on the dominant comorbidities.

References

Bachmann GA, Moeller TP, Benett J (1988) Childhood sexual abuse and the consequences in adult woman. Obstet Gynecol 71: 631–642

Basile KC, Chen J, Black MC, Saltzman LE (2007) Prevalence and characteristics of sexual violence victimization among U.S. adults, 2001–2003. Violence Vict 22: 437–448

Borsig B, Niemeier V, Kupfer J, Gieler U (2000) Urticaria and the recall of a sexual trauma. Dermatol Psychosom 1: 53–55

Egle T, Hoffmann SV, Joraschky P (1997) Sexualer Mißbrauch, Misshandlung, Vernachlässigung. Schattauer, Stuttgart

Feldman W, Feldman E, Goodman JT, McGrath PJ, Pless RP, Corsini L, Bennett S (1991) Is childhood sexual abuse really increasing in prevalence? An analysis of the evidence. Pediatrics 88: 29–33

Gross G (1992) Condylomata acuminata in der Kindheit – Hinweis für Sexualen Mißbrauch. Hautarzt 43: 120–125

Gupta MA, Gupta AK (1993) Dermatitis artefacta and sexual abuse. Int J Dermatol 32: 825–826

Harth W, Linse R (2000) Dermatological symptoms and sexual abuse: a review and case reports. J Eur Acad Dermatol Venereol 14: 489–494

Lowy G (1992) Sexually transmitted diseases in children. Pediatr Dermatol 9: 329–334

Moffaert M van (1991) Localization of self-inflicted dermatological lesions: what do they tell the dermatologist? Acta Derm Venereol Suppl (Stockh) 156: 23–27

Polizeiliche Kriminalstatistik 2006 (2007) Bundeskriminalamt Wiesbaden

Satin AJ, Paicurich J, Millman S, Wendel GD (1992) The prevalence of sexual assault: a survey of 2404 puerperal woman. Am J Obstet Gynecol 167: 973–975

Spencer MJ, Dunklee P (1986) Sexual abuse of boys. Pediatrics 78: 133–138

Further Reading

Adams JA, Harper K, Knudson S, Revilla J (1996) Examination findings in legally confirmed child sexual abuse. Pediatrics 97: 148–150

Bays J, Jenny C (1990) Genital and anal conditions confused with child sexual abuse trauma. Am J Dis Child 144: 1319–1322

Davies AG, Clay JC (1992) Prevalence of sexually transmitted disease infection in woman alleging rape. Sex Transm Dis 19: 298–300

Folland DS, Burke RE, Hinman AR, Schaffner W (1977) Gonorrhea in preadolescent children: an inquiry into source of infection and mode of transmission. Pediatrics 60: 153–156

Jenny C, Hooton TM, Bowers A, Copass K, Krieger JN, Hiller SL, Kiviat N, Corey L, Stamm WE, Holmes KK (1990) Sexually transmitted diseases in victims of rape. N Engl J Med 322: 713–716

Siegel RM, Schubert CJ, Myers PA, Shapiro RA (1995) The prevalence of sexually transmitted diseases in children and adolescents evaluated for sexual abuse in Cincinnati: rationale for limited STD testing in prepubertal girls. Pediatrics 96: 1090–1094

Stalder JF, Picherot G (1994) The dermatologist and sexual abuse of children. Ann Dermatol Venereol 121: 451–453

12 Special Psychosomatic Concepts in Dermatology

Psychosomatic Theories

The theories listed in Table 12.1 summarize the basic psychosomatic concepts.

Freud described the concept of *conversion* as transformation of the sum of excitation of intolerable emotional processes to the physical realm. He explained the connection between the physical and emotional levels as an expression process in which somatic processes take on symbolic meaning (Freud 1923/1994).

Alexander's *specificity theory* comprises the theory of disease-specific psychodynamic conflicts. Physical syndromes are understood in the sense of functional secondary presentations of chronic suppressed emotional tensions and are interpreted as organ neuroses (Alexander 1971).

Mitscherlich described the concept of *two-phase repression*. Chronic stress leads first to mobilization of emotional defenses and is in part accompanied by formation of neurotic symptoms. In the second step, there is repression with transferral to physical defense processes, which leads to the onset of a physical symptom. In this concept, the onset of organic symptoms in an attempt to solve the conflict is preceded by emotional repressional conflict solving (Mitscherlich 1968).

Schur described the concept of *resomatizing*. This comprises the idea that regression to an earlier developmental phase of the psychophysiological entity occurs during an emotional conflict. Because there is no distinction in this regression between psyche and soma, traumatic influences can lead directly to pathophysiologic processes or symptoms (Schur 1955).

In the *alexithymia model*, psychosomatic illnesses show a specific personality structure in which the patients are incapable of perceiving their feelings and describing them in words (emotional blindness; Acklin and Alexander 1988; Nemiah and Sifneos 1970; Nemiah et al. 1976; Pasquini et al. 1997).

The psychophysiologic concept was described especially by Selye (1907–1982) in the *stress concept*. In this concept, there is coupling between the psyche and physiological processes, which are coupled as key functions, especially at the hormonal level (Selye 1936, 1973).

Other concepts of behavior therapy focus on the terms *conditioning* (Pavlov 1927) and *reinforcement* (Skinner 1985), whereby the purely behavioristic responses arise according to congenital and acquired coupling and programs. The *learning theory* assumes emotional disorders with learned and maladjusted behavior patterns.

The results of the *bonding theory* appear to have especially close correlation to problems in psychosomatic dermatology. The skin is a contact and sexual organ, and bonding disorders may take on a central key function.

Bonding theory addresses early childhood experiences, close reference persons, and the effects on later personality and thus the person's tendency to develop close intensive feelings to other people or partners. The proximity to the reference person corresponds to the innate need of the infant for a safe base, which is constructed as a strategy crucial to survival and which exerts underlying influence on later bonding behavior. In this way, a lack of emotional support in early childhood can lead to long-lasting emotional distancing and impairments in the natural need for contact and proximity.

Often, only insecure avoidance bonds can be established to other persons, whereby a proximity–distance conflict may result. This can be mutually potentiated by the onset of stigmatizing skin diseases or serious generalized chronic dermatoses. The three main types of bonding variants are

1. Secure or autonomic bonding
2. Insecure, avoiding bonding
3. Insecure ambivalent bonding

Classification manual. Further development of the classification systems ICD-10 (World Health Organization 1995) and DSM-IV-R (American Psychiatric Association 2000) have made it possible to ascribe emotional disorders to an improved scientific classification and thus make them more comparable. The classification is made side by side for emotional as well as somatic findings.

A multiaxial diagnosis system requires evaluation on various axes, of which five are defined in the DSM-IV-R.

12

Table 12.1 Psychosomatic concepts

Concept/model	Author/describer
1. Psychoanalytic theories	
Conversion and actual neurosis	Freud
Specificity theory	Alexander
De- and resomatization	Schur
Two-phase repression	Mischerlich
Symbol models	Groddeck
Alexithymia	Nemiah, Sifneos
Situation circle	Uexküll
Bonding theory	Bowlby
2. Behavior-medical theories	
Stress model	Selye
Transactional stress model	Lazarus
Learning theory	Pavlov, Skinner
Cognitive behavioral model	Beck and others

References

Acklin M, Alexander G (1988) Alexithymia and somatization. J Nerv Ment Dis 176: 343–350
Alexander F (1971) Psychosomatische Medizin. Grundlagen und Anwendungsgebiete. de Gruyter, Berlin
American Psychiatric Association (2000) Diagnostic and statistical manual of mental disorders, 4th edn: DSM-IV. American Psychiatric Association, Washington, DC [Diagnostisches und Statistisches Manual Psychischer Störungen DSM–IV. Hogrefe, Göttingen]
Freud S (1923) Das Ich und das Es. In: Freud S (1994) Psychologie des Unbewussten. Studiensausgabe Bd III, 7. Aufl, Fischer, Frankfurt
Freud S (1994) Abriß der Psychoanalyse. Fischer, Frankfurt
Mitscherlich A (1968) The mechanism of biphasic defence in psychosomatic diseases. Int J Psychoanal 49(2): 236–240
Nemiah JC, Sifneos PE (1970) Affects and fantasy in patients with psychosomatic disorders. In: Modern trends in psychosomatic medicine, vol 2. Butterworth, London, pp 26–34
Nemiah JC, Freyberger H, Sifneos PE (1976) Alexithymia: a view of the psychosomatic process. Psychosom Med 3: 430–439
Pavlov IP (1927) Conditioned reflexes. Dover, Baltimore
Pasquini M, Bitetti D, Decaminada F, Pasquini P (1997) Insecure attachment and psychosomatic skin disease. Ann Ist Super Sanita 33(4): 605-608
Schur M (1955) Comments on the metapsychology of somatization. Psychoanal Study Child 10: 119–164
Selye H (1936) A syndrome produced by diverse noxious agents. Nature 38: 26–32
Selye H (1973) The evolution of the stress concept. Am Sci 61: 692–699
Skinner BF (1985) Cognitive science and behaviourism. Br J Psychol 76(Pt 3): 291–301
World Health Organization (1995) International statistical classification of diseases and related health problems, 10th revision, vol 1. WHO, Geneva [Internationale statistische Klassifikation der Krankheiten und verwandter Gesundheitsprobleme. 10. Rev, Bd 1, Deutscher Ärzteverlag, Köln]

Stress

The importance of stress and coping with stress are important for the manifestation or deterioration of chronic diseases in the expanded viewpoint of the biopsychosocial model. There is a close chronological association between stress and the onset of skin changes in a number of psychosomatic diseases in dermatology. Among these are atopic dermatitis, psoriasis vulgaris, seborrheic eczema, dyshidrosiform eczema, hyperhidrosis, and herpes genitalis and labialis.

This close association of stress and various dermatoses does not, however, apply to all patients with skin diseases but usually to subgroups (clusters), which should be identified by more detailed diagnostics.

In general, it has become customary to differentiate between the group of stress responders and non-stress-responders for better understanding.

Central Nervous System – Skin Interactions: Role of Psychoneuroimmunology and Stress

Psychoneuroimmunology

The notion that the mind is an integral part of the healing process is not new. Although mainstream Western medicine appears to have rediscovered the idea of mind–body integration in the last few decades, it has been a central tenet of health care in medical practices in the Far East, such as in Chinese and Ayurvedic medicine, for more than 2,000 years. Hippocrates (ca. 460–360 BC) believed that disease was caused by imbalance of body, mind, and the environment.

The discipline of psychoneuroimmunology can be traced to the seminal work of Ader and Cohen, who showed that behavioral conditioning, in a similar manner as described by Pavlov, could modify the immune response. These concepts were met with skepticism by immunologists because at that time scientists were resistant to accept that immune responses could occur in the context of nerves and neurohormones. Since then, numerous lines of evidence have emerged to support the notion of tight communication between the central nervous system (CNS) and the immune system.

- Classical conditioning paradigms are capable of enhancing or impairing immune responses in laboratory animals.

Table 12.2 Comparison of sympathetic and parasympathetic stimulation

Organ	Sympathetic stimulation	Parasympathetic stimulation
Skin: sweat secretion	Increase	Decrease
Skin vessels	Constriction	Dilatation
Heart (rate)	Elevation	Reduction
Coronary vessels	Dilatation	Constriction
Pupils	Dilatation	Narrowing
Bronchia	Dilatation	Constriction
Esophagus	Relaxation	Contraction
Stomach (peristalsis and gland activity)	Inhibition	Stimulation
Small and large intestine (peristalsis)	Inhibition	Stimulation
Liver	Promotion of glycogen breakdown	Activation of glycogenesis
Bladder	Urinary retention, inhibition of the detrusor, stimulation of the sphincter	Urinary evacuation, stimulation of the detrusor, relaxation of the sphincter
Genitals	Vasoconstriction	Vasodilatation and erection
Adrenals (adrenalin secretion)	Stimulation	Inhibition
Pancreas (insulin secretion)	Inhibition	Stimulation
Thyroid (secretion)	Stimulation	Inhibition
Metabolism	Increased dissimilation	Increased assimilation
Immune system	Inhibition	Stimulation

- CNS (hypothalamic) interventions alter immunologic reactivity, and the elicitation of an immune response alters CNS activity.
- There is sympathetic innervation of the spleen and other lymphoid organs, including the skin (Table 12.2).
- Immune cells express receptors for a variety of hormones and transmitters and can also secrete these hormones.
- Changes in hormone or transmitter levels produce changes in immune function, and vice versa.
- Products of the CNS (hormones, neurotransmitters, neuropeptides) have effects on immune cells.
- Cytokines produced by immune cells have effects on the CNS.

It makes sense for the brain to transmit to the immune system signs of impending danger. In such manner, the CNS can activate the defense mechanisms in the presence of a predator and redistribute, for example, lymphoid cells to organs such as the skin, which may be injured by a predator. The communication is bidirectional; the information goes back to the brain in the form of cytokines or through the vagus nerve.

Stress

A stressor represents an internal or external force that threatens to disrupt the homeostatic balance of the organism, and the stress response reflects a physiologic adaptation for survival of the individual. The organism has the ability to adapt to acute homeostatic challenges; however, chronicity leads to exhaustion, distress and disease, as originally described by Hans Selye. During thousands of years of evolution, organisms developed a systematic defense mechanism to confront acute danger to life, which mostly came in the form of a predator. As soon as an animal perceives the proximity of immediate threat (frequently a predator), heart rate and blood pressure increase, and blood is diverted to the CNS and the limbs in order to help the animal escape. However, the human organism has not yet been able to adapt to the chronic stressors of the modern daily lives of our civilization because the mechanisms to deal with adversity have not evolved accordingly. Indeed, chronic stress has been shown to adversely affect health and life expectancy.

Stressors activate two major neural pathways: the hypothalamopituitary adrenal (HPA) axis and the sympathetic nervous system.

Neurosensory signals perceived by the cerebral cortex are ultimately processed in the paraventricular nucleus (PVN) of the hypothalamus and the locus ceruleus noradrenergic center.

In response to stressors,

- The hypothalamus secretes corticotropin-releasing hormone (CRH) and arginine vasopressin.
- CRH release further activates the HPA axis, leading to release of peptides from the pituitary: adrenocorticotropic hormone (ACTH), enkephalins, and endorphins.
- ACTH induces downstream release of glucocorticoids from the adrenal cortex.
- CRH and noradrenergic neurons in the CNS innervate and stimulate each other. Activation of the noradrenergic pathways by CRH results in secretion of norepinephrine by the peripheral sympathetic nervous system and release of norepinephrine and epinephrine from the adrenal medulla.
- The activation of these two neurochemical pathways and release of hormones and transmitters can have profound downstream effects on immune function.

Stress and Immunity

Stress hormones regulate inflammatory diseases through their effects on the balance between cell-mediated and humoral immunity and on neurogenic inflammation in peripheral tissues such as the skin (Fig. 12.1).

Adaptive immunity may be divided into two major pathways:

- Cell-mediated immunity, represented by a Th1 response
- Th2-mediated humoral immunity, which is closely associated with allergy

Each subset of T cells (Th1 and Th2) is mutually exclusive.

Homeostasis within the immune system is largely dependent on cytokines, the chemical messengers between immune cells, which play crucial roles in mediating inflammatory and immune responses.

- Th1 cells primarily secrete interferon (IFN)-γ, interleukin (IL)-2, and tumor necrosis factor (TNF)-beta, which promote cell-mediated immunity.
- Th2 cells primarily secrete IL-4, IL-10, and IL-13, which enhance humoral immunity (Fig. 12.2).

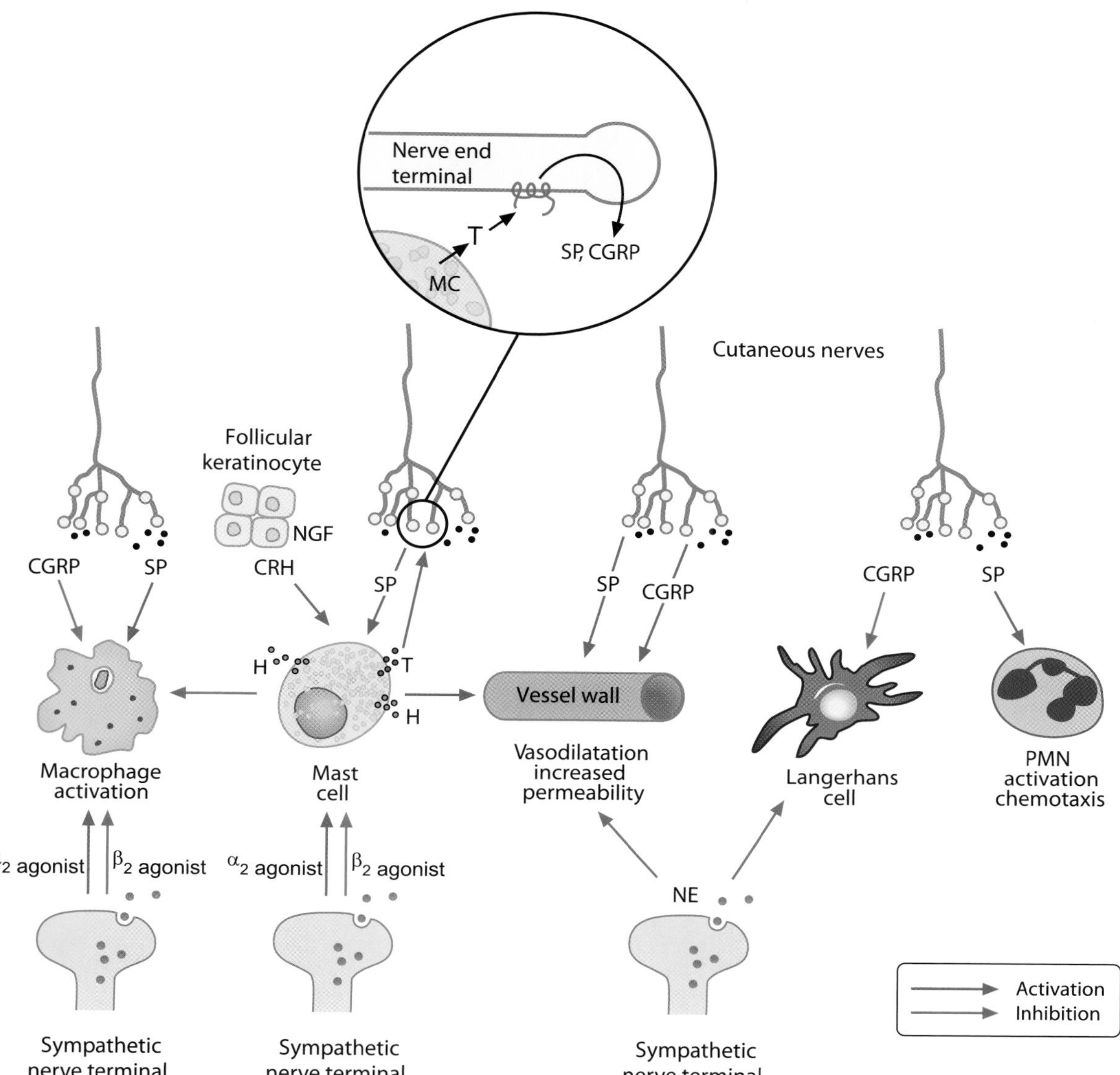

Fig. 12.1 Neurogenic inflammation. Nerve terminals present in cutaneous sensory nerves release neuropeptides such as calcitonin gene-related peptide (CGRP) and substance P (SP), which have numerous effects on local inflammation. SP activates macrophages; induces keratinocyte proliferation and nerve growth factor (NGF) release; releases histamine (H), tryptamine (T), and tumor necrosis factor-alpha from mast cells; and enhances blood vessel permeability, attracting neutrophils to areas of inflammation and enhancing phagocytosis. Tryptamine secreted from mast cells acts on nerve end terminals, enhancing the secretion of additional SP and CGRP. In this manner, neurogenic inflammation expands, and local peptidases such as neutral endopeptidase contribute to the inactivation of SP, allowing for control of the indiscriminate expansion of inflammation. CGRP, on the other hand, inhibits macrophage activation, induces prolonged blood vessel dilatation, and has a strong inhibitory function on Langerhans cells. The latter function is shared by norepinephrine (NE). This neurotransmitter decreases blood vessel dilatation and permeability. Sympathetic nerve end terminals have contradictory effects on mast cells and macrophages depending on their beta or alpha agonist functions. Additionally, keratinocyte-derived corticotropin-releasing hormone (CRH) and NGF participate in neurogenic inflammation by contributing to mast cell activation

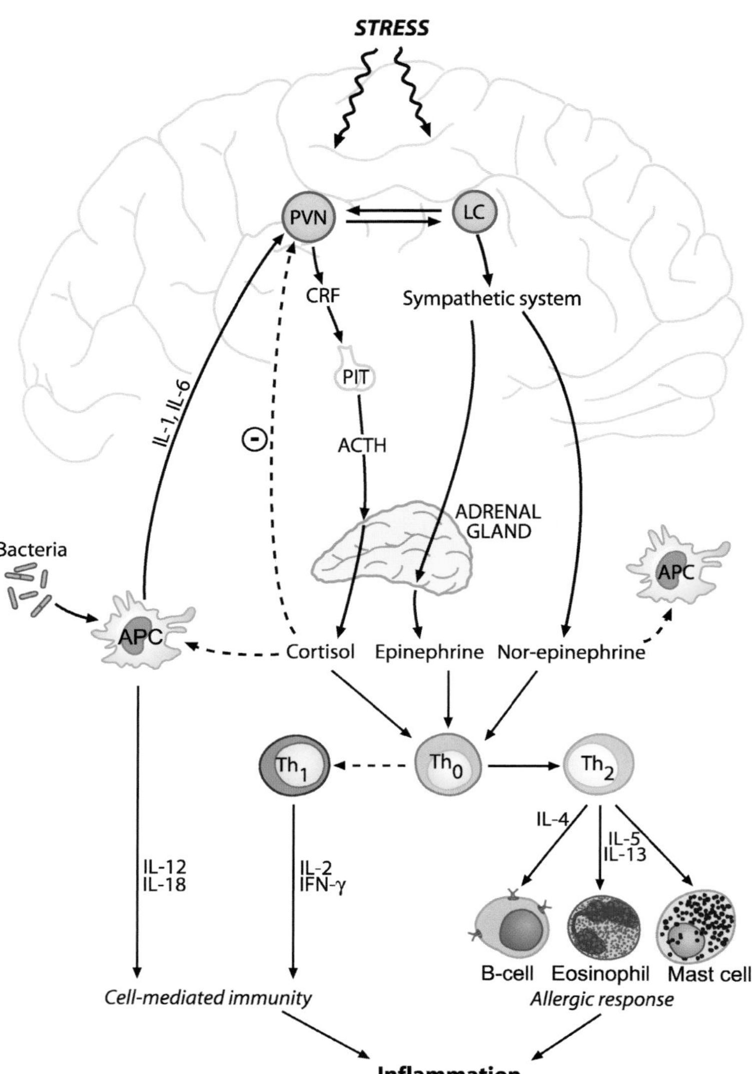

Fig. 12.2 The hypothalamopituitary adrenal (HPA) axis and immunity. The identification of an external perceived stressor by the brain results in activation of the paraventricular nucleus (PVN) of the hypothalamus and the closely interconnected locus ceruleus (LC). Corticotropin-releasing factor (CRF) is secreted from the hypothalamus and transported through the portal circulation to the pituitary, where it induces the release of adrenocorticotropic hormone (ACTH) from the anterior pituitary into the general circulation. The effect of this molecule results in the secretion of glucocorticosteroids and, to a lesser extent, catecholamines from the adrenal gland. Cortisol acts as negative feedback on the hypothalamus, inhibiting the further release of CRF. The cells of the locus ceruleus have a rich neuronal connection with the PVN and activate the sympathetic system, which results in the secretion of epinephrine and norepinephrine. Both catecholamines and cortisol have a potent effect on the immune system. They modulate antigen-presenting cells and macrophages, inhibiting their activity and the production of IL-12 and IL-18, and they mediate the differentiation of naïve T helper cells toward the TH2 constellation, in detriment of the development of TH1-mediated immunity. This results in tilting the balance toward humoral immunity by increasing the production of IL-4, IL-5, and IL-13, which activate B cells, mast cells, and eosinophils, increasing the allergic inflammatory response. The chronic dampening of cell-mediated immunity could result in an impaired ability to effectively confront the development of infectious or tumoral insults.

On the other hand, internal stressors are exemplified here by bacterial infections. The released bacterial lipopolysaccharides (LPS) bind to toll-like receptors on macrophages, and through nuclear factor kappa B induce the production of IL-1 and IL-6. These cytokines are able to cross the blood–brain barrier and reach the hypothalamus, where they stimulate the secretion of CRF, initiating the activation of the HPA axis. In this manner, infections have the potential to shift the immune balance favoring the humoral TH2-mediated response. Diseases that involve this arm of the immune system, such as autoimmune or allergic diseases, would deteriorate with the presence of stressors of the internal as well as the external kind. Modified from Tausk et al. (2008) Psychoneuroimmunology. Dermatologic therapy, vol. 21, pp 22–31.

The precursor naive T cells (Th0) may differentiate toward either Th1 or Th2 lymphocytes, depending on the cytokines present in the immediate milieu.

- IL-12 secreted by macrophages is the main molecule that will induce TH0 differentiation toward the Th1 phenotype, and in combination with IFN-γ inhibit Th2 cell activity.
- IL-4 and IL-10 inhibit Th1 and promote humoral immunity by stimulating the growth and activation of mast cells and eosinophils, the differentiation of B cells, and IgE production. Importantly, these cytokines also inhibit macrophage activation, T cell proliferation, and the production of pro-inflammatory cytokines.

As mentioned above, stress-mediated activation of the HPA axis results in the secretion of catecholamines and glucocorticosteroids. These have a profound influence on immunity, inducing a Th2 shift by upregulating Th2-cytokine production and also by suppressing macrophage and Th1-cytokine production. Thus, glucocorticosteroids and catecholamines suppress the production of IL-12, the main inducer of Th1 responses. Glucocorticosteroids also have a direct effect on Th2 cells by upregulating their IL-4, IL-10, and IL-13 production. In this manner, stress inhibits cell-mediated immunity, favoring antibody-mediated and allergic responses.

This combined effect on the TH1–TH2 balance may explain why the activity of some diseases appears to fluctuate during periods of stress. Autoimmune diseases, including pemphigus or conditions with TH2 predominance, such as atopic eczema, may deteriorate if the immunity is shifted toward the humoral TH2 response during periods of psychological stress or concurrent infections.

Inherited Alterations of the HPA Axis and Skin Diseases

Some patients have a genetic dysfunction of the hypothalamus that is responsible for an inappropriate secretion of glucocorticosteroids in the presence of stressors. This phenomenon, initially studied in rodents by Sternberg (Sternberg et al. 1992), Aksentijevich (Aksentijevich et al. 1992), and colleagues, was subsequently found to operate in patients with rheumatoid arthritis. Later it was observed to be present in some skin diseases:

- Children and adults with atopic dermatitis respond to common stressors with a significantly lower peak of cortisol compared with healthy controls.
- Patients with psoriasis whose course fluctuates with stress were found to have the same lowered steroid secretion when exposed to experimental stressors.
- These observations suggest that these patients have inflammatory diseases that may flare when they are unable to sustain normal levels of corticosteroids when confronted with adverse stimuli.

Stress and Cutaneous Immunity

Recent studies have shown that skin immunity is modulated by stress:

- Chronic stressors inhibit cell-mediated immunity.
- Acute stressors enhance cell-mediated immunity.

Following chronic (daily for 21 days) restraint sessions, delayed-type hypersensitivity (DTH) responses were suppressed compared with control mice; however, after a single session of restraint prior to challenge, DTH responses in skin were enhanced, and this effect was abrogated by adrenalectomy, suggesting that glucocorticosteroids and epinephrine may mediate these effects. Dhabhar and McEwen (1997) proposed that acute stress may induce "redeployment" of peripheral blood lymphocytes to the skin and that this would be an adaptive response during the fight-or-flight response.

Stress and Wound Healing

- Marucha et al. (1998) initially reported that experimental mucosal wounds healed significantly slower in healthy students during periods of examinations compared with nonstressful times.
- More recently, these investigators studied the relationship between the quality of marital relationships and the partners' time to heal a blister wound. Those with hostile interactions had wounds that healed significantly later.
- Cardiovascular exercise in older adults (mean age 65 years) accelerated the rate of experimental wound healing very significantly.
- Thus, the process of wound healing is affected by stressful life conditions and can be improved through intervention and/or changes in lifestyle. It remains to be determined, however, through what specific mechanisms the nervous system, both central and peripheral, can alter innate and cellular immunity in the skin in response to a wound.

Stress and the Skin Function as a Barrier

- The barrier function of the skin is altered in stressed mice, showing increased transepidermal water loss; this is reversed by treatment with anxiolytics.

- Healthy students have impaired barrier function during episodes of psychological stress.
- Altered skin barrier function creates increased susceptibility to cutaneous inoculation with environmental agents (e.g., allergens such as dust mites, dander, bacteria, and viruses) that are potential precipitants of atopic flares.

Stress and Skin Diseases
Diseases of the skin, more than any other organ, appear to be influenced by emotional factors, and most dermatologists encounter patients who report a temporal relationship between disease flares and stressful life events. Emotional stressors have been linked to the development or evolution of a variety of cutaneous diseases, including acne, vitiligo, alopecia areata, lichen planus, seborrheic dermatitis, herpes simplex infections, pemphigus, urticaria, psoriasis, and atopic eczema.

Psoriasis

! Stress affects the evolution of psoriasis.

- Emotional stressors have been reported to precede the onset of psoriasis, as well as precipitate flares.
- Psoriatic patients who suffered traumatic section of sensory innervation had resolution of the plaques in the areas innervated by the sectioned nerves; the disease reappeared when nerve fibers regenerated and the sensitivity returned. This observation highlights the role played by sensory cutaneous nerves in the maintenance of psoriatic disease.
- Psoriatic plaques display increased nerve fiber density and altered content of neuropeptides such as calcitonin gene-related peptide (CGRP), substance P (SP), vasoactive intestinal peptide, and nerve growth factor (NGF).
- High expression of NGF mediates T cell and keratinocyte proliferation, mast cell migration, degranulation, and memory T cell chemotaxis, which are all hallmarks of psoriasis.

Stress reduction and psoriasis. The following observations have been noted:
- Psychosocial interventions aimed at stress reduction have proven to be successful in the treatment of psoriasis.
- Mindfulness meditation during phototherapy sessions decreased the length of phototherapy; the subjects in the intervention group cleared their psoriasis 50% faster than those receiving phototherapy only.
- Psoriatic patients improved significantly during hypnosis sessions in which they received suggestions that they were being exposed to "whatever they believed would ameliorate their condition."
- This observation, in addition to the high rates of placebo responses in some clinical trials for psoriasis drugs, may suggest that the placebo effect could be harnessed and utilized in the pharmacotherapy of these patients.

Atopic Dermatitis

Atopic dermatitis (AD) exemplifies the relationship of the delicate balance between genetic, environmental, and psychosocial factors and evolution of a skin disease.
- Patients with AD have severe impairment in their quality of life, resulting in significant emotional distress.
- This relationship is bidirectional because stressors are important contributors to the flares and exacerbation of the disease.
- AD patients have upregulation of glucocorticoid receptors on peripheral leukocytes, making them hyperreactive to steroid stimulation. Thus, despite a blunted HPA axis response to stress, effector cells that are exquisitely sensitive to systemic glucocorticoid release may respond in a hyperreactive fashion to stress-induced cortisol elevations, accentuating the cytokine shift from Th1 to the Th2 immune response.
- Elevated levels of norepinephrine found in these individuals leads to the secretion of IL-13 and IL-4 and to Th2 differentiation.
- Stress-induced local and systemic secretion of epinephrine or its metabolites may also play a role in the worsening of AD, since these patients have increased mononuclear cell activation of intracellular type 4 phosphodiesterases (PDE4).
- Stressors shift the immune response, impairing TH1 and favoring the Th2 humoral immune response and a redistribution of lymphocytes and eosinophils.
- Pharmacologic doses of corticosteroids are also able to suppress the production of IL-4, which is an agent of differentiation toward Th2 cells, explaining the beneficial effect of systemic or topical application of these agents.

Stress-reducing interventions in AD. The following have been reported to be effective in improving the skin manifestations of AD patients:

- Insight-oriented psychotherapy
- Cognitive behavioral therapy
- Psychoeducation
- Hypnosis
- Biofeedback

Urticaria

- Patients suffering from adrenergic urticaria report that their symptoms invariably follow acute stressful events.
- The finding that stress mediates the degranulation of mast cells via CRH and neuropeptides and the upregulation of mast cell CRH receptors supports its role in the pathogenesis of urticaria.

Infections

Numerous studies have demonstrated the deleterious effects of stressors on the evolution of infections:

- Stress affects experimental bacterial infections of the skin.
- Recurrent herpetic infection can be precipitated by psychiatric illness, life events, and disgust.
- Stress appears to significantly modulate the evolution of human infection with herpes simplex virus (HSV).
- Experimental restraint stress correlates with the reactivation of latent HSV infection in the dorsal root ganglion neuron of rats.
- Human studies show that persistent, but not single or acute, stressors are associated with the frequency of recurrences.
- The above is in agreement with findings that chronic, but not acute, stress correlates with the development of experimental viral infections in normal volunteers.
- Psychosocial interventions have been shown to decrease the frequency of recurrence of HSV infections.

Cancer

Studies have suggested that natural or experimental stressors can modulate the evolution of malignancies in humans as well as in other animals, suppressing lymphocyte proliferation and natural killer cell activity.

- We recently reported a model of stress-induced carcinogenicity in which mice treated with ultraviolet (UV) light that were exposed repeatedly to the presence of a predator scent developed squamous cell carcinomas significantly earlier (week 8) than nonstressed controls (week 21), an observation that was subsequently confirmed by others.
- Stress reduction interventions have been shown to significantly prolong the survival of individuals with metastatic neoplasms. For example, patients with metastatic melanoma were found to benefit from limited sessions of psychosocial interventions, thereby significantly increasing their 6-year survival rate.
- One possible explanation for the benefit of these interventions could be the modulatory effect of stress and stress reduction on natural killer cell function, which is presumed to represent one of the first innate lines of immune defense against foreign (including cancerous) cells.
- Another example is relaxation training, which significantly increased older adults' cytotoxic function, even though chronic stress has been shown to suppress natural killer cell activity.

Psychoneuroimmunology is an evolving area of science that will help us understand the relationship between the mind and the body. The past 30 years of research in the field of psychoneuroimmunology have validated the close relationship between the CNS and the immune system. A growing body of evidence supports the effect of the psyche – stress, in particular – on immune responses and a multitude of skin conditions. The effects of stress on shifting the immune response are not completely understood; however, researchers are aware that stress modifies the delicate balance between health and disease. Just as interesting are the numerous studies demonstrating that a nonpharmacologic approach can ameliorate certain dermatologic diseases. Seeking alternative interventions can only enhance our ability to treat patients.

References

Aksentijevich S, Whitfield HJ Jr, Young WS 3rd, Wilder RL, Chrousos GP, Gold PW, Sternberg EM (1992) Arthritis-susceptible Lewis rats fail to emerge from the stress hyporesponsive period. Brain Res Dev Brain Res 65(1): 115–118

Dhabhar FS, McEwen BS (1997) Acute stress enhances while chronic stress suppresses cell-mediated immunity in vivo: a potential role for leukocyte trafficking. Brain Behav Immun 11(4): 286–306

Marucha PT, Kiecolt-Glaser JK, Favagehi M (1998) Mucosal wound healing is impaired by examination stress. Psychosom Med 60(3): 362–365

Sternberg EM, Glowa JR, Smith MA, Calogero AE, Listwak SJ, Aksentijevich S, Chrousos GP, Wilder RL, Gold PW (1992) Corticotropin releasing hormone related behavioral and neuroendocrine responses to stress in Lewis and Fischer rats. Brain Res 570(1-2): 54–60

Further Reading

Ader R, Cohen N (1975) Behaviorally conditioned immunosuppression. Psychosomatic Med 37(4): 333–40

Altemus M, Rao B, Dhabhar FS, Ding W, Granstein RD (2001) Stress-induced changes in skin barrier function in healthy women. J Invest Dermatol 117(2): 309–317

Barisic-Drusko V, Rucevic I (2004) Trigger factors in childhood psoriasis and vitiligo. Coll Antropol 28(1): 277–285

Ben-Eliyahu S (2003) The promotion of tumor metastasis by surgery and stress: immunological basis and implications for psychoneuroimmunology. Brain Behav Immun 17(Suppl 1): S27–S36

Benhard JD, Kristeller J, Kabat-Zinn J (1988) Effectiveness of relaxation and visualization techniques as an adjunct to phototherapy and photochemotherapy of psoriasis. J Am Acad Dermatol 19(3): 572–574

Biondi M, Zannino LG (1997) Psychological stress, neuroimmunomodulation, and susceptibility to infectious diseases in animals and man: a review. Psychother Psychosom 66(1): 3–26

Buske-Kirschbaum AGA, Hollig H, Morschhauser E, Hellhammer D (2002) Altered responsiveness of the hypothalamus-pituitary-adrenal axis and the sympathetic adrenomedullary system to stress in patients with atopic dermatitis. J Clin Endocrinol Metab 87(9): 4245–4251

Buske-Kirschbaum A, Jobst S, Psych D, et al (1997) Attenuated free cortisol response to psychosocial stress in children with atopic dermatitis. Psychosom Med 59(4): 419–426

Buske-Kirschbaum AGA, Wermke C, Pirke KM, Hellhammer D (2001) Preliminary evidence for herpes labialis recurrence following experimentally induced disgust. Psychother Psychosom 70(2): 86–91

Charmandari E, Tsigos C, Chrousos G (2005) Endocrinology of the stress response. Ann Rev Physiol 67: 259–284

Chaudhary S (2004) Psychosocial stressors in oral lichen planus. Aust Dent J 49(4): 192–195

Chiu A, Chon SY, Kimball AB (2003) The response of skin disease to stress: changes in the severity of acne vulgaris as affected by examination stress. Arch Dermatol 139(7): 897–900

Chrousos GP (1995) The hypothalamic-pituitary-adrenal axis and immune-mediated inflammation. N Engl J Med 332(20): 1351–1362

Cohen F, Kemeny ME, Kearney KA, Zegans LS, Neuhaus JM, Conant MA (1999) Persistent stress as a predictor of genital herpes recurrence. Arch Intern Med 159(20): 2430–2436

Cohen S, Tyrrell DA, Smith AP (1991) Psychological stress and susceptibility to the common cold. N Engl J Med 325(9): 606–612

Cremniter D, Baudin M, Roujeau JC et al. (1998) Stressful life events as potential triggers of pemphigus [letter]. Arch Dermatol 134: 1486–1487

Cupps TR, Gerrard TL, Falkoff RJ, Whalen G, Fauci AS (1985) Effects of in vitro corticosteroids on B cell activation, proliferation, and differentiation. J Clin Invest 75(2): 754–761

Delgado M F-AM, Fuentes A (2002) Effect of adrenaline and glucocorticoids on monocyte cAMP-specific phospodiesterase (PDE4) in a monocyte cell line. Arch Dermatol Res 294: 190–197

Dhabhar FS, McEwen BS (1999) Enhancing versus suppressive effects of stress hormones on skin immune function. Proc Natl Acad Sci U S A 96(3): 1059–1064

Dunn A (1995) Psychoneuroimmunology, stress and infection. In: Friedman K (ed) Psychoneuroimmunology, stress, infection. CRC, Boca Raton, pp 25–45

Elenkov IJ, Chrousos GP (1999) Stress hormones, Th1/Th2 patterns, pro/anti-inflammatory cytokines and susceptibility to disease. Trends Endocrinol Metab 10(9): 359–368

Elenkov IJ WR, Chrousos GP, Vizi ES (2000) The sympathetic nerve – an integrative interface between two supersystems: the brain and the immune system. Pharmacol Rev 52(4): 595–638

Emery CF, Kiecolt-Glaser JK, Glaser R, Malarkey WB, Frid DJ (2005) Exercise accelerates wound healing among healthy older adults: a preliminary investigation. J Gerontol 60(11): 1432–1436

Farber EM, Nall L (1993) Psoriasis: a stress-related disease. Cutis 51(5): 322–326

Faulstich ME, Williamson DA, Duchmann EG, Conerly SL, Brantley PJ (1985) Psychophysiological analysis of atopic dermatitis. J Psychosom Res 29(4): 415–417

Fawzy FI, Fawzy NW, Hyun CS, et al (1993) Malignant melanoma. Effects of an early structured psychiatric intervention, coping, and affective state on recurrence and survival 6 years later. Arch Gen Psychiatry 50(9): 681–689

Fearon DT, Locksley RM (1996) The instructive role of innate immunity in the acquired immune response. Science 272(5258): 50–53

Fortune DG RH, Griffiths CEM, Main CJ (2002) Psychological stress, distress and disability in patients with psoriasis: consensus and variation in the contribution of illness perceptions, coping and alexithymia. Br J Dermatol 41: 157–174

Fortune DG RH, Griffiths CEM, Main CJ (2005) Psychologic factors in psoriasis: consequences, mechanisms, and interventions. Dermatol Clin 4: 681–694

Ginsburg IH (1996) Coping with psoriasis: a guide for counseling patients. Cutis 57(5): 323–325

Glaser R, Kiecolt-Glaser JK, Speicher CE, Holliday JE (1985) Stress, loneliness, and changes in herpesvirus latency. J Behav Med 8(3): 249–260

Glaser R, Rice J, Speicher CE, Stout JC, Kiecolt-Glaser JK (1986) Stress depresses interferon production by leukocytes concomitant with a decrease in natural killer cell activity. Behav Neurosci 100(5): 675–678

Goldberg I IA, Brenner S (2004) Pemphigus vulgaris triggered by rifampin and emotional stress. Skinmed 3(5): 294

Gulec AT, Tanriverdi N, Duru C, Saray Y, Akcali C (2004) The role of psychological factors in alopecia areata and the impact of the disease on the quality of life. Int J Dermatol 43(5): 352–356

Kabat-Zinn J, Wheeler E, Light T, et al. (1998) Influence of a mindfulness meditation-based stress reduction intervention on rates of

12

skin clearing in patients with moderate to severe psoriasis undergoing phototherapy (UVB) and photochemotherapy (PUVA). Psychosom Med 60(5): 625–632

Kagi MK, Wutrich B, Montano E, Barandun J, Blaser K, Walker C (1994) Differential cytokine profiles in peripheral blood lymphocyte supernatants and skin biopsies from patients with different forms of atopic dermatitis, psoriasis and normal individuals. Int Arch Allergy Immunol 103: 332–340

Kamarck TW, Everson SA, Kaplan GA, et al (1997) Exaggerated blood pressure responses during mental stress are associated with enhanced carotid atherosclerosis in middle-aged Finnish men: findings from the Kuopio Ischemic Heart Disease Study. Circulation 96(11): 3842–3848

Khansari DN, Murgo AJ, Faith RE (1990) Effects of stress on the immune system. Immunol Today 11(5): 170–175

Kiecolt-Glaser JK, Glaser R (1999) Chronic stress and mortality among older adults. JAMA 282: 2259–2260

Kiecolt-Glaser JK, Garner W, Speicher C, Penn GM, Holliday J, Glaser R (1984) Psychosocial modifiers of immunocompetence in medical students. Psychosom Med 46(1): 7–14

Kiecolt-Glaser JK, Loving TJ, Stowell JR, et al (2005) Hostile marital interactions, proinflammatory cytokine production, and wound healing. Arch Gen Psychiatry 62(12): 1377–1384

Korte SM, Koolhaas JM, Wingfield JC, McEwen BS (2005) The Darwinian concept of stress: benefits of allostasis and costs of allostatic load and the trade-offs in health and disease. Neurosci Biobehav Rev 29(1): 3–38

Langan SM, Bourke JF, Silcocks P, Williams HC (2006) An exploratory prospective observational study of environmental factors exacerbating atopic eczema in children. Br J Dermatol 154(5): 979–980

Levite M (1998) Neuropeptides, by direct interaction with T cells, induce cytokine secretion and break the commitment to a distinct T helper phenotype. Proc Natl Acad Sci U S A 95(21): 12544–12549

McEwen BS (2004) Protection and damage from acute and chronic stress: allostasis and allostatic overload and relevance to the pathophysiology of psychiatric disorders. Ann NY Acad Sci 1032:1–7

Mosmann TR, Sad S (1996) The expanding universe of T-cell subsets: Th1, Th2 and more. Immunol Today 17(3): 138–146

Moynihan JA SS (2001) Mechanisms of stress-induced modulation of immunity in animals. In: Ader R FD, Cohen (eds) Psychoneuroimmunology. Academic Press, New York, pp 227–249

Naldi L, Peli L, Parazzini F, Carrel CF (2001) Family history of psoriasis, stressful life events, and recent infectious disease are risk factors for a first episode of acute guttate psoriasis: results of a case-control study. J Am Acad Dermatol 44(3): 433–438

Panina-Bordignon P, Mazzeo D, Lucia PD, et al. (1997) Beta2-agonists prevent Th1 development by selective inhibition of interleukin 12. J Clin Invest 100(6): 1513–1519

Papadopoulos L, Bor R, Legg C, Hawk JL (1998) Impact of life events on the onset of vitiligo in adults: preliminary evidence for a psychological dimension in aetiology. Clin Exper Dermatol 23(6): 243–248

Parker J, Klein SL, McClintock MK, et al (2004) Chronic stress accelerates ultraviolet-induced cutaneous carcinogenesis. J Am Acad Dermatol 51(6): 919–922

Raychaudhuri SP, Jiang WY, Farber EM (1998) Psoriatic keratinocytes express high levels of nerve growth factor. Acta Derm Venereol 78(2): 84–86

Raychaudhuri SP, Jiang WY, Smoller BR, Farber EM (2000) Nerve growth factor and its receptor system in psoriasis. Br J Dermatol 143(1): 198–200

Reiche EM, Morimoto HK, Nunes SM (2005) Stress and depression-induced immune dysfunction: implications for the development and progression of cancer. Intl Rev Psychiatry (Abingdon, England) 17(6): 515–527

Richards HL, Ray DW, Kirby B, et al (2005) Response of the hypothalamic-pituitary-adrenal axis to psychological stress in patients with psoriasis. Br J Dermatol 153(6): 1114–1120

Rojas IG, Padgett DA, Sheridan JF, Marucha PT (2002) Stress-induced susceptibility to bacterial infection during cutaneous wound healing. Brain Behav Immun 16(1): 74–84

Sanders VM, Baker RA, Ramer-Quinn DS, Kasprowicz DJ, Fuchs BA, Street NE (1997) Differential expression of the beta2-adrenergic receptor by Th1 and Th2 clones: implications for cytokine production and B cell help. J Immunol 158(9): 4200–4210

Saraceno R, Kleyn CE, Terenghi G, Griffiths CE (2006) The role of neuropeptides in psoriasis. Br J Dermatol 155(5): 876–882

Schmid-Ott G, Jacobs R, Jäger B, et al (1998) Stress induced endocrine and immunological changes in psoriasis patients and healthy controls. Psychother Psychosom 67: 37–42

Schmid-Ott G, Jäger B, Adamek C, et al (2001) Levels of circulating CD8(+) T lymphocytes, natural killer cells, and eosinophils increase upon acute psychosocial stress in patients with atopic dermatitis. J Allergy Clin Immunol 107(1): 171–177

Schmid-Ott G, Jäger B, Meyer S, Stephan E, Kapp A, Werfel T (2001) Different expression of cytokine and membrane molecules by circulating lymphocytes on acute mental stress in patients with atopic dermatitis in comparison with healthy controls. J Allergy Clin Immunol 108(3): 455–462

Schulz R, Beach SR (1999) Caregiving as a risk factor for mortality: the Caregiver Health Effects Study [see comments]. JAMA 282: 2215–9

Selye H (1936) A syndrome produced by diverse nocuous agents. Nature 138:32

Selye H (1946) The general adaptation syndrome and the disease of adaptation. J Clin Endocrinol 6: 117–230

Singh LK, Pang X, Alexacos N, Letourneau R, Theoharides TC (1999) Acute immobilization stress triggers skin mast cell degranulation via corticotropin releasing hormone, neurotensin, and substance P: a link to neurogenic skin disorders. Brain Behav Immun 13(3): 225–239

Spiegel D, Bloom JR, Kraemer HC, Gottheil E (1989) Effect of psychosocial treatment on survival of patients with metastatic breast cancer [see comments]. Lancet 2(8668): 888–891

Stone R (2000) Social science. Stress: the invisible hand in Eastern Europe's death rates. Science 288: 1732–1733

Tamir A, Ophir J, Brenner S (1994) Pemphigus vulgaris triggered by emotional stress [letter]. Dermatology 189:210

Tausk F, Whitmore SE (1999) A pilot study of hypnosis in the treatment of patients with psoriasis. Psychother Psychosom 68(4): 221–225

Theoharides TC, Donelan JM, Papadopoulou N, Cao J, Kempuraj D, Conti P (2004) Mast cells as targets of corticotropin-releasing factor and related peptides. Trends Pharmacol Sciences 25(11): 563–568

Trinchieri G (2003) Interleukin-12 and the regulation of innate resistance and adaptive immunity. Nature Reviews 3(2): 133–146

Yang EV, Glaser R (2003) Stress-induced immunomodulation: implications for tumorigenesis. Brain Behav Immun 17(suppl 1): S37–S40

Zane L (2003) Psychoneuroendocrinimmunodermatology: pathophysiological mechanisms of stress in cutaneous disease. In: Koo JYM, Lee CS (eds) Psychocutaneous medicine. Dekker, New York, pp 65–95

Central Nervous System – Skin Interactions: Role of Neuropeptides and Neurogenic Inflammation

In 1912 Ninian Bruce observed that the cutaneous erythema secondary to irritation of the skin could be abolished by severing the sensory nerve between the dorsal root ganglion and the skin. He concluded that cutaneous inflammation requires intact nerves. Since then, numerous studies have shown that sensory nerves play a significant role in the maintenance of cutaneous physiology. Many of these functions are mediated through the release of neuropeptides from free nerve end terminals, which have a regulatory role on blood vessels and cells such as keratinocytes, Langerhans cells, mast cells, and leukocytes (Fig. 12.3). The advent of antibodies to the neuronal marker PGP-9.5 has evidenced the presence of a rich network of peripheral nerves that extends through the dermis all the way to the superficial layers of the epidermis.

Neurogenic inflammation is the term that describes the participation of products of sensory nerves in the cutaneous inflammatory response that provides the link between the CNS and the skin. Recent studies have also provided evidence that various mediators of the stress response traditionally known to be present in the endocrine and CNS are produced by cutaneous cells. In such manner, CRH, proopiomelanocortin (POMC), ACTH, alpha-melanocyte-stimulating hormone (αMSH), PC1, PC2, and cortisol, among others, are secreted from keratinocytes and other cells, thus creating a parallel network in the skin that mirrors the HPA axis.

12

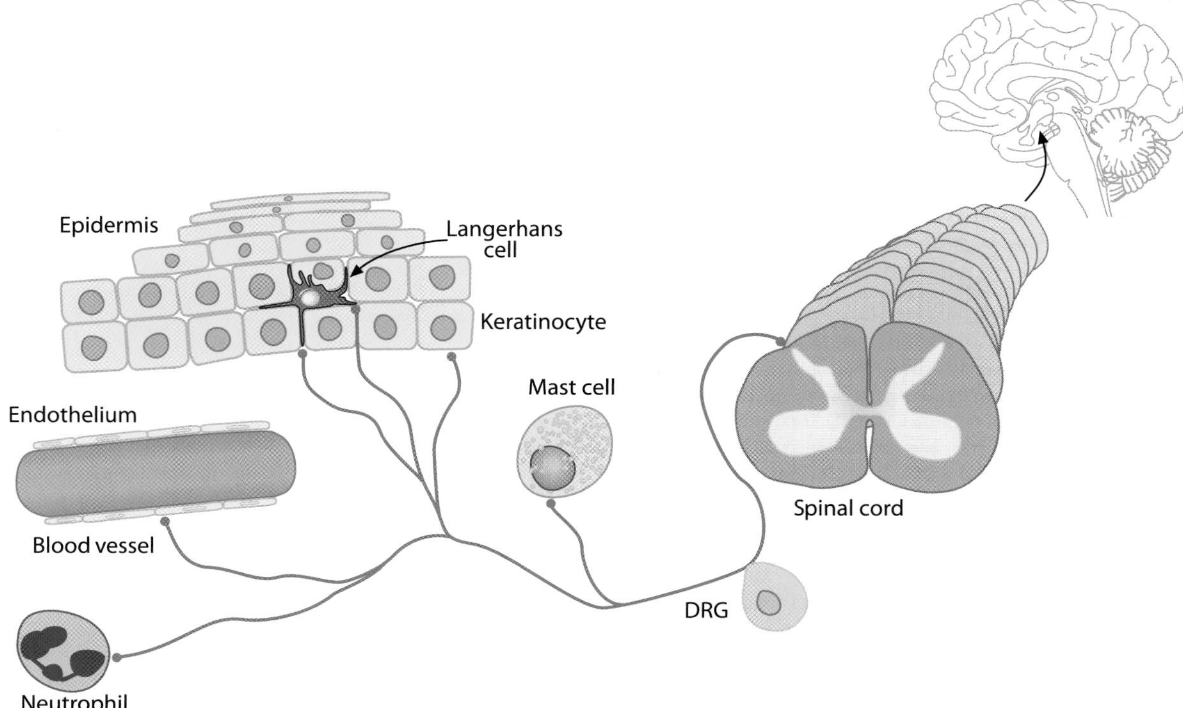

Fig. 12.3 Slow-conducting cutaneous nerve fibers transmit sensory information to the central nervous system through projections in the spinal cord. However, antidromic transmission allows impulses to be delivered to the skin. These fibers appear to innervate numerous skin structures and release neuropeptides that have profound effects on the cutaneous inflammatory response

Cutaneous Neuropeptides

Neurons utilize a variety of molecules to transmit information, including neurotransmitters (such as epinephrine), gases (such as nitric oxide), and neuropeptides. The latter are small peptides originally found to be secreted by neural tissue. They have potent effects not only on the CNS but also on peripheral tissues such as the skin. Small, slow-conducting C- and Aδ-fibers innervate the skin and reach the superficial layers of the epidermis. Neuropeptides synthesized in the dorsal root ganglion are transported through the nerves, reaching the free nerve end terminals, where they are stored in vesicles and may be released under different conditions. Neuropeptide-containing nerves have been found in close proximity to a variety of cells, including mast cells, endothelial cells, keratinocytes, and Langerhans cells, all of which express receptors for neuropeptides; in this manner, a network with a shared language is created that allows communication between the CNS and the cutaneous immune system, modulating the cutaneous inflammatory responses. Impulses are transmitted in an antidromic fashion (that is, from the center to the peripheral nerve ending, which is opposite to the normal orthodromic conduction in sensory nerves), and when they reach the cutaneous free nerve endings, they may release peptides such as SP and CGRP.

Substance P. Substance P (SP) is an 11-amino-acid peptide that belongs to the family of the tachykinins. Its release from peripheral C-nerve fibers results in vasodilatation through the production of endothelial nitric oxide, and it induces increased vascular permeability. This, in conjunction with the upregulation of vascular adhesion molecules, allows the rolling and extravasation of neutrophils. The chemotactic and activating effects of SP subsequently allow neutrophils to participate in cutaneous inflammation. Other functions of SP in the skin are

- Activation of keratinocytes, inducing their proliferation, and secretion of chemokines such as IL-1 as well as NGF
- Activation of mast cells to release histamine, TNFα, leukotriene B4, and prostaglandins
- Mediation in addition to erythema, edema, and pain

CGRP. Calcitonin gene-related peptide (CGRP) is a 37-amino-acid peptide that is the prevalent neuropeptide in the skin. CGRP is the most potent physiologic vasodilator, mediating prolonged erythema. CGRP-immunoreactive nerve fibers are found in close apposition to Langerhans cells, influencing their function. Some of the cutaneous functions of CGRP are to

- Mediate erythema
- Induce keratinocyte and melanocyte proliferation
- Potentiate the activity of SP, having a significant role in immunomodulation; CGRP inhibits the antigen-presenting function of Langerhans cells in part by inducing the autocrine secretion of IL-10

Nerve growth factor. Nerve growth factor (NGF) belongs to a family of neurotropic growth factors that include neurotrophin-3 and brain-derived nerve growth factor (BDNF).

NGF plays a critical role during embryogenesis, stimulating nerve growth and the direction of sensory nerve fibers to the skin. However, following the neonatal period, the growth and guidance of sensory nerves that become severed is under the influence of BDNF.

Adult skin exhibits NGF and its receptors on cutaneous nerves as well as in keratinocytes, melanocytes, and mast cells, and its expression appears to be enhanced by the presence of SP and CGRP. It is increased in the skin of patients with AD and psoriasis.

The cutaneous functions of NGF include the following:

- Keratinocyte proliferation
- Protection of melanocytes from UV-induced apoptosis through the Bcl-2 mechanism
- Maintenance of the tropism of cutaneous nerves
- Induction of degranulation of mast cells
- Mast cell proliferation
- Stimulation of IL-1 production
- Activation of B cells

Neurogenic Inflammation

The skin is innervated primarily by sensory C-fibers that extend to the very superficial layers of the epidermis. Their free nerve endings contain neuropeptides such as SP, CGRP, and pituitary adenylate cyclase-activating polypeptide (PACAP), whose release may initiate cutaneous inflammation. These bind to receptors on cutaneous blood vessels, inducing vasodilatation, increased vessel permeability, exocytosis, chemotaxis, and activation of neutrophils. These peptides, in conjunction with keratinocyte-derived CRH and NGF, also act on mast cells, resulting in the degranulation of these cells and secreting TNFα, histamine, and tryptamine. The latter has a proteolytic action on proteinase-activated receptor 2 (PAR2) on the nerve end surface. The cleavage of the tethered portion of this receptor results ultimately in the release of additional SP and CGRP. In this manner, neurogenic inflammation has the potential to extend beyond the original area. In order to control the generalization of the inflammatory response, proteases such as neutral endopeptidase are present in the tissue to mediate the degradation of the neuropeptides and thus end their activity.

Further Reading

Ding W, Wagner JA, Granstein RD (2007) CGRP, PACAP, and VIP modulate Langerhans cell function by inhibiting NF-kappa-B activation. J Invest Dermatol 127(10): 2357–2367

Hosoi J, Murphy GF, Egan CL, et al (1993) Regulation of Langerhans cell function by nerves containing calcitonin gene-related peptide. Nature 363(6425): 159–163

Peters EM, Ericson ME, Hosoi J, Seiffert K, Hordinsky MK, Ansel JC, Paus R, Scholzen TE (2006) Neuropeptide control mechanisms in cutaneous biology: physiological and clinical significance. J Invest Dermatol 126(9): 1937–1947

Roosterman D, Goerge T, Schneider SW, Bunnett NW, Steinhoff M (2006) Neuronal control of skin function: the skin as a neuroimmunoendocrine organ. Physiol Rev 86(4): 1309–1379

Rousseau K, Kauser S, Pritchard LE, Warhurst A, Oliver RL, Slominski A, Wei ET, Thody AJ, Tobin DJ, White A (2007) Proopiomelanocortin (POMC), the ACTH/melanocortin precursor, is secreted by human epidermal keratinocytes and melanocytes and stimulates melanogenesis. FASEB J 21(8): 1844–1856

Seiffert K, Granstein RD (2006) Neuroendocrine regulation of skin dendritic cells. Ann NY Acad Sci 1088: 195–206

Steinhoff M, Vergnolle N, Young SH, et al (2000) Agonists of proteinase-activated receptor 2 induce inflammation by a neurogenic mechanism. Nat Med 6(2): 151–158

Ziegler CG, Krug AW, Zouboulis CC, Bornstein SR (2007) Corticotropin releasing hormone and its function in the skin. Horm Metab Res 39(2): 106–109

Coping

Every attack of a disease is accompanied by psychosocial reactions, which in turn also have an effect on the disease process. Dealing with these processes is known in Anglo-American usage as coping. Coping with disease is the entirety of all processes to control, offset, or master existing or anticipated stress in connection with a disease emotionally, cognitively, or by actions.

In dermatology, coping is in the focus of the expanded treatment strategy, especially in the case of chronic-recurrent, disfiguring, and prognostically unfavorable diseases, and also under the aspect of improving quality of life. One example of this is metastasis-free long-term survival in malignant melanoma (see Chap. 2), which is associated with an effective coping style (Drunkenmölle et al. 2001).

Questions of coping and quality of life are also in the foreground of therapy concepts in incurable virus diseases, such as HSV infections, due to their chronic course (Spencer et al. 1999).

In dermatology, the following central mechanisms can repeatedly be observed: disease – adjustment disorder – anxiety – depression – social withdrawal.

Every physical disease is accompanied by emotional coping. Disease can not only be elicited by stress, but it also generates in stress, which in turn potentiates the symptoms. Successful coping thus affects the disease process itself and vice versa.

Coping refers both to the individual and to the social structure. Psychosocial coping (Heim 1988) is oriented

- To the individual disease model – that is, the subjective theory of disease, which includes all pertinent personal experience and knowledge as well as family and sociocultural values
- To the objective state of disease in a given stage of the disease
- To the current illness situation, whether in outpatient, family, or inhospital care
- To personal resources

Differentiation is made between favorable and unfavorable coping strategies (Heim 1988; Lazarus and Folkmann 1984).

***Negative* passive coping comprises recurrent fears, depressive moods, acceptance of the disease, and passive-resigned behavior with social withdrawal and self-accusation.**

In passive coping, control is transferred to others, the symptoms influence all areas of life, and helplessness and hopelessness result. In turn, unfavorable coping can lead to exacerbation of the symptoms.

***Positive* active strategies consist of vigor, dedication, problem analysis, rebellion, and emotional relief.**

Positive coping mechanisms are necessary to adequately deal with rapidly changing emotional and sociocultural stress and altered life conditions.

Overcoming the problem proceeds through five stages:
- Shock
- Denial
- Intrusion
- Working out
- Closure

Close primary relationships are a central component of the coping strategy in a potentially threatening underburdening or overburdening environment (Lazarus 1966; Lazarus and Folkmann 1984). Social support is especially important here; it elicits subjective relief and reduces anxiety and depression (Biondi and Picardi 1999).

Aspects of social support consist primarily of the following:
- Emotional support – giving the feeling of proximity, support, and protection
- Support in solving problems – including offers of discussion, encouragement, and feedback
- Practical/material support – including financial and tactical help
- Social integration – a network of social relationships; support from common convictions and community
- Relational security – reliability in partnership, friendship, and family

Modern therapy concepts must thus promote individual coping strategies with positive coping in addition to indication-appropriate effective internal and local drug therapy in order to reduce the frequency of recurrence of attacks of the illness or to overcome serious traumatization.

The Doctor's Promotion of Positive Coping

The doctor must first gain insight into the patient's coping with respect to biopsychosocial aspects. This usually depends essentially on the stage of the disease and the patient's psychosocial situation. For example, hospitalization should be made as pleasant as possible. It is important to know whether the patient can accept the disease and is emotionally stable or decompensated. Conclusions concerning the effectiveness of coping can be drawn from this and an adequate procedure deduced. The offer of discussion, in the sense of psychosomatic primary care, takes priority. The doctor, as a reliable discussion partner, also serves as a source of relief for the patient.

Measures for Positive Coping

- Identification and promotion of personal coping strategies
- Permission for emotional display
- Cognitive restructuring
- Involvement of the social environment
- Creation of a pleasant framework for treatment
- Occupational rehabilitation

Disruptions in the family should be relieved by involving the family early and by holding discussions with family members. A climate should be created in which fears and questions can be voiced openly to give the patient a sense of security.

Supportive measures with promotion of intact personality traits are foremost for offering help in dealing with problems. If this is not adequate, specialist psychotherapeutic intervention should be initiated.

References

Biondi M, Picardi A (1999) Psychological stress and neuroendocrine function in humans: the last two decades of research. Psychother Psychosom 68(3): 114-150

Drunkenmölle E, Helmbold P, Kupfer J, Lübbe D, Taube KM, Marsch WC (2001) Metastasenfreies Langzeitüberleben bei malignem Melanom ist mit effektivem Copingstil assoziiert. Z Hautkr 76(Suppl 1): 47

Heim E (1988) Coping und Adaptivität: Gibt es geeignetes und ungeeignetes Coping? Psychother Psychosom Med Psychol 38: 8–18

Lazarus RS (1966) Psychological stress and the coping process. McGraw-Hill, New York

Lazarus RS, Folkmann S (1984) Stress, appraisal and coping. Springer, New York

Spencer B, Leplege A, Ecosse E (1999) Recurrent genital herpes and quality of life in France. Qual Life Res 8(4): 365–371

Further Reading

Heim E, Augustiny K, Blaser A (1983) Krankheitsbewältigung (Coping) – ein integratives Modell. Psychother Psychosom Med Psychol 33: 34–40

Quality of Life

Quality of life consists of the partial areas of physical well-being, emotional well-being, social relationships, and functional capacity (Bullinger 1997). The quality of life in the sense of the patient's experience is determined these days by standardized questionnaires for self-rating (Fig. 12.4). Increased limitations in quality of life refer to the areas of the person's job, family, nutrition, financial situation, and social relationships (Bullinger 1997).

In all dermatological studies, the greatest limitation in quality of life was found in patients with AD. These patients feel significantly more limited in their quality of life than patients with urticaria, alopecia androgenetica/diffusa, glossodynia, alopecia areata, or dermatitis artefacta (Niemeier et al. 2002).

Quality of life is more frequently taken into account in dermatological therapy studies, such as in oncology as a further assessment and comparison criterion in studies on chemotherapy. Broad application in practical patient care has, however, proven useful only in individual cases.

A number of questionnaires are currently available for self-rating of quality of life (AWMF 2000):

Cardiff Acne Disability Index (Motley and Finlay 1992), Dermatology Life Quality Index (Finlay and Khan 1994), Dermatology-Specific Quality of Life Instrument (Anderson and Rajagopalan 1997), Eczema Disability Index (Salek 1993), Freiburg Quality of Life Assessment (Augustin 1997), *Lebensqualitätsfragebogen bei arterieller Verschlusskrankheit*-86 (Bullinger et al. 1996), Marburg Skin Questionnaire (Stangier et al. 1996), Psoriasis Disability Index (Finlay and Kelly 1987), Recurrent Genital Herpes Quality of Life Questionnaire (Doward 1998), Rhinitis Quality of Life Questionnaire (Juniper 1993), Skindex (Chren et al. 1996, 1997), *Tübinger Fragebogen zur Messung der Lebensqualität von CVI-Patienten* (Klyscz 1998), and for children, the Children Dermatology Life Quality Index (Lewis-Jones and Finlay 1995) and Pediatric Symptom Checklist (Rauch et al. 1991).

More detailed literature on the questionnaires is available from Hogrefe-Verlag, Göttingen (see Chap. 14).

References

Anderson RT, Rajagopalan R (1997) Development and validation of a quality of life instrument for cutaneous diseases. J Am Acad Dermatol 37(1): 41–50

12

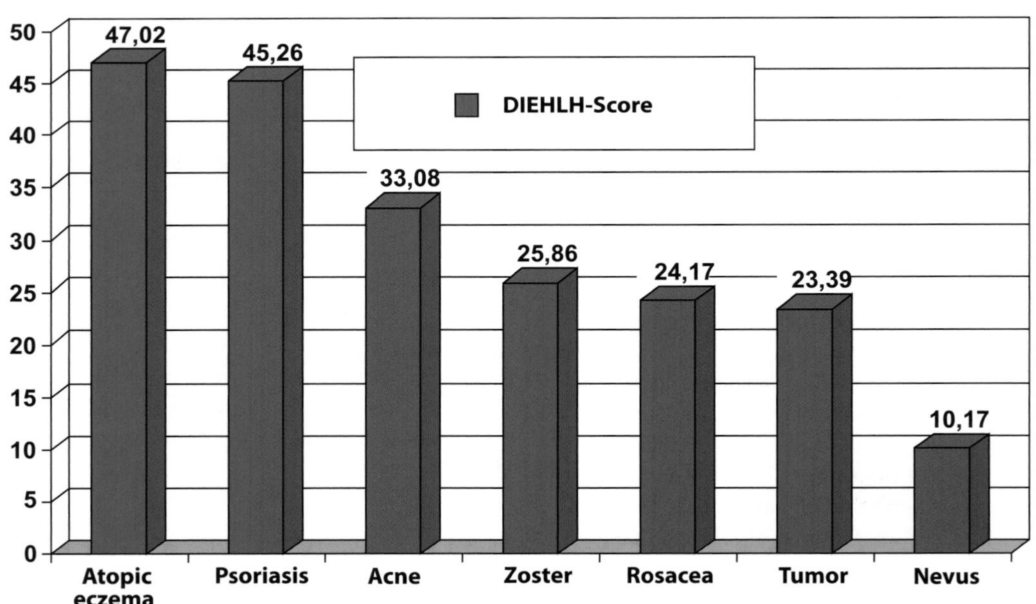

Fig. 12.4 Quality of life in dermatology (high scores correspond to high limitations). From Staudt et al. (2002)

Augustin M, Dieterle W, Zschocke I, Brill C, Trefzer D, Peschen M, Schöpf E, Vanscheidt W (1997) Development and validation of a disease-specific questionnaire on the quality of life of patients with chronic venous insufficiency. Vasa 26(4): 291–301

AWMF (2000) Erfassung von Lebensqualität in der Dermatologie. http://www.AWMF-Leitlinien.de

Bullinger M (1997) Gesundheitsbezogene Lebensqualität und subjektive Gesundheit. Überblick über den Stand der Forschung zu einem neuen Evaluationskriterium in der Medizin. Psychother Psychosom Med Psychol 47: 76–91

Bullinger M, Cachovan M, Creutzig A, Diehm C, Gruss J, Heidrich H, Kirchberger I, Loeprecht H, Rogatti W (1996) Development of an illness-specific instrument for assessment of quality of life in patients with arterial occlusive disease (Peripheral Arterial Occlusive Disease 86 Questionnaire). Vasa 25(1): 32–40

Chren MM, Lasek RJ, Quinn LM, Mostow EN, Zyzanski SJ (1996) Skindex, a quality-of-life measure for patients with skin disease: reliability, validity, and responsiveness. J Invest Dermatol 107(5): 707–713

Chren MM, Lasek RJ, Flocke SA, Zyzanski SJ (1997) Improved discriminative and evaluative capability of a refined version of Skindex, a quality-of-life instrument for patients with skin diseases. Arch Dermatol 133(11): 1433–1440

Doward LC, McKenna SP, Kohlmann T, Niero M, Patrick D, Spencer B, Thorsen H (1998) The international development of the RGHQoL: a quality of life measure for recurrent genital herpes. Qual Life Res 7(2): 143–153

Finlay AY, Kelly SE (1987) Psoriasis – an index of disability. Clin Exp Dermatol 12(1): 8–11

Finlay AY, Khan GK (1994) Dermatology Life Quality Index (DLQI) – a simple practical measure for routine clinical use. Clin Exp Dermatol 19(3): 210–216

Juniper EF, Guyatt GH, Andersson B, Ferrie PJ (1993) Comparison of powder and aerosolized budesonide in perennial rhinitis: validation of rhinitis quality of life questionnaire. Ann Allergy 70(3): 225–230

Klyscz T, Jünger M, Schanz S, Janz M, Rassner G, Kohnen R (1998) Quality of life in chronic venous insufficiency (CVI). Results of a study with the newly developed Tübingen Questionnaire for measuring quality of life of patients with chronic venous insufficiency. Hautarzt 49(5): 372–381

Lewis-Jones MS, Finlay AY (1995) The Children's Dermatology Life Quality Index (CDLQI): initial validation and practical use. Br J Dermatol 132: 942–949

Motley RJ, Finlay AY (1992) Practical use of a disability index in the routine management of acne. Clin Exp Dermatol 17: 1–3

Niemeier V, Harth W, Kupfer J, Mayer K, Linse R, Schill WB, Gieler U (2002) Prävalenz psychosomatische Charakteristika in der Dermatologie. Hautarzt 53: 471–477

Rauch PK, Jellinek MS, Murphy JM, Schachner L, Hansen R, Esterly NB, Prendiville J, Bishop SJ, Goshko M (1991) Screening for psychosocial dysfunction in pediatric dermatology practice. Clin Pediatr (Phila) 30(8): 493–497

Salek MS (1993) Measuring the quality of life patients with skin disease. In: Walker SR, Rosser RM (eds) Quality of life assessment; key issues in the 1990 s. Kluwer Academic, Lancester, pp 355–370

Stangier U, Ehlers A, Gieler U (1996) Fragebogen zur Bewältigung von Hautkrankheiten (FBH), Manual. Hogrefe, Göttingen

Further Reading

Finlay AY (1997) Quality of life measurement in dermatology: a practical guide. Br J Dermatol 136: 305–314

Sociocultural Influence Factors and Culture-Dependent Syndromes

The spectrum of dermatology – especially venereology – has shifted over the centuries because of social and cultural developments (Hindson 1982; Spitzer 1967).

A transcultural comparison of various habitats brings a particular gain in knowledge concerning the influence of sociocultural aspects (Guarnaccia and Rogler 1999). Comparative studies of various cultures and social systems are particularly helpful in revealing pathogenic and psychosocial causes and comorbidities.

Migration

Migrations of ethnic groups have taken place for thousands of years. The causes have usually been hunger, epidemics, war, climate, and religious or economic difficulties. Currently, the spectrum of disease is influenced by general mobility in seeking work and increasing travel activities (Hausen et al. 2000), which give new and greater importance to vacation dermatoses, including tropical dermatoses.

The altered environmental conditions, with separation of foreigners from their accustomed home environment, and the social factors of emigration, as well as job

Table 12.3 Diagnosis spectrum of Germans and foreigners (*STD* sexually transmitted disease)

Frequent diagnoses	Foreigners (*n*=369)	German control group (*n*=200)
Urticaria	16.5%	3.5%
STD	11.7%	4.0%
Eczema	10.6%	11.0%
Psoriasis	9.8%	9.0%
Erysipelas	6.0%	11.0%
Malignant melanoma	3.0%	11.0%
Leg ulcers	1.1%	8.0%

loss or dissatisfaction, poverty, malnutrition, and grief may elicit a state of adaptive failure and contribute to the onset of psychosomatic illnesses (Weiner 1983).

In Germany, marked differences were found in the diagnosis spectrum of Germans and foreigners in the example of hospitalized patients at the dermatology clinic of the Free University Berlin (Harth 1991; see Table 12.3). Among the foreigners, urticaria and sexually transmitted diseases dominated the diagnoses reached, while leg ulcers, erysipelas, and malignant melanomas were rather rare.

References

Guarnaccia PJ, Rogler LH (1999) Research on culture-bound syndromes: new directions. Am J Psychiatry 156(9): 1322–1327

Harth W (1991) Haut- und Geschlechtserkrankungen in einem ausländischen Patientenkollektiv. Med Dissertation, Freie Universität Berlin

Hausen BM, Stephan U, Heidbreder G (2000) p-Phenylendiamin-Kontaktallergie als Urlaubssouvenir. Akt Dermatol 26: 230–234

Hindson TC (1982) Skin diseases of immigrants. Practitioner 226: 1271–1274

Spitzer R (1967) Geographische Verteilung der Hautkrankheiten. In: Gottron (Hrsg) Handbuch der Haut- und Geschlechtskrankheiten. Ergänzungswerk Bd VIII, Springer, Berlin, S 24

Weiner H (1983) Gesundheit, Krankheitsgefühl und Krankheit; Ansätze zu einem integrativem Verständnis. Psychother Psychosom Med Psychol 33: 15–34

12

Further Reading

Graham-Brown RA, Berth-Jones J, Dure-Smith B, Naafs B, Pembroke AC, Harth W, Gollnick H, Orfanos C, Kurwa A, Bowry V (1990) Dermatologic problems for immigrant communities in a Western environment. Int J Dermatol 29: 94–101

Classification Problems in Culture-Dependent Syndromes

Culture-dependent syndromes (ICD-10: F48.8) are limited to specific societies and cultural areas and show close association with locally accepted sociocultural beliefs and behavior patterns. They are thus a prime example for the decisive influence of sociocultural causality in the biopsychosocial model.

Differential-diagnostically, local variations of anxiety and panic disorders, depressive disorders, and, especially, somatoform disorders must be clarified.

Because the discussion is still ongoing, the culture-dependent syndromes are listed separately in the appendix to the DSM-IV (American Psychiatric Association 2000). Among these are amok, ataque de nervios, bilis/cholera (muina), bouffée délirante, brain fag, dhat, falling-out/blacking out, ghost sickness, hwa-byung/wool-hwa-byung, koro, latah, locura, mal de ojo, nervios, pibloktoq, qi-gong, rootwork, sangue dormido, shenjing shuairuo, shen-k'uei, shin-byung, spell, susto, taijin kyofusho, and zar.

Latah is (as a special form of posttraumatic stress disorder) a fear-laden reaction to sudden stress situations (war, natural disasters, or social changes), which is expressed in hypersuggestibility, automatic obedience, and various echo phenomena (echolalia and echopraxia).

Susto is the fear in certain South American areas that the soul could temporarily leave the body because of stress.

The *Koro syndrome* (ICD-10: F48.8) is a culture-dependent syndrome that occurs epidemically and suddenly in Asia (Chap. 5).

These syndromes occur only sporadically as comorbidities in Germany (Kraeplin 1913). There is no specific culture-dependent syndrome for Western industrial nations. In our culture, however, the classification of eating disorders, especially anorexia nervosa (ICD-10: F50.0), is discussed as a culture-dependent syndrome. Anorexia nervosa is defined as an intentionally caused or maintained loss of weight.

References

American Psychiatric Association (2000) Diagnostic and statistical manual of mental disorders, 4th edn: DSM-IV. American Psychiatric Association, Washington, DC [Diagnostisches und Statistisches Manual Psychischer Störungen DSM–IV. Hogrefe, Göttingen]

Kraeplin E (1913) Psychiatrie Lehrbuch, 8. Aufl. Barth, Leipzig

Part IV

From the Practice for the Practice

13 Psychosomatic Psychodermatologic Primary Care and Psychosomatic Diagnostic

Psychosomatic psychodermatologic primary care is the professional term for the procedures and basic treatment of psychosomatic problems in dermatology.

The goal of psychosomatic psychodermatologic primary care is to enable every doctor to apply psychosomatic models in his or her diagnostic and therapeutic activities and as a component of insurance contract/ medical services.

According to a statement issued by the Quality Control Commission of the Federal Medical Boards in Germany (AWMF), the care of psychosomatic problems in primary care should achieve the following:

- Recognize psychosocial aspects of a disease in frequently occurring problems
- Create knowledge of interactionary access to the patient, enhancing attention to the importance of the practitioner–patient interaction
- Provide extended services, including systems to accommodate the psychosocial care of patients

The first contact with the patient must serve to provide an empathetic and accepting context leading to increased cooperation between the patient and the doctor, including implementing a structured interview and taking a psychosomatically oriented history. Initially the dermatologist needs to create a context with sufficient privacy, signaling and creating a willingness for discussion, including eliciting the patient's explanations and beliefs regarding his or her disease as well as subjective experience, with verbalization of emotional experiences; this is often a basic prerequisite to providing psychodermatologic somatic primary care in this field.

A positive attitude that basically accepts the patient's views and beliefs, including his or her nonsomatic problems, is critical. This may be expressed by verbal and nonverbal behavior. In principle, a benevolent composure should exist. Acceptance of the suffering that the patient subjectively experiences because of his or her skin disease must also be accepted, even if it appears exaggerated to the doctor (such as in the case of body dysmorphic disorder) or without foundation (as in delusions of parasitosis).

Due to the lack of an exclusive linear causality between the dermatological condition acting as a syndrome and the underlying psychiatric cause, the psychiatric diagnosis is crucial for developing an effective treatment plan.

The diagnosis of the underlying psychiatric conditions in psychodermatology involves several dimensions. Evaluating each of these provides the psychodermatologist with more opportunities to develop an effective treatment:

1. Establish the level of functioning
2. Evaluate the different physical and psychosocial stressors influencing the level of functioning
3. Evaluate concurrent affective components
4. Weight the presence of secondary gain
5. Consider the bona fide quality of the consultation

Establishing the Level of Functioning

For assessing the level of functioning, a broad approximation can operatively orient toward treatment (1. psychosis/confusional, 2. borderline/dissociative, 3. neurotic/repressive). Useful tools for assessing functioning include preliminary information and systematic clinical tools, which can be contributory. Each practitioner needs to become proficient in using an appropriate set of these.

Using Preliminary Information

The information in the chart at the time of the interview can give important clues to the psychodermatologist. The psychosocial information can suggest probable difficulties with compliance with treatment and keeping of appointments, particularly in cases of homelessness. Medical records, particularly psychiatric and dermatological records, can provide a history of previous providers and treatments (doctor-hopping, shopping for the "right" treatment). The chief complaint motivating the consultation is an important issue, although there is no certainty regarding the causality of a condition. For example, with dermatitis artefacta and factitious disorder, more often than not the dermatitis artefacta is caused by factitious disorder, so the presence of complaints consistent with dermatitis artefacta orients the clinician to rule out or confirm the presence of factitious disorder.

More often, the discovery of the need for a psychodermatologic approach is evidenced by findings in the consultation itself, or while encountering difficulties in treatment compliance or unexplainable obstacles for resolving the condition while treating patients in a busy institutional or private practice.

Using Systematic Clinical Tools

Examples of clinical tools are specific questionnaires to be filled out by the patient, structured interviews, and psychosomatically oriented history taking.

Classic Psychosomatically Oriented History vs. Structured Interview

History taking can stem the anxiety of both the patient and the practitioner (particularly if a resident) because it falls within the classic expectations, giving an active role to the practitioner and a passive role to the patient.

On one hand, classic history taking is content-oriented, collects more data, and is good for decreasing stress, but it tends to prevent evaluation of the patient's functioning in the interview itself. On the other hand, the process-oriented structured interview obtains information by observing the patient's presentation and his or her reactions to the psychodermatologist's exploration, giving a very reliable picture of the patient's level of functioning including the level of anxiety and the patient's reactions to stress; thus, the structured interview provides a sample of the patient's current functioning.

The methodical classic history-taking model is reliable and can be performed by someone with little training. The structured interview needs supervised practice in order to facilitate the clinician's proficiency.

Several structured psychiatric interviews are effective and reliable and can be adapted to the dermatological consultation.

One Example of a Structured Interview Following the Kernberg Structural Interview

The usefulness of Kernberg's structural interview applied to the psychodermatologic situation lies in giving the practitioner the opportunity to establish the current psychiatric level of functioning (neurotic/repressive, borderline/dissociative, psychotic/confusional, organic brain syndrome) while evaluating and assessing the patient's treatment of the chief complaint, in this case the dermatological symptoms.

Kernberg suggests inviting the patient to present an outline of the reasons for the consultation, including his or her expectations of the treatment, and to describe the symptoms, problems, and predominating difficulties.

The patient's answers are evaluated in two different ways, one passive: The patient's answers are evaluated for their capability to comprehend and describe himself/herself and the current circumstances, the type of defenses used – dissociative defenses (in polarities, idealized or denigrated; black or white or repressive where a more integrated set of attributions in which desired and undesirable traits coexist) – and the reality testing.

This passive qualifying of the patient presentation is probed by the clinician in a dynamic way, with three types of progressive interventions:

1. **Clarifications** are used for discriminating contradictory or unclear material (dates, places, temporal sequences, use of neologisms, and so on).
2. **Confrontation/integration** probes the patient with regard to dissociated or alternating attribution of qualities (this can be in regard to himself/herself or to significant others, or eventually the previous dermatologist or other figures perceived as all good or all bad).

3. **Interpretations** challenge the patient to acknowledge some of the usually partially repressed ambivalent feelings regarding the practitioner (for example, the patient's concern before the consultation that it will not resolve the problem).

As is easy to predict, **psychotics** will have initial difficulty following the multiple-level initial questioning and will need recurrent prompts from the interviewer (taking into account the patient's educational level and cultural factors). Very often they may show difficulties for **resolving clarifications** related to data, time, causality, and chronological sequence, and their confusional functioning will worsen as the stress of the interview increases by performing clarifications. The capability of these patients to describe themselves and significant others is often markedly limited, stereotyped, and shallow. Depending on the seriousness of the psychotic phenomenon, the reality testing is impaired in one or several areas, and internal delusions often replace common sense. If confusional/psychotic functioning is predominant, exploration of other areas of the mental status examination (attention, orientation, memory, judgment, etc.) may be indicated to rule out organicity.

Patients with borderline/dissociative functioning will be more able to follow some of the levels of the initial questions; they will be able to resolve clarifications except in circumstances of high stress. (Even if the statements are untrue, the patient will be generally able to avoid making his or her lies contradictory.) The patient will be able to have some capability to describe himself/herself and significant others, often with dissociated attributes (all good or all bad). It is not unusual for those attributes to not be fixed, and the patient may refers to a significant other as being wonderful but two sentences later says the opposite. Using gentle confrontations, the psychodermatologist can explore the degree to which the borderline/dissociative patient can **integrate the dissociated attributions**; this gives the doctor an idea of the seriousness of the disorder as well as the degree to which the patient can tolerate frustration. Confrontations are interventions that increase anxiety and can be implemented only when supported by a very solid alliance with the patient. The practitioner's reactions to the dissociating patient are often intense, positively affective, or hostile, indicating to the physician the presence of "projective identification," a dissociative defense.

Neurotic/repressive functioning has several areas in common with "normal" patients. Clarifications and confrontations will not be challenging for them, and they will have the capability to describe themselves to a better extent. Most of the time, the description may allow the practitioner to have appropriate empathy for these patients. The higher level of functioning of these patients is probed with interpretations related to acknowledging some ambivalence (or appropriate lack of confidence) in the practitioner at the time or before the consultation. For some neurotic patients, the interpretation may be stressful, and they may regress to a dissociative functioning and duel in an idealization of the dermatologist that is not based on reality.

Because of its probing, a structured interview is as valuable in dermatology as it is in psychiatry. The psychiatric information obtained will furnish the clinician with valuable data regarding the patient's cognitive abilities, which is essential for planning psychoeducation. It clarifies the differential diagnosis between psychotic and borderline (dissociative) functioning, and it is also informative regarding the patient's capability for self-examination. Finally, it provides an opportunity to assess the degree of motivation that the patient is bringing to the treatment. The results of the structured interview are a good complement to the information obtained through questionnaires, psychosomatically oriented history taking, and other instruments.

Using the Findings

Exploring the patient's perceptions regarding previous dermatologists or medical practitioners opens the door to exploring the patient's perception of the dermatologist in the present consultation, giving very good clues about how to proceed. Self-observation of the psychodermatologist's own reactions with regard to the patient can inform the psychodermatologist about the type of interaction being attempted by the patient. Patients with underlying dissociative pathologies of the group of borderline personality disorder often generate in the practitioner more intense reactive affects than those with other underlying constellations.

While the perceptive psychodermatologist may at times rapidly establish a dermatological diagnosis and as well as a good psychiatric estimation of the underlying psychic pathology, a rigorous diagnostic process for establishing the level of psychic functioning is just the beginning.

The First Step

The first step is to clarify the patient's cognitive distortions with regard to the pathophysiology of the skin disease. In the case of delusional beliefs, it will be very difficult to reduce them. Showing the patient skin findings under a microscope, using a dermatology atlas, psychoeducation, digital photography for measuring progression and so on may be necessary and at times insufficient, requiring persistence at this level of work while using medication until the patient can sufficiently reduce the cognitive distortions. Irreducible delusions in the absence of intense stressors indicate a more severe psychotic underlying condition. Going further in trying to overcome confusion may increase anxiety and decrease the level of functioning in psychotic patients.

The Second Step

After completing the previous step, the patients themselves often start to elicit and correct the distortions of the relations with the dermatologist, equivalent to transference and countertransference in psychodynamic psychotherapy. First they discuss their unhappiness with previous practitioners and in some cases are able to elicit the mistrust they had with the psychodermatologist at the beginning of the treatment. The psychodermatologist must respect the pace of the patient to approach each of these aspects, not going to the next step until some results are achieved in the previous one, so that smooth acceptance of the appropriate dermatological interventions is not endangered.

The eliciting of the concerns regarding the current interview and the lack of hope and the distrust the patient had when coming to the interview are very positive indicators of high-level neurotic functioning that reveals awareness. Describing a poorly trusted previous practitioner and a very idealized version of the current provider is more suggestive of the use of dissociations.

When the level of functioning is established (psychosis/confusional, borderline/dissociative, neurotic/repressive) by using the structured interview or other clinical tools, it is particularly important to relate the determined level of functioning with the intensity of the stressors, taking into account that the concurrent stressors can be the cause of a worsening of the level of functioning (also called regression). Stressors are often caused by psychosocial pressures (economic, job- or school-related, familial, romantic, etc.) or by direct action of a disease or the burden of coping with it. Reaction to stressors may include regression and different types of anxiety.

It is important to consider that these concerns for contextualizing the psychiatric disease by including the presence of different stressors are well reflected by the diagnostic structure of the DSM-IV-TR and previous versions, in which five axes need to be specified in order to convey a full diagnostic psychiatric picture:

Axis I and axis II are used for coding the principal diagnosis and/or the cause of the consultation and the personality of the patient, respectively. In the case of children, axis II also codes developmental disorders such as mental retardation. Axis III codes the presence of general medical conditions, axis IV includes the psychosocial and environmental stressors, and axis V concerns a global assessment of functioning.

Weighting the Affective Component

Another dimension to relate with the level of functioning is evaluation of the affective dimensions, particularly the presence of depressive mood, which can also worsen the level of functioning, at times leading to a psychotic level. When addressing the affective components, discriminating the characteristics of the depressive components requires exploration of the history in order to rule out the presence of a bipolar disorder. In this case, it is particularly important to avoid prescribing antidepressants because of the risk of inducing a manic/hypomanic episode. Using mood stabilizers and antipsychotic medication with mood-stabilizing properties is the appropriate approach. In cases in which the underlying pathology is more psychoaffective, the mood component may require appropriate treatment.

Evaluating Secondary Gain

This is a crucial area to evaluate in order to identify or rule out underlying factitious disorder and malingering. In factitious disorder, the secondary gain that the patient is pursuing is to obtain the role of the sick person; there are no material, economic, legal, job-related, or other benefits, which is always the case in malingering. The underlying functioning is dissociative in factitious disorder, and awareness fluctuates. In malingering, the person is completely aware and can be better understood as a malingering.

Conducting the Treatment

Ideally, the phenomena of transference and countertransference and perception of cognitive structures should be incorporated. Time management and structures must be clarified so that smooth operation of the dermatological practice is not endangered.

Specific case management and psychosocial resources must be considered for patients unable to perform their treatment due to psychosocial stressors. At times it may be necessary to enlist the help of family, friends, or involved neighbors. Psychosocial stressors require psychosocial solutions.

Practical Intervention Techniques: Outlining the Process

- Be empathetic and establish cooperation, even with difficult patients.
- Explore the subjective theory of disease and life situation (stress, life events).
- Diagnose dermatological, medical and underlying psychiatric conditions.
- Diagnose basic circular patterns such as itching–scratching, excoriation–anxiety relief, etc.
- Begin with clarification of the subjective theory of disease.
- Obtain cooperation and compliance with treatment.
- Cautiously correct irrational expectations.
- Provide a biopsychosocial model of disease, giving information and knowledge about the disease (psychoeducation).
- Provide compliance assurance and clarification of individual therapy goals (help patient to self-help).
- Promote coping.
- Strive for mutual development of biopsychosocial treatment.
- Follow with clarification of distortion of interactions with the provider/s.
- Evaluate other stressors.
- Evaluate concurrent disease.
- Evaluate and treat affective components.
- Develop a multilevel intervention plan.
- Further techniques include thematization, possibly enhancement of further motivation, indication, initiation of special treatment procedures, relaxation techniques, and differential indication for psychotherapy and/or psychopharmacotherapy.

Other Therapeutic Implementations

Family inclusion. Long before the conceptualization of family therapies, families were the ones most commonly taking care of individuals with medical and psychiatric problems. Obtaining the patient's consent to include his or her family in the treatment plan is something for the psychodermatologist to consider. The initial goals of obtaining better compliance with treatment, appointment keeping, and/or disrupting the itching–scratching cycle are some of the many indications for including the patient's family.

In some cases, exploring the existence of family conflict that adds stress to the patient or the existence of disruption in family relations due to the patient's skin condition can be considerations for a referral to family therapy.

Factors that are decisive include the doctor's continued education and knowledge about the diagnosis and differential diagnosis of psychosomatic disorders; psychosomatic treatment concepts; various psychotherapeutic procedures, including relaxation procedures; differential indication for psychotherapy; and initiation of special treatment procedures.

In the biopsychosocial approach, a change in the doctor–patient relationship can motivate the patient to initiate psychotherapy. This can often be achieved when the dermatologist sees through the distortions of the perception of the dermatologist by the patient (also called transference) and the practitioner's own reactions (called countertransference phenomena in dynamic psychology) in dealing with problem patients.

Catamnestic studies after a period of 12 months or more especially confirm that more has been achieved and elicited by psychosomatic primary care than was initially apparent. Some psychological problems are probably improved after the dermatological ones are successfully resolved.

Supportive Procedures and Crisis Intervention

Supportive psychotherapy as part of psychosomatic primary care, strengthening of coping (see Chap. 12, section on coping), and acute crisis intervention comprise primarily supportive techniques, for example, in reactive adjustment disorders. Supportive psychotherapy is the application of psychoanalytical principles to patients who would not find interpretive psychotherapy helpful. Supportive psychotherapy is a collective term for various techniques and procedures aimed at correcting or relieving acute emotional decompensations. This procedure does not aim primarily, however, at supporting insight and knowledge or at initiating maturation steps.

Strengthening of the stable and intact personality traits is especially used to support the overcoming of difficulties. In addition, supportive interventions such as sedation, instruction, and consultation are used. The transition to short-term therapy or focal therapy is often fluid. In crisis intervention, the therapist's activity and guidance in structuring are more pronounced than in other supportive measures.

Deep-Psychological Focal Therapy/Short-Term Therapy

It is often necessary to perform psychotherapy as focal therapy, in which only the current main conflict in the symptoms is addressed. The main conflict can usually be identified as the elicitor, for example in acute urticaria. The conflict is recalled to currency in therapy and set in the focus of in-depth treatment without addressing other related areas.

Tips and Tricks for Psychosomatic Dermatology in Clinical Practice

The practicing physician is often caught between the main task of making an objective, quick somatic decision and providing the necessary empathy with patients in the area of psychosomatic dermatology. The expanded initial access is first made via the psychosomatic anamnesis, possibly in a setting outside the routine office appointment or ward rounds (Chap. 19).

A structured doctor–patient relationship, structured scheduling of appointments, and patience are primary.

> **Initial Structuring of Cooperation in the Practice (Stepwise Plan)**
>
> - Structuring of the doctor–patient relationship
> - Clarification of the setting
> - Structured appointment schedule, created by making concrete appointments (2–4 week intervals, time limits)
> - Complaint diary
> - Psychoeducation

Acceptance of psychosocial aspects or psychotherapy motivation is initially rare, yet it can be promoted by scheduling concrete appointments (2–4 week intervals) and long-term and regular follow-up appointments. Attention should be paid to the time frame and limits. This point has proven useful in practice because it can reduce pressure in dealing with problem patients.

A complaint diary can also promote biopsychosocial understanding of the disease (see Chap. 14), as can psychoeducation.

Psychoeducation

Patients with dermatitis artefacta syndrome, somatoform disorders including body dysmorphic disorder, hypochondria, or delusional diseases are frequently not open to biopsychosocial concepts, and especially not to psychotherapy. These patients usually have a purely somatic concept of disease or desire somatic therapy.

If the diagnosis of a psychological disorder has been confirmed by the practitioner, but the patient is not motivated for psychotherapy, there is often a doctor–patient conflict.

If no tenable doctor–patient relationship can be established under expanded biopsychosocial aspects – with primary emotional causality of the dermatosis – structured psychoeducation is often the best step and the only possible procedure to create a working relationship with these otherwise hard-to-treat problem patients.

The basis of psychoeducation is teaching psychosomatic concepts by providing information and knowledge about the disease, thereby teaching a biopsychosocial model of the disease.

For this, the following information and topics are helpful as "soothing assurances" and can contribute to the reduction of anxiety, even in nonmotivated patients.

> **Practical Theme-Centered Psychoeducation Using Biopsychosocial Aspects**
>
> - The patient's problem is not a rare case.
> - The genesis of the disease is known (psychosomatic).
> - The disease is unpleasant but not dangerous.
> - Help and treatment are available and successful.
> - Deteriorations will be dealt with in therapy.
> - Relate patient successes.
> - Refer to earlier experiences (life experiences, therapy experiences).

Additional topics are those that focus on coping with everyday stress and the patient's psychosocial situation, the intent being to later enable access to central conflicts.

The minimal form of psychoeducation is initially helpful (e.g., body dysmorphic disorder) and should contain the following basic topics:

- Body dysmorphic disorder is a widespread illness.
- It is well studied and responds well to treatment.
- A number of patients suffer from it.

A viewpoint oriented to biopsychosocial aspects can be promoted by thematizing emotional contents, even in initially nonmotivated patients.

Training

Patients with chronic skin diseases, somatopsychic disorders, and others that need intensive dermatological treatment require additional therapeutic alternatives, such as the training that is currently broadly offered as part of the model project for atopic dermatitis patient training and education. Training centers have now been established throughout Germany and Europe. Other single training programs are offered regionally for patients with psoriasis and malignant melanoma.

Patient training should provide knowledge and the ability to improve self-management. This includes long-term improvement of the skin disease by increasing therapy motivation, adequate coping with somatic and psychosocial aspects of the disease, and strengthening of the patient's own competence.

The enhanced control of the disease should ideally lead to improvement in psychosocial adjustment, better ability to cope with the disease, reduced complications, enhanced compliance, reduced hospitalizations, and improved quality of life.

Training Usually Consists of Three Central Components

1. Education about the disease and knowledge for self-management
2. Working out of new emotional experiences and modification of behavior (social education)
3. Training in relaxation techniques

Auxiliary Tools for Psychodermatological Evaluation Diagnosis and Treatment

The previous sections described two different pathways for evaluating the psychological and psychosomatic level of functioning, using clinical approaches centered in the interview with the patient. Similar information can be gleaned by using tests and self-assessment questionnaires.

Several areas of psychopathology are well covered by self-assessment questionnaires, particularly psychotic symptoms; manic, hypomanic, and depressive symptoms; and psychosocial and familial conflicts. Also, insights may be obtained regarding the level of stress and anxiety as well as psychotic symptoms that otherwise are often masked.

It is important for each clinic and practitioner to find a set of self-assessment questionnaires and/or tests and become familiar with them. The more familiar the dermatologist becomes in administering and/or evaluating the test and self-reporting questionnaires, the easier it will become to identify and treat the different psychiatric conditions that underlie, aggravate, or are reactive to the dermatological disease. When the dermatologist becomes experienced in diagnosing these conditions, the use of standardized tools may no longer be necessary.

Each of the standardized assessment tools includes scales demarcating when the symptomatology is abnormal, and even though the diagnosis is not secured by the test, a strong presumption may orient the diagnosis by the psychodermatologist and indicate the appropriate therapeutic intervention.

Extreme values may be indicative of postponing the dermatological therapeutic approach and referring the patient urgently to the psychiatric service.

Self-assessment questionnaires and tests can be administered without the assistance of an experienced clinician.

Additionally, self-reporting questionnaires are routinely used in the United States for tracking service satisfaction and psychosocial needs and can bring light to housing, environmental, familial crisis, or other conflicts that are amplifying or influencing mood or psychotic disorders. Inconsistencies throughout the questionnaires can document and clarify issues related to secondary gain as well.

Advantages of the tests and self-assessment questionnaires:

1. They standardize evaluation.
2. They allow extensive review of the patient's psychopathologic and psychosocial characteristics.
3. They systematically document the information, and the information is ready for further review and research.
4. They are impersonal; asking questions personally about psychiatric symptoms can be interpreted in different fashions by the patient, particularly the paranoid patient who may interpret the questions as the clinician's assuming that the patient has that symptom, particularly in the case of hallucinations or psychotic symptoms.

5. Suicidal risk and exploration of past attempts can be evaluated with less charge or chance of being construed with suspicion or suggestion.
6. Some of the questionnaires can be filled out by family members, furnishing complementary information.

Psychological Test Diagnostics

Psychological self-rating instruments can support the clinical diagnostics and indication decision for psychotherapy in dermatology. Special dermatological as well as general questionnaires for self-rating and rating by others can be used.

The questionnaire on coping with skin diseases (*Marburger Hautfragebogen*, MHF, Stangier et al. 1997) and the Symptom Checklist SCL-90-R (Franke 1995) have proven beneficial in the framework of liaison services in Germany.

Frequently Used Psychological Test Instruments in Dermatology

- General self-rating questionnaires
  - Symptom checklist: SCL-90-R
  - Beck Depression Inventory (BDI)
  - Hospital Anxiety and Depression Scale (HADS)
  - Dysmorphic Concern Questionnaire (DCQ)
- Special dermatological questionnaires
  - Dermatology Life Quality Index (DLQI; Finlay & Khan 1994)
  - Skindex
  - Marburg Skin Questionnaire (MHF)

13

Questionnaires for Practical Use in Dermatology

Many international questionnaires relating to skin diseases have been developed in recent years. Most of the publications address quality of life, but sporadic studies of other aspects of skin diseases, such as coping, itching, skin disfigurement, have also been conducted and published. General questionnaires for patients with skin diseases have also been used in studies. Here we present first the best-known questionnaires on quality of life in skin diseases, followed by questionnaires on specific skin diseases, and finally a few general questionnaires that have also been used in patients with skin diseases.

Quality of Life in Skin Diseases

Information on the specific quality of life in patients with skin diseases represents the greatest proportion of the published articles, since quality of life has particular importance under the aspect of coping with a skin disease. The term "quality of life" is often interpreted very differently. The concept of health-related quality of life has become established in international questionnaires. It takes into account physical, mental, and social aspects as they relate to dealing with skin disease.

Dermatology Life Quality Index (Finlay and Khan 1994) The best-known of all international questionnaires on quality of life is undoubtedly the Dermatology Life Quality Index (DLQI), published by Finlay and Khan (1994) and standardized on 120 patients with 33 different skin diagnoses. The questionnaire is short and concise, which makes it particularly well suited for use in clinical routine. However, due to its brevity, it has low variance, and the emotional effects of skin diseases are not given sufficient attention. The questionnaire consists of 10 items, which are answered on a scale from 0 to 3. A general index is formed from this scale. The questionnaire has been used and tested in numerous clinical studies (Badia et al. 1999; Harlow et al. 2000; Mazotti et al. 2003; Williams et al. 2001; Zachariae et al. 2000). A random sample with 200 consecutive patients of a normal population taken at a city dermatology clinic in the United States has also been published (Hahn et al. 2001). Metaanalyses have also found the DLQI to be a very useful instrument for use in clinical practice (Skoet et al. 2003).

Dermatology Quality of Life Scales (Morgan et al 1997). This questionnaire is widely used in England and was based originally on 50 consecutive polyclinic patients (Morgan et al. 1997). It consists of a total of 41 items, divided into 17 items with psychosocial dimension, 12 items concerning physical activity, and 12 items concerning severity.

Dermatology Specific Quality of Life (Anderson and Rajagopalan 1997). This quality of life questionnaire developed in the United States was developed from information in the literature and the reports of seven young acne patients and is based on the authors' clinical experience (Anderson and Rajagopalan 1997). The questionnaire consists of 43 items and contains two scales of the SF-36, thus covering the typical aspects of physical, emotional, and social quality of life.

UK Sickness Impact Profile (Salek et al 1996). The UK Sickness Impact Profile contains 132 questions divided into 12 dimensions of life quality: sleep and relaxation, nutrition, work, household matters, hobbies and recreation, mobility, freedom of movement, personal hygiene and everyday living, social life, concentration, emotional behavior, and communication. The questionnaire has been used in patients with psoriasis, AD, and acne, and the sum value was considerably higher in the sense of limitation compared with a healthy control group (Finlay et al. 1990; Salek et al. 1993, 1996).

Dermatitis Family Impact (Lawson et al 1998). Continuing the development of quality-of-life questionnaires, Finlay's team in Cardiff also developed this questionnaire to address burdens for parents of atopic dermatitis children.

Children's Dermatology Life Quality Index (Lewis-Jones and Finlay 1995). This questionnaire on quality of life in children with skin diseases was standardized using already existing questionnaires, such as the DLQI. It consists of 10 items and can be used with children about 7 years of age or older.

Infant Dermatology of Life Quality Index (Lewis-Jones et al 2001). This questionnaire was developed as a version of the DLQI especially to record health-related quality of life in parents of children with skin diseases, and in particular children under 4 years of age. The questionnaire contains 10 items and was validated on a sample of 102 parents of atopic dermatitis children younger than 4 years of age.

Skindex (Chren et al 1996). This questionnaire was developed to measure the effects of skin diseases on the patient's quality of life. The original version of the Skindex consisted of 61 items, arranged in eight scales (Chren et al. 1996). The improved, revised version of the questionnaire by Chren et al. (1997) is shorter and shows good reliability and validity. This version, like the German translation, has 29 items arranged in three scales: symptoms, with seven items; emotions, with 10 items; and functioning, with 12 items. Patients select the statements that apply to them from a five-step scale (never/rarely/sometimes/often/always).

The terminology of the scales in the English original by Chren (1996, 1997) is used in the following description. The scale for "symptoms" primarily covers the somatic symptoms of the skin disease (e.g., the items "My skin hurts," "My skin burns or stabs"). The scale for "emotions" covers the emotional area (e.g., "The condition of my skin is depressing"), and the scale for "functioning" covers the area of social interaction/function (e.g., "The condition of my skin affects my social life," "I tend to stay home more often because of my skin disease"). It is more useable than the DLQI especially because of the inclusion of the emotional dimension. Like the DLQI, the Skindex has been used in many clinical studies (Renzi et al. 2002; Picardi et al. 2001) and has been rated as very useful in metaanalyses as well (Skoet et al. 2003).

General Questionnaires for Skin Patients

Adjustment of Chronic Skin Disorders (Stangier et al 2003). The adjustment of chronic skin disorders (ACS) is a questionnaire that assesses problems in adapting to chronic skin disorders. The original item pool was completed by 442 patients with different skin disorders. Principal-component analysis suggested a six-factor solution that was largely replicated with two additional samples of 192 patients with psoriasis or atopic dermatitis and 165 patients with atopic dermatitis. Four of the factors showed very good internal consistencies, retest reliabilities, and sufficient correlations with expert ratings: social anxiety/avoidance, itch–scratch cycle, helplessness, and anxious-depressive mood. Two short additional scales, impact on quality of life and deficit in active coping, showed moderate internal consistencies but good retest reliabilities. Correlations of the subscales with measures of depression, anxiety, and coping and meaningful differences between dermatological subgroups support the construct validity of the scales. A treatment study showed that changes in some of the subscales correlated with changes in the severity of the skin condition. The questionnaire is available in English, German, French, Italian, and Dutch.

Skin Satisfaction Questionnaire – an Instrument for Recording Attitudes Toward the Skin in Healthy Persons and Patients (Grolle et al 2003). The purpose of the Skin Satisfaction Questionnaire (SSQ, or HautZuf in German) was to construct a questionnaire on skin satisfaction suitable for recording satisfaction and attitudes toward one's own skin that can be used by dermatology and other patients, as well as by healthy subjects. In this sense, the goal was to expand the existing spectrum of dermatological-psychosomatic/psychological questionnaires, which primarily address the areas of coping with disease, quality of life, stigmatization in skin diseases, and disease-specific problems, to include underlying deep-psychological aspects, such as the role of the skin in the regulation of closeness–distance.

The SSQ has a five-factor solution, which explained 38.3% of the variance. Finally, an item pool of 30 items crystallized out; these were arranged in the following five areas: partnership touching, shame, family touching, disgust, and self-touching.

The scales all showed a high degree of internal consistency and reliability (Cronbach's alpha 0.73–0.80; split-half reliability 0.71–0.78). The scale intercorrelations were low except for correlations between the touching scales. Correlations with the Giessen test, a personality questionnaire established in Germany that was recorded in parallel, showed reconstructable correlations of the scales, but also the difference that apparently relates to the recording of a special spectrum of psychological characteristics by the SSQ.

The SSQ is thus a practicable test instrument that records a broad range of parameters in five scales with 30 items on specific psychosocial aspects of skin perception and satisfaction and on the attitudes toward the skin. It can be used by both healthy persons and (skin) patients. The SSQ is available in English, German, French, Italian, Polish, and Japanese.

Questionnaire on Experience with Skin Complaints (Schmid-Ott et al 1996). The Questionnaire on Experience with Skin Complaints (QES), which is especially for psoriasis and atopic dermatitis, was developed along the lines of the Stigmatization Questionnaire by Ginsburg and Link (1989). An English version is available (Schmid-Ott et al. 1998, 1999). Feelings of stigmatization in skin patients can be distinguished using the QES, which is a self-reporting instrument consisting of six scales and 38 items in total; the scoring system used was a Likert scale. High scores on the scale for interference of skin symptoms and self-esteem ("self-esteem") are related to frequent perceptions of worthlessness, loneliness, and uncleanliness, and high scores on the scale for outward appearance and situation-caused retreat ("retreat") are related to a lack of physical attractiveness or sexual desirability within the context of the skin disease.

Additional items question special ways of dressing or avoiding public situations. High scores on the rejection and devaluation ("rejection") scale correspond to intense anticipated or perceived reactions of others, and high scores on the composure scale describe calmness and confidence in a satisfactory life in spite of the skin disease. High scores on the concealment scale are related to frequent tendencies for hiding the diagnosis and keeping the disease a secret, and high scores on the "experienced refusal" scale are related to having frequent feelings of stigmatization in very specific situations, such as shopping or using public transportation. In a previous study, the reliability of the six QES scales was demonstrated through split-half analyses (n=384), in which Cronbach's alpha fell between 0.89 and 0.59.

Questionnaires for Specific Skin Diseases

The questionnaires that refer to specific skin diseases have the basic disadvantage that they cannot be compared with other diseases. Instead, they are designed specifically for the skin disease to be recorded and can be used very specifically for that disease.

Acne Disability Index (Motley and Finlay 1989). The Acne Disability Index (ADI) consists of 48 items arranged in eight scales: psychological aspects, physical, relaxation, job, self-perception, social reactions, skin treatment, and finances. Girman et al. (1996) developed a very similar test, which contains only 24 items based on four scales (perception, social life, emotional status, and acne symptoms).

Allergic Rhinitis (Juniper et al 1991, 1993). Juniper's team developed several questionnaires configured especially for rhinitis allergica in adults (Juniper et al. 1991) and adolescents (Juniper et al. 1993).

Allergic Rhinitis LQ (Kupfer et al 2001). This questionnaire by Kupfer et al. has not only items that address quality of life but also includes questions on coping with allergic rhinitis. It was developed, validated, and used in a therapy study.

Atopic Dermatitis (Herd et al 1997). Herd et al. (1997) developed a specific life-quality questionnaire for atopic dermatitis.

Cardiff Acne Disability Index (Salek et al 1996). The Cardiff Acne Disability Index (CADI) is a short form of the Acne Disability Index and contains only five items.

Itching Questionnaire (Yosipovitch et al 2002). Yosipovitch and his team (2002) developed a specific itching questionnaire, derived from the well-known McGill Pain Questionnaire and validated it on 100 patients with AD. A German questionnaire to record cognitions in itching has been developed (Ehlers et al. 1993), and an English version is also available. This itching cognition questionnaire has also been standardized in Japan (Tsutsui et al. 2003).

Leg Ulcer Questionnaire (Hyland 1994). With this questionnaire, Hyland introduced an instrument to record quality of life in ulcer patients. It was validated with other life-quality instruments.

Melasma Quality of Life Scale (Balkrishnan et al 2003). This questionnaire to record life quality in melasma is a 10-item questionnaire that was standardized along with the Skindex and the Melasma Area and Severity Index in 102 women with melasma.

MIMIC Questionnaire (Leu 1985). This multidimensional questionnaire uses psoriasis as an example to record disease-related quality of life, and it also takes the costs of disease into account in the recording. Due to its multidimensional structure, it is better applicable to scientific studies and has not become established in clinical studies since its publication.

MM Module (Sigurdardotti et al 1993). This life-quality questionnaire designed for melanoma patients consists of 13 items. The disease-specific symptoms are recorded, as are the consequences of chemotherapy.

Psoriasis Disability Index (Finlay and Kelly 1987). The Psoriasis Disability Index was one of the first questionnaires to record a specific aspect of psoriasis. It consists of only 10 items and describes the limitations of life quality in psoriasis. This questionnaire has been used in several important clinical studies and has proven valuable (Richards et al. 2003; Fortune et al. 2002).

Psoriasis Life Stress Inventory (Gupta and Gupta 1995). The questionnaire developed by the husband and wife team of Gupta and Gupta addresses the daily stressors for patients with psoriasis in the sense of daily hassles.

Psoriasis Specific Measure of Quality of Life (McKenna et al 2003). The PSORIQoL was tested on 62 patients with psoriasis in England, Italy, and the Netherlands. It consists of 25 items and shows good validity.

Scalpdex (Chen et al 2002). The Scalpdex was developed to record the quality of life in patients with diseases of the scalp. It contains 23 items and was validated in a study with 52 skin patients. Three scales of quality of life are differentiated: symptoms, functioning, and emotions.

Vespid Allergy Quality of Life Questionnaire (Oude Elberink et al 2002). This questionnaire was developed especially to address quality of life in patients with allergies to insect toxins. It contains 14 items covering health-related quality of life in those with allergies to bee and wasp stings. It was validated in both England and the Netherlands.

General Questionnaires Also Used for Skin Diseases

Questionnaires that do not especially address skin diseases have been repeatedly used in skin diseases. Numerous other questionnaires have also been used in skin diseases, but reference is made here only to a study by Lu et al. (2003), which, using two questionnaires on quality of life, identified helplessness as a predictor of a sense of stigmatization. Mention is made here only of particular queries in adolescents, such as the use of the Youth Self Reports and the Child Behavior Check List. If questionnaires for adolescents and their parents are of interest, a study by Berg-Nielsen et al. (2003) showed interesting correlations between self-acceptance of appearance in adolescents and depression in the mothers.

SF-36 (Bullinger 1995). The SF-36 questionnaire from Bullinger et al. (1995) was developed interculturally, and in its actual form contains 36 items. It contains questions about health-related life quality and the subjective impairment of health. It has been used primarily in internal medicine and has been standardized in several countries. Studies on dermatological samples are, however, also available (Bingefors et al. 2002).

Nottingham Health Profile (Hunt et al 1981). This questionnaire from England was developed in the 1970s and contains 38 dichotomous questions arranged in six different scales: sleep, energy, pain, physical mobility, emotional reactions, and social isolation (Kind and Care-Hill 1978). It is controversial as a sensitive instrument because it differentiates poorly in various diseases and cannot be used well for health screening.

General Health Questionnaire (Goldberg 1972). The General Health Questionnaire consists of 12 items and was developed by Goldberg as early as 1972 for the differentiation of psychiatric diseases. It has been used in various studies in dermatology (Picardi et al. 2001; Renzi et al. 2002).

Dysmorphic Concern Questionnaire. The Dysmorphic Concern Questionnaire (DCQ), used to assess dysmorphic concern and to establish correlations with clinical variables, is based on the General Health Questionnaire

(Goldberg 1972). The seven items are rated on a four-point scale. The DCQ showed strong correlations with distress and work and social impairment, lending face validity to the questionnaire. It is a good screening instrument for body dysmorphic disorder in dermatology.

Psychosocial Adjustment of Illness Scale (Derogatis 1986). The Psychosocial Adjustment of Illness Scale (PAIS), which is used worldwide to estimate psychological and psychiatric aspects in all kinds of patients, has also been used for skin patients, especially those with alopecia areata (Ruiz-Doblado et al. 2003). It is known in Germany as the SCL-90. The English version consists of 46 items and differentiates in several aspects.

SCL-90-R (Symptom Checklist). The SCL-90-R is a symptom checklist that serves to record emotional and psychovegetative complaints and takes psychopathological aspects into account. The German version was developed by Franke and Rief (Franke 1995; Rief et al. 1991). The 90 questions are arranged on scales for somatization, compulsiveness, insecurity in social contact, depressiveness, anxiety, aggressiveness/animosity, phobias, paranoid thinking, and psychoticism.

13

Three global parameters are covered in the assessment: the general symptomatic index, the positive symptom total, and the positive symptom distress index.

The SCL-90R fills the diagnostic gap between temporally extremely variable well-being and the personality structure that lasts over time. It measures the subjectively experienced impairment caused to the person being examined using 90 listed physical and emotional symptoms (Rief et al. 1991).

Beck Depression Inventory (BDI). The BDI is a self-rating instrument to record the severity of depressive symptoms and has been successfully used for more than 30 years (Hautzinger et al. 1995). It consists of 21 items, which result in sum values between 0 and 63. The contents of the items refer to sad mood, pessimism, failure, dissatisfaction, feelings of guilt, need for punishment, self-loathing, self-accusation, suicidal impulse, crying, irritability, social withdrawal and isolation, ability to make decisions, negative body image, work disability, sleep disorder, resistance to fatigue, loss of appetite, weight loss, hypochondria, and loss of libido.

General Depression Scale (ADS). The ADS (Hautzinger and Bailer 1993) asks about depressive traits: lack of self-confidence, exhaustion, hopelessness, self-denegration, despondency, loneliness, sadness, lack of energy, feeling of rejection by others, crying, ability for enjoyment, withdrawal, fear, gladness, lack of reactivity, sleep disorders, appetite disorders, trouble concentrating, and pessimism.

The ADS sum scores are formed from a 20-item version, whereby a plausibility criterion is still calculated with negative-poled items (four items).

Well-Being Scale (Zerssen and Koeller 1976). The well-being scale is a list of characteristics developed as a test to record well-being at the given moment. The test scores reflect the current subjective well-being and the state in a global sense, which is expressed in the term well-being. The contents of the items are characterized by opposites; the characteristics comprise opposite states of feeling.

Stress Coping Questionnaire (SVF 120). The SVF 120 serves to record the individual tendency to apply various means of coping under stress. These coping methods are defined by 20 subtests of six items each (Janke et al. 1997).

The subtests contain trivialization, playing down, defense against guilt, diversion, vicarious satisfaction, self-affirmation, relaxation, situation control, reaction control, positive self-instructions, need for social support, avoidance, flight, social withdrawal, brooding, resignation, self-pity, self-accusation, aggression, and taking of drugs. The assessment of the subtests is made by positive strategies and negative strategies; positive strategies are in the first 10 subtests, and negative strategies are in subtests 13–18.

Hospital Anxiety and Depression Scale – German version (HADS-D). The HADS-D is one of the most common screening-self-rating questionnaires for anxiety and depression in somatic medicine. The questionnaire has proven useful in practice, especially in functional disorders and reactive adjustment disorders. The main disorders are covered briefly with 14 items in two subscales of anxiety and depression (Herrmann et al. 1995).

Giessen test (GT). The Giessen test is a test procedure for rating oneself and others according to real-image and self-image (Beckmann et al. 1991). The responses are recorded in six scales (social resonance, dominance, control, basic mood, perviousness, social power). The test is especially well suited for control of therapeutic success.

Freiburg Personality Inventory (FPI-R). The FPI-R (Fahrenberg et al. 2001) is a factor-analytical personality procedure in questionnaire form with 138 items and the scales of satisfaction with life, social orientation, performance orientation, inhibition, excitability, aggressiveness, strain, physical complaints, worry about health, openness, and extraversion and emotionality.

Psychological Test Questionnaire for Rating by Others

Hamilton Depression Scale. The Hamilton Depression Scale is the most widely used procedure for rating by others for estimating the severity of a diagnosed depression (Hamilton 1967). The entire scale consists of 21 items, each assessed in multilevel category scales referring to the intensity of symptoms. The categories contain verbal descriptions. Information from relatives, caregivers, or friends may be used in the assessment.

References

Anderson R, Rajagopalan R (1997) Development and validation of a quality of life instrument for cutaneous disease. J Am Acad Dermatol 37: 41–50

Badia X, Mascaro JM, Lozano R (1999) Measuring health-related quality of life in patients with mild to moderate eczema and psoriasis: clinical validity, reliability and sensitivity to change of the DLQI. Brit J Dermatol 141: 698–02

Beckmann D, Brähler E, Richter HE (1991) Der Gießen-Test (GT), 4. Aufl. mit Neustandardisierung 1990. Huber, Bern

Balkrishnan R, McMichael AJ, Camacho FT, Saltzberg F, Housman TS, Grummer S, Feldman SR, Chren MM (2003) Development and validation of a health-related quality of life instrument for women with melasma. Brit J Dermatol 149: 572–577

Berg-Nielsen TS, Vika A, Dahl AA (2003) When adolescents disagree with their mothers: CBCL-YSR discrepancies related to maternal depression and adolescent self-esteem. Child Care Health Dev 29: 207–213

Bingefors K, Lindberg M, Isacson D (2002) Self-reported dermatological problems and use of prescribed topical drugs correlate with decreased quality of life: an epidemiological survey. Brit J Dermatol 147: 285–290

Bullinger M (1995) German translation and psychometric testing of the SF-36 Health Survey: preliminary results from the IQOLA Project. International quality of life assessment. Soc Sci Med 41: 1359–1366

Chen SC, Yeung J, Chren MM (2002) Scalpdex – a quality of life instrument for scalp dermatitis. Arch Dermatol 138: 803–807

Chren MM, Lasek RJ, Quinn LM, Mostow EN, Zyzanski SJ (1996) Skindex, a quality-of-life measure for patients with skin disease: reliability, validity, and responsiveness. J Invest Dermatol 107: 707–713

Chren MM, Lasek RJ, Flocke SA, Zyzanski SJ (1997) Improved discriminative and evaluative capability of a refined version of Skindex, a quality-of-life instrument for patients with skin diseases. Arch Dermatol 133: 1433–1440

Derogatis LR (1986) The psychosocial adjustment to illness scale (PAIS). Psychosom Res 30: 77–91

Ehlers A, Stangier U, Dohn D, Gieler U (1993) Kognitive Faktoren beim Juckreiz: Entwicklung und Validierung eines Fragebogens [Cognitive factors in itching: Development and validation of a questionnaire]. Verhaltenstherapie 3: 112–119

Fahrenberg J, Hampel R, Selg H (2001) Freiburger Persönlichkeitsinventar, 7. Aufl. Hogrefe, Göttingen

Finlay AY, Kelly (1987) Psoriasis – an index of disability. Clin Exp Dermatol 12: 8–11

Finlay AY, Khan GK, Luskombe DK, Salek MS (1990) Validation of Sickness Impact Profile and Psoriasis Disability Index in psoriasis. Brit J Dermatol 123: 751–756

Finlay AY, Khan G (1994) Dermatology Life Quality Index (DLQI) – a simple practical measure for routine clinical use. Clin Exp Dermatol 19: 210–216

Fortune DG, Richards HL, Main CJ et al (2002) A cognitive-behavioural symptom management programme as an adjunct in psoriasis therapy. Brit J Dermatol 146: 458–465

Franke G (1995) Die Symptom-Checkliste von Derogatis – Deutsche Version – Manual. Beltz, Weinheim

Ginsburg IH, Link BG (1989) Feelings of stigmatization in patients with psoriasis. J Am Acad Dermatol 20: 53–63

Girman CJ, Hartmeaier S, Thiboutot D, et al (1996) Evaluating health-related quality of life in patients with facial acne: development of a self-administered questionnaire for clinical trials. Qual Life Res 5: 481–490

Goldberg DP (1972) The detection of psychiatric illness by questionnaire. Oxford University Press, London

Grolle M, Kupfer J, Brosig B, Niemeier V, Hennighausen L, Gieler U (2003) The Skin Satisfaction Questionnaire – an instrument to assess attitudes toward the skin in healthy persons and patients. Dermatol Psychosom 4: 14–20

Gupta MA, Gupta AK (1995) The Psoriasis Life Stress Inventory: a preliminary index of psoriasis-related stress. Acta Derm Venereol (Stockh) 75: 240–243

Hahn HB, Melfi CA, Chuang TY, Lewis CW, Gonin R, Hanna MP, Farmer ER (2001) Use of the Dermatology Life Quality Index (DLQI) in a midwestern U.S. urban clinic. J Am Acad Dermatol 45: 44–48

Hamilton M (1967) Die Hamilton Depressionsskala. In: Collegium Internationale Psychiatriae (Hrsg) "Internationale Skalen für Psychiatrie". 4. Aufl, Beltz, Weinheim, S 93–96

Harlow D, Poyner T, Finlay AY, Dykes PJ (2000) Impaired quality of life of adults with skin disease in primary care. Brit J Dermatol 143: 979–982

Hautzinger M, Bailer M (1993) ADS. Beltz, Weinheim

Hautzinger M, Bailer M, Worall H, Keller F (1995) BDI. Huber, Bern

Herd RM, Tidman MJ, Ruta DA, Hunter JAA (1997) Measurement of quality of life in atopic dermatitis: correlation and validation of two different methods. Brit J Dermatol 136: 502–507

Herrmann Ch, Buss U, Snaith RP (1995) HADS-D – Hospital Anxiety and Depression Scale. (German version: Ein Fragebogen zur Erfassung von Angst und Depressivität in der somatischen Medizin) Huber, Bern

Hunt SM, McKenna SP, McEven J, Williams J, Papp E (1981) The Nottingham health profile: subjective health status and medical consultations. Soc Sci Med 15: 221–229

Hyland ME (1994) Quality of life of leg ulcer patients: questionnaire and preliminary findings. J Wound Care 3: 294–298

Janke W, Erdmann G, Kallus W (1997) Stressverarbeitungsfragebogen (SVF) mit SVF 120. Hogrefe, Gottingen

Juniper EF, Guyatt GH (1991) Development and testing of a new measure of health status for clinical trials in rhinoconjunctivitis. Clin Exp Allergy 21: 77–83

Juniper EF, Guyatt GH, Ferrie PJ, Griffith LE (1993) Measuring quality of life in adolescents with allergic rhinoconjunctivitis: development and testing of a questionnaire for clinical trials. J Allergy Clin Immunol 93: 413–423

Kind P, Carr-Hill R (1987) The Nottingham health profile: a useful tool for epidemiologists? Soc Sci Med 25: 905–910

Kupfer J, Brosig B, Gottwald B, Niemeier V, Gieler U (2001) Questionnaire of life quality in patients with allergic rhinitis. Allergologie 24: 300–308

Lawson V, Lewis-Jones MS, Finlay AY, et al (1998) The family impact of childhood atopic dermatitis: Dermatitis Family Impact Questionnaire. Brit J Dermatol 138: 107–113

Leu RE (1985) Economic evaluation of new drug therapies in terms of improved life quality. Soc Sci Med 10: 1153–1161

Lewis-Jones MS, Finlay AY (1995) The Children's Dermatology Life Quality Index (CDLQI): initial validation and practical use. Brit J Dermatol 132: 942–949

Lewis-Jones MS, Finlay AY, Dykes PJ (2001) The Infants' Dermatitis Quality of Life Index. Brit J Dermatol 144: 104–110

Lu Y, Duller P, van der Valk PGM, Evers AWM (2003) Helplessness as predictor of perceived stigmatization in patients with psoriasis and atopic dermatitis. Dermatol Psychosom 4

Mazzotti E, Picardi A, Sampogna F, Sera F, Pasquini P, Abene D (2003) Sensitivity of the Dermatology Life Quality Index to clinical change in patients with psoriasis. Brit J Dermatol 149: 318–322

McKenna SP, Ciook SA, Whalley D, Doward LC, Richards HL, Griffiths CEM, Van Assche D (2003) Development of the PSORIQoL, a psoriasis-specific measure of quality of life designed for use in clinical practice and trials. Brit J Dermatol 149: 323–331

Morgan M, McReedy R, Simpson J, Hay R (1997) Dermatology quality of life scales – a measure of the impact of skin diseases. Brit J Dermatol 136: 202–206

Motley RJ, Finlay AY (1989) How much disability is caused by acne? Clin Exp Dermatol 14: 194–198

Oude Elberink JNG, de Monchy JGR, Golden DBK, Brouwer JLP, Guyatt GH, Dubois AEJ (2002) Development and validation of a health-related quality of life questionnaire in patients with yellow jacket allergy. J Allergy Clin Immunol 109: 162–170

Picardi A, Abeni D,Pasquini P (2001) Assessing psychological distress in patients with skin diseases: reliability, validity and factor structure of the GHQ-12. J European Acad Dermatol Venereol 15: 410–417

Renzi C, Picardi A, Abeni D, Agostini E, Baliva G, Pasquini P, Puddu P, Braga M (2002) Association of dissatisfaction with care and psychiatric morbidity with poor treatment compliance. Arch Dermatol 138: 337–342

Richards HL, Fortune DG, Main CJ, Griffiths CEM (2003) Stigmatization and psoriasis. Brit J Dermatol 149: 209–211

Rief W, Greitemeyer M, Fichter MM (1991) Die symptom check list SCL-90-R: überprüfung an 900 psychosomatischen Patienten. Diagnostika 37: 58–65

Ruiz-Doblado S, Carrizosa A, Garcia-Herandez MJ (2003) Alopecia areata: psychiatric comorbidity and adjustment to illness. Int J Dermatol 42: 434–437

Salek MS, Khan GK, Finlay AY (1996) Questionnaire techniques in assessing acne handicap: reliability and validity study. Qual Life Res 5:131–138

Salek MS, Finlay AY, Luscombe DK, et al (1993) Cyclosporin greatly improves the quality of life of adults with severe atopic dermatitis. A randomized, double-blind, placebo-controlled trial. Brit J Dermatol 129: 422–430

Schmid-Ott G, Jäger B, Künsebeck HW, Ott R, Lamprecht F (1996) Dimensions of stigmatization in patients with psoriasis in a "questionnaire on experience with skin complaints." Dermatology 193: 304–310

Schmid-Ott G, Jäger B, Künsebeck HW, Ott R, Wedderer K, Lamprecht F (1998) Psychosocial influences on the illness experience of psoriasis-patients. A study with the "Questionnaire on Experience with Skin Complaints" (QES). ZKPP (Zeitschrift für Klinische Psychologie, Psychiatrie und Psychotherapie) 46: 330–343

Schmid-Ott G, Künsebeck HW, Jäger B, Werfel T, Frahm K, Ruitmann J, Kapp A, Lamprecht F (1999) Validity study for the stigmatization experience in atopic dermatitis and psoriasis patients. Acta Derm Venereol 79: 443–447

Sigurdardotti V, Bolund C, Brandberg Y (1993) The impact of generalized malignant melanoma on quality of life evaluated by the EORTIC questionnaire technique. Qual Life Res 2: 193–203

Skoet R, Zachariae R, Agner T (2003) Contact dermatitis and quality of life: a structured review of the literature. Brit J Dermatol 149: 452–456

Stangier U, Ehlers A, Gieler U (2003) Measuring adjustment of chronic skin disorders: validation of a self-report measure. Psychological Assessment 15: 532–549

Stangier U, Heidenreich T, Gieler U (1997) Stadien der Psychotherapymotivation in der psychosomatischen Versorgung von Hautkranken. Z Hautkr 5(72): 341–348

Tsutsui J, Miyoshi H, Yoshii K, Hashiro M, Kanzaki T, Nozoe S, Tetsuro Naruo T (2003) Validation of the Japanese version of the itch-related cognition questionnaire for atopic dermatitis. Dermatol Psychosom 4: 21–26

Williams TL, May CR, Esmail A, Griffiths CEM, Shaw NT, Fitzgerald D, Stewart E, Mould M, Morgan M, Pickup L, Kelly S (2001) Patient satisfaction with teledermatology is related to perceived quality of life. Brit J Dermatol 145: 911–917

Yosipovitch G, Goon AT, Wee J, Chan YH, Zucker I, Goh CL (2002) Itch characteristics in Chinese patients with atopic dermatitis using a new questionnaire for the assessment of pruritus. Int J Dermatol 41: 212–216

Zachariae R, Zachariae C, Ibsen H, Touborg Mortensen J, Wulf HC (2000) Dermatology Life Quality Index: data from Danish inpatients and outpatients. Acta Derm Venereol 80: 272–276

Zerssen D, Koeller DM (1976) Die Befindlichkeitsskala (Bf). Beltz, Weinheim

Further Reading

Finlay AY (1997) Quality of life measurement in dermatology: a practical guide Brit J Dermatol 136: 305–314

Finlay AY (1998) Quality of life assessments in dermatology. Semin Cutan Med Surg 17: 291–296

Halioua B, Beumont MG, Lunel F (2000) Quality of life in dermatology. Int J Dermatol 39: 801–808

13

Oosthuizen P, Lambert T, Castle DJ (1998) Dysmorphic concern: prevalence and associations with clinical variables. Aust N Z J Psychiatry. 32(1): 129–132

Radloff LS (1977) The CES-D scale: a self-report depression scale for research in the general population. Applied Psychol Measurements 1: 385–401

Renzi C, Abeni D, Picardi A, Agostini E, Melchi CF, Pasquini P, Puddu P, Braga M (2001) Factors associated with patient satisfaction with care among dermatological outpatients. Brit J Dermatol 145: 617–623

Ware JE, Sherbourne CD (1992) The MOS 36-item short form health survey (SF-36). Conceptual framework and item selection. Med Care 30: 473–483

Complaint Diary

The use of complaint diaries in dermatology, sometimes in a modified form, has proven useful and versatile. Keeping a diary can be used for long-term course control of all subjectively experienced or even objective complaints. Moreover, it is also helpful when no complaints are present at the time of consultation (negative presentation effect). Classic areas of use are the allergy diary, such as in chronic-recurrent urticaria, or pain diaries for patients with chronic pain or chronic itching.

In psychosomatic dermatology, a diary is also meaningful to slowly bring a patient with purely monocausal somatic understanding of disease and treatment expectations to an expanded psychosocial understanding of the disease. In addition to the time, site, and duration of the complaints, the place, situation, and emotional state can be noted, along with any particular features (Fig. 13.1).

The complaint diary can be used to record when exacerbations or clear improvements in the complaints occur and what changes in behavior or habits are connected with the complaints. Central to this is instructing the patient to also notice and record the emotional importance or effect of the complaints. This information can help to better structure the circumstances of the complaints. The intensity of the complaint can be made more specific by additionally using a visual analog scale.

In psychosomatic dermatology, diaries are used in itching, scratching, tearing, erythrophobia, and body dysmorphic disorders. Recording self-observations or observations by others in a diary can also help in paraartefacts (such as a tearing diary in trichotillomania or manipulation diaries) to restore impulse control of the act and often achieve a cure.

Visual Analog Scale (VAS)

The visual analog scale (VAS) is a scale on which patients can rate their personal perception of their complaints (disfiguration, pain, itching, etc.). The scale ranges, for example, from 0 "no pain" to 10 "most severe pain" (Fig. 13.2).

Using the ratings given by the patient, the doctor obtains a score and thus information for dosing pain relievers or antihistamines as well as information on therapeutic success. The extent of pain, itching, or other complaints from the patient's point of view can be recorded by means of the VAS. These ratings should, however, also be checked in the interview.

Rating Scales in Body Dysmorphic Disorders

In body dysmorphic disorder, the patient is excessively preoccupied with an imagined deficiency or subjective disfiguration of his or her outward appearance. If there is a slight physical anomaly, the afflicted person's concern is greatly exaggerated.

Date	**- Complaints (VAS)** **- Skin symptoms**	**Situation** **a) Circumstances** **b) Emotions**
–....................................... –....................................... –.......................................	–....................................... –....................................... –.......................................	–....................................... –....................................... –.......................................

Fig. 13.1 Basic form of a psychosomatic complaint diary

There is a difference between the doctor's objective and the patient's subjective rating, which may lead to disruptions in the doctor–patient relationship. Diagnostically, body dysmorphic disorder is characterized primarily by a great discrepancy between the disfiguration as rated by the examiner and the disfiguration as experienced by the patient.

The VAS from 1 to 10 has proven useful in practice as a quick (2-min) diagnostic and rating scale of body dysmorphic disorders to determine this discrepancy and also to serve as a course control.

The patient is given a VAS from 1 to 10 and indicates on this how greatly he or she feels disfigured. At the same time, the examiner independently rates the quasi-objective disfiguration. If there is a discrepancy of more than 4 units on the VAS, a body dysmorphic disorder can be suspected, which should then be more closely examined and confirmed.

The different subjective rating of the presumed anomaly can be quantified with this rating scale, and therapeutic success can be assessed later in the course (Fig. 6.3).

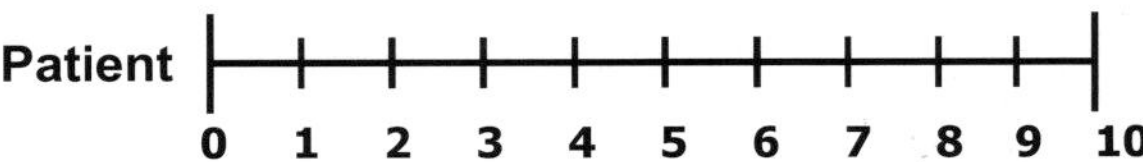

Fig. 13.2 Example of the visual analog scale (VAS)

Procedure: The doctor and patient each independently rate and document the severity of the item by marking on a scale between 0 and 10.

Question for the patient: How strongly are your feelings about yourself affected by your apperance?

Question for the doctor: How strongly is the patient affected by his or her appearance?

Assessment: If there is a difference of more than 4 points in the result, a suspected diagnosis of body dysmorphic disorder can be confirmed with high probability.

14 Psychotherapy

Indication For and Phases of Psychotherapy

As in somatic diseases, attention must be paid to indications and contraindications for psychotherapy. Moreover, there is the additional important factor of patient motivation, so reaching a decision can sometimes take years. Overall, however, the less time that elapses between the onset of emotional symptoms and adequate therapy, the better the prognosis.

Before referring the patient to a mental health provider, the psychodermatologist needs to address a number of issues. A dermatologic and psychiatric diagnosis must be performed and treatment attempted. If the treatment resolves the condition, the psychotherapy that was needed (if any) has been done. If the treatment does not resolve the psychodermatologic condition, then the psychotherapist, as a consultant or as a referral, may bring some help.

The following aspects are also discussed in the previous chapter:

- How the psychodermatologist performs a psychiatric evaluation while performing the dermatologic consultation
- How confusional (psychotic), dissociative (borderline), and neurotic functioning are evidenced in the dermatologic consultation
- How to structure the interview in order to ascertain the patient's level of functioning without creating violent situations

DSM-IV-TR
Axis 1 Psychiatric condition
Axis 2 Personality
Axis 3 Significant medical issues
Axis 4 Psychosocial stressors
Axis 5 Current level of functioning vs. previous level of functioning

Evaluating each axis clarifies the difficulties present and opens avenues for multiple levels of intervention on each level.

The psychodermatologist's interventions may progress as follows:

- Extending the joining, thereby deepening and developing the alliance
- Paying attention to the patient's theory of the disease and complaints
- Reframing and extending/enlarging the perceived causes of the disease
- Introducing dermatological interventions and treatments as appropriate, focusing on resolving the patient's complaints

The pertinent psychodermatologic evaluation will include assessment of the fund of knowledge, the abstracting level of the patient, and the psychologic/psychiatric level of functioning by walking the patient through psychoeducation, clarification, and confrontation.

Frequent Indications for Psychotherapy in Dermatology

- Deterioration of skin symptoms under emotional stress (acute or chronic)
- Pronounced social anxieties or avoidance behavior due to the skin disease (sociophobia)
- Disfiguration syndrome (body dysmorphic disorder)
- Excessive manipulation of the skin

Reaching a decision for psychotherapy depends on numerous factors. The individual's concept of disease, as well as already existing experience with therapy, is of far-reaching importance (Bassler 1995).

The severity of the core symptoms and chronification processes, which depend especially on the duration of the disease, are also involved. In individual cases, a specific eliciting situation can be identified on the basis of the patient's life history. The following central questions should be clarified during the decision-making process in dermatological consultations:

> **What kind of help is the patient seeking? What concrete support can the doctor offer in self-restructuring?**

The treating physician can thus support reflection on the problem by offering information and neutral explanations of psychotherapy; otherwise, early confrontation of the patient may lead him or her to terminate the doctor–patient relationship. The liaison interview is often the decisive building block in introducing psychotherapy in practical dermatology (Chap. 19).

The indication for psychotherapy is generally not a polarized yes–no decision but proceeds through several distinguishable phases in the course of treatment (Table 14.1).

The indication for psychotherapy is a decisional process that may last for years in dermatology. The prognosis in psychosomatic/psychiatric illnesses, as in other organic diseases, is more favorable the earlier that diagnosis and therapy are begun (Ormel et al. 1990). On average, skin patients consult a liaison service 8.7 years after onset of their disease (Niemeier et al. 2002).

A time period of 8.7 years to the possibility of a psychotherapeutic offer must be assumed to be unfavorable, since unfavorable chronification mechanisms may become manifest during that time. Shortening of this time can be achieved by the doctor's taking psychosocial factors into account and by generally creating widespread availability of liaison services as routine.

Table 14.1 Phases of psychotherapy motivation (Stangier et al. 1997)

Phase	Patient	Doctor
Prephase of problem consciousness	Denial of emotional factors	Empathy
	Monocausal concept of disease	Proposal of self-observation
		Cautious questioning
Problem reflection	Perception	Information: explanation of advantages and disadvantages of change
	Concepts of disease more precise	
Reaching a decision	Active search for change	Concrete indication
	Decision to change oneself	Referral to psychotherapy
Change	Active cooperation in therapy	Psychotherapist: psychotherapy
	Practicing new modes of behavior	Doctor: somatic therapy
		Supporting psychotherapist
Maintenance	Retention of what has been gained Change Consolidation	Doctor: somatic therapy, renewed referral to psychotherapist
		Psychotherapist: relapse prophylaxis, cooperation with the doctor

References

Bassler M (1995) Prognosefaktoren für den Erfolg von psychoanalytisch fundierter stationärer Psychotherapy. Z Psychosom Med Psychoanal 41: 77–97

Niemeier V, Harth W, Kupfer J, Mayer K, Linse R, Schill WB, Gieler U (2002) Prävalenz psychosomatischer Charakteristika in der Dermatologie. Hautarzt 53: 471–477

Ormel J, van den Brink W, Koeter MWJ, Giel R, van der Meer K, van der Willige G, Wilmink FW (1990) Recognition, management and outcome of psychological disorders in primary care: a naturalistic follow-up study. Psychol Med 20: 909–923

Further Reading

Stangier U, Heidenreich T, Gieler U (1997) Stadien der Psychotherapymotivation in der psychosomatischen Versorgung von Hautkranken. Z Hautkr 5(72): 341–348

Limitations of Psychotherapy

In initiating or recommending psychotherapy, as in somatic specialties, attention must be paid to its limitations.

The most important limitations are the following.

> **Limitations (Patient) in Psychosomatic Dermatology**
>
> - Acute psychoses
> - Brain-organic psychosyndrome
> - Acute suicidal intent
> - Alcoholism (withdrawal treatment is primary)
> - Lack of motivation for therapy (motivation phase first)
> - Malingering
> - Inadequate time resources

In the case of acute danger of suicide or acute psychoses, and also in addictions, emergency psychiatric treatment is usually in the foreground. Emergency treatment when danger to self or others is present, adherence to reporting laws, and mandatory commitment take precedence over referrals and long-term treatment. Neurological diagnostics should be made or given precedence in brain-organic changes.

The presence of organic symptoms needs to be diagnosed and considered, particularly impairments of attention, understanding, or memory of the issues important for successful treatment. Cognitive, memory, and attention deficits make verbal interventions markedly ineffective. Auxiliary methods can be implemented for compensating or can be accommodated to these impairments.

On the other hand, it is also important that a patient with low motivation not be talked into psychotherapy (refer to the information on avoidable medical treatment errors in Chap. 17).

Psychotherapy Procedures

Worldwide, there are about 2,000 therapy procedures in the area of psychosomatics, with various approaches and content. In Germany, deep-psychologically-based psychotherapy and psychoanalysis and behavior therapy are currently recognized by the medical council and thus belong to the therapeutic procedures reimbursable by the insurance system. Supplementary relaxation procedures, including autogenic training and progressive muscle relaxation in the Jacobsen method, are also included.

Determination of the indication and choice of adequate therapeutic procedure depends on the target problem, the diagnosis reached, the time frame, the patient's motivation, interaction behavior on the part of the patient, and the goal of therapy (Table 14.2).

Establishing a workable doctor–patient relationship for positive strengthening of coping and relief is always the first step (Fig. 14.1).

Behavior Therapies

Every instance of behavior therapy must be preceded by an analysis of the problematic behavior.

The SORC scheme is the central foundation for understanding this analysis:

- Stimulus (S)
- Organism variable (O)
- Reaction (R): experienced/described behavior
- Consequence (C): positive/negative reward – direct/indirect punishment

The efficacy of cognitive behavior therapy and behavior therapy interventions has been confirmed in several metaanalyses of randomized controlled studies.

The current forms of behavior therapy comprise a number of special procedures including conditioning techniques, systematic desensitization (hyposensitiza-

Table 14.2 Differential psychotherapy indication in skin diseases (adapted from Stangier and Gieler 2000)

	Behavior therapy	Deep-psychology-based psychotherapy and psychoanalysis
Target problem	Delimitable problematic behavior	General problems of life
Time frame	Definable	More likely open (exception focal therapy)
Motivation	Change-oriented explanatory model and expectations from treatment	Examination of childhood development and its influences
Interaction behavior	Willingness to cooperate	Transference relationship
Therapy goal	Mastery	Understanding and reexperiencing emotional reactions

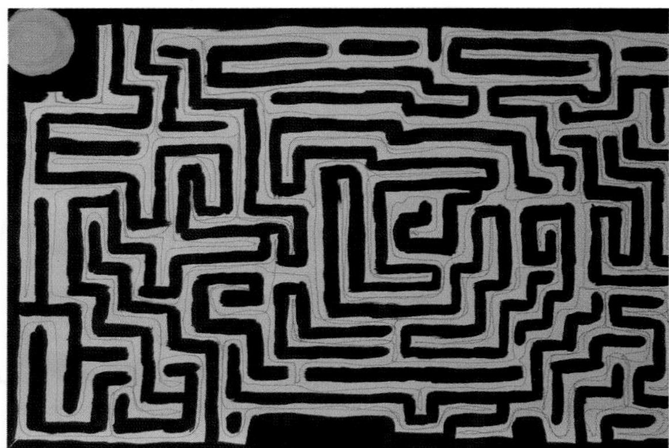

Fig. 14.1 Depressive patient: light at the end of the labyrinth in art therapy

tion), stimulus flooding, confrontation, counterconditioning, negative exercises (extinction-related reflexes), aversion techniques, learning by success, model learning, cognitive restructuring, and methods to improve self-management with promotion of self-observation and self-reward, including biofeedback as well as the inclusion of relaxation procedures.

Central behavior therapy procedures in dermatology include cognitive restructuring, especially for depressive patients. Once a therapeutic relationship has been established and the patient informed about the illness, the automatic dysfunctional cognitive strategies are identified and dealt with. In cognitive restructuring, the patient learns to better recognize his or her personal successes and to think more highly of them.

Habit-Reversal Technique (Atopic Dermatitis and Acne Excoriée)

One of the prerequisites for breaking through the itching–scratching cycle in atopic dermatitis is interrupting the automatized process of scratching and achieving self-control. A behavior therapy process for this is the habit-reversal technique.

The basis is, first, conscious recognition of the impulse to scratch, and second, interrupting the act of scratching with internal warning signals as a stop technique.

The process consists of exercises under supervision, which proceed as follows:

- First the hand moves toward the itching area on the skin.
- The patient says to himself/herself, “Don’t scratch.”
- The movement is then interrupted.
- The patient then thinks of how the scratched skin would look.
- The patient presses his or her hand firmly on the skin area for 1 min.
- Then a brief relaxation exercise is performed, and the patient remains in the relaxed phase.

For additional information on behavior therapy group programs, we refer the reader to the extensive literature, especially *Neurodermitis Bewältigen* by Stangier et al. (1996).

Reference

Stangier U, Gieler U, Ehlers A (1996) Neurodermitis bewältigen. Springer, Berlin

Further Reading

Kent A, Drummond LM (1989) Acne excoriée – a case report of treatment using habit reversal. Clin Exp Dermatol 14: 163–164

Rosenbaum MS, Ayllon T (1981) The behavioral treatment of neurodermatitis through habit-reversal. Behav Res Ther 19: 313–318

Stangier U, Gieler U (2000) Hauterkrankungen. In: Senft W, Broda M (Hrsg) Praxis der Psychotherapy, 2. Aufl. Thieme, Stuttgart, S 566–581

Deep-Psychological Psychotherapies

The psychodynamic point of view assumes the skin disease to be an expression of an unmanageable disorder at the emotional level. The skin is viewed and charged with different meanings, becoming an organ of expression that reveals deficits, in part symbolically ["My scaly armor protects me!" (Gieler et al. 1986)] and with many dissociated ambivalences.

Work is undertaken to overcome and resolve developmental/psychologically important conflicts and deficits, taking transference and countertransference into account.

! Psychoanalytical therapies are indicated if serious persistent personality problems contribute to disease as a consequence of traumatizations in the patient's life history.

During psychodynamic psychotherapy, typical personality problems related to perceiving a dissociated and ambivalent world are integrated and worked out.

For example, early childhood molding of a skin patient by a mother who, in the framework of her own depressive mood, repeatedly withheld herself emotionally, may be relevant. The patient has not experienced that he can (co)establish a stable inner relationship to an important reference person, although he longs to do so. In this way, he was torn as a child between his need for proximity and his experience that he is better protected emotionally when he keeps a certain distance. Even as an adult, he cannot – without therapeutic help – resolve this conflict.

Predominant in treatment is, first of all, empathy, understanding measures, patience, and thinking over longer periods of time.

The motive for one's own acts and the determinants of one's own experience are often not clear and only partially conscious. They are often of a conflicting nature, and a subjective, hard-to-resolve inner proximity–distance conflict is often relevant.

Examples of Unresolved Dissociated Ambivalent Conflicts in Dermatology

- Proximity–distance conflict
- Dependence–autonomy conflict
- Provision–independence conflict
- Control–submission/helplessness
- Power–powerlessness
- Good–bad
- Friend–foe
- Safety–menace
- Narcissistic conflict, self-esteem conflict
- Disgust–symbiosis
- Guilt–shame
- Desire–lack of desire
- Here–there
- Now–never

Often the patients are torn between the poles and cannot resolve the conflict because of developmental delays, marked impulsivity, inhibitions, defense mechanisms, or difficulty postponing satisfaction grounded on past experiences, or because they are too afraid of the possible consequences. In dermatology, a focus is on integrating with affect the experience, aspects of guilt and shame, disgust, and proximity and distance conflicts and at times ventilating disrupted parent–child relationships.

Longer-term psychodynamic psychotherapies may aim at enabling a revival of conflict-laden interaction patterns in the therapeutic relationship or may use present interactions and/or transference to work these out therapeutically and, if possible, to change them and so achieve better mastery of central inner conflicts.

In the framework of psychoanalytical psychotherapy, the central conflict (between two inner, apparently incompatible tendencies) is restaged. During the restaging, the patient can modify the underlying tendencies and maladjustments, and challenge his/her life history experiences and moldings, as well as working out the current eliciting situation. Ideally, an integrated view and thus a (partial) resolution of the inner conflict can then be reached and better alternative possible solutions found.

Supporting interventions and classical psychoanalytical interventions with analysis, confrontations, and interpretations are used. The intensive therapeutic relationship with conflicts and transference constellations that arise in this framework represent a new experience and also contain long-term learning mechanisms.

Relaxation Therapies

A number of relaxation therapies have been successfully applied in dermatology. Among the main procedures are autogenic training, progressive muscle relaxation in the Jacobsen method, and hypnosis. Progressive muscle relaxation achieves relaxation on both the physical and emotional levels. In progressive muscle relaxation, learning exercises are used in which tensing (of muscles) and relaxation alternate. The most important procedure for attaining emotional relaxation is autogenic training, which can be used especially in dermatology in a modified form.

Autogenic Training

After extensive experience with hypnosis, Heinrich Schultz developed autogenic training in the 1920s. In this procedure, self-relaxation is practiced by concentrated inner recitation (Schultz 2003).

The starting point is the fact that body and soul are never separated but always act together. By continuous exercise and inner recitation of relaxing words or formulae, relaxation is also attained at the physical level. Mantra-like formulations may be used, which are constructed especially for the individual and individual diseases.

In performing the exercise, differentiation is made between the basic formula and specific exercises with mantra-like formulations:

Basic Formulas

General basic formulas
- I feel calm.
- All noises are unimportant.

Heaviness exercises
- My right arm is getting heavy.
- My left arm is getting heavy.
- My right leg is getting heavy.
- My left leg is getting heavy.
- Both arms and legs are getting heavy.

Warmth exercises
- My right arm is getting warm.
- My left arm is getting warm.
- My right leg is getting warm.
- My left leg is getting warm.

Final formulas
- Breathe deeply.
- Bend the arms firmly and stretch them out.
- Open your eyes.

Basic formulas are done 6–8 times at the beginning. Final formulas are always done 1–2 times at the end.

Organ exercises
- My breathing is calm and even.
- My abdomen (solar plexus, stomach) is getting soft and warm.
- My heart is beating calmly and steadily.
- My forehead is cool and smooth.

See also: http://www.guidetopsychology.com/autogen.htm

In addition to the general AT formula, certain formulas adapted for dermatology should be added.

Special Formulas for Dermatology

General formulas for the skin may be as follows:
- The skin is completely quiet and pleasantly cool.
- The skin will stay healthy.
- I will do my skin only good.

Special formulas for itching skin may be as follows:
- The itching is getting weaker and weaker.
- The itching is disintegrating.
- The itching is melting.
- The itching doesn't bother me.
- The itching is getting weaker and weaker with every breath I take.
- I don't need to scratch.
- I am in control of myself.
- I can exhale the itching, etc.

Further Psychotherapy Procedures

Depending on the therapeutic school, there are a number of additional psychotherapy procedures, some of which show well-confirmed therapeutic benefits but are not presently reimbursable.

Active imagination. Active imagination is a concept introduced by Carl Jung of actively establishing contact with one's own soul. In active imagination, images are supposed to rise from the subconscious and be dealt with.

Breathing therapy. Breathing therapy is one of the oldest healing arts, with a focus on respiration.

Family therapy. In family therapy, psychological work is undertaken with the entire family present instead of just with the individual alone. The family is viewed as an entity, a system in which individual behavior is alternately influenced and mutually caused among the family members.

Feldenkrais method. The Feldenkrais method attains consciousness through movement and functional integration between body and psyche, especially with respect to the developmental history and understanding and relief of pain.

Conversational psychotherapy. Carl Rogers developed conversational psychotherapy in the United States. This procedure is also called client-centered psychotherapy, of which the most important elements are sensitivity, empathy, acceptance, and congruence. The client and his or her self-concept are the focal point.

Gestalt therapy. With the help of nonverbal forms of expression and identity switching in role playing, an experience-oriented entry into a conflict-laden power play is worked out in order to track down and perceive an emotional conflict potential and then work it out.

Creative therapy. In creative therapy, repetition of experience is made possible during a creative process, such as art therapy, pottery making, or music. There are various processing levels, whereby the creative results, such as pictures, are subsequently discussed for their possible meaning.

Hypnosis. Hypnosis is probably the oldest psychotherapeutic procedure. A transient state of altered attention is elicited in the patient, and an elevated susceptibility for suggestion or thoughts is present.

Catathymic image experience. This is an imaginative procedure in which images are seen with the inner eye and worked out, taking into consideration the content and possible aspects of symbolic character to resolve unresolved conflicts and fears. It is assumed that the images or symbols are a means of expressing what is repressed and hidden and that interpretation enables better understanding of unconscious mechanisms.

Concentrative movement therapy. This form of treatment is based on the perception of the body in the "here and now." In concentrative movement therapy (CMT), the aim is to open body–mind relationships to experience by attentive concentration on one's own body, such as heart palpitations and sweating in the experience of fear. In dermatology, CMT is a very good procedure for establishing contact with one's own skin organ and for restoring and experiencing emotional relationships, especially in chronic diseases such as psoriasis and AD. CMT can also be helpful in alexithymia disorders, in which patients are incapable of perceiving their feelings and describing them in words.

CMT starts with exercising and training of regular movement processes with sensitivity and awareness of posture and movement. In expanded CMT for skin patients, there should be awareness and self-experience of one's own skin organ and emotional pathways (for example, the sensation of itching) tracked.

In psychosomatic-dermatological patients with loss of skin–mind continuity (conversion disorder, dissociative disorder, somatoform disorder, hypochondria, fibromyalgia), CMT may contribute to restitution of the wholeness of the body. CMT is a voyage of discovery of the skin organ in order to create an emotional relationship to the skin through intensive attention (concentration).

Neurolinguistic programming. Neurolinguistic programming attempts to decipher mental thinking processes and emotional experience. This is a complex communication model and training program that comprises various concepts and methods of behavior, learning, and perception psychology as well as cognition psychology, linguistics, and parts of hypnosis.

Transactional analysis. It is assumed in transactional analysis that there are various adult-ego and parent-ego interaction levels. In transactional analysis, a change in the human personality is to be promoted under aspects of communication theories, development theories, and experience and behavior patterns that characterize our lives.

References

Gieler U, Ernst R, Fritz J (1986) "My scale armor protects me"! The personality image and physical disability of psoriasis patients. [Article in German] Z Hautkr 61(8): 572–576

Schultz JH (2003) Das autogene Training. Thieme, Stuttgart
Stangier U, Gieler U (2000) Hauterkrankungen. In: Senft W, Broda M (Hrsg) Praxis der Psychotherapy, 2. Aufl. Thieme, Stuttgart, S 566–581

Further Reading

Anzieu D (1991) Das Haut-Ich. Suhrkamp, Frankfurt
Beck AT, Rush AJ, Shaw BF, Emery G (1996) Kognitive Therapie der Depression. PVU, Weinheim
Detig C (1989) Hautkrank: Unberührbarkeit aus Abwehr? Psychodynamische Prozesse zwischen Nähe und Distanz. Vandenhoeck & Ruprecht, Göttingen
Gieler U, Stangier U, Ernst R (1988) Psychosomatische Behandlungsansätze im Rahmen der klinischen Therapie von Hauterkrankungen. Prax Klin Verhaltensmed Rehabilitation 1: 50–84
Gieler U, Detig-Kohler C (1994) Nähe und Distanz bei Hautkranken. Psychotherapeut 39: 259–263
Hautzinger M (2000) Kognitive Verhaltenstherapie bei Depressionen, 5. Aufl. PVU/Beltz, Weinheim
Hoegl L, Fichter M, Plewig G (1998) Stationäre Verhaltensmedizin chronischer Hautkrankheiten. Hautarzt 49: 270–275
Hoffmann N, Schauenburg H (2000) Psychotherapy der Depression. Thieme, Stuttgart
Hornstein OP (1980) Was kann die Dermatologie von der Psychotherapy erwarten? Ein Plädoyer. Z Hautkr 55: 913–928
Marty P (1958) La relation objectale allergique. Rev Fr Psychoanal 22: 5–35
Niebel G (1995) Verhaltensmedizin der chronischen Hautkrankheit. Huber, Bern Göttingen
Niemeier V, Kupfer J, Köhnlein, Schill WB, Gieler U (1996) Der psychosomatische Therapieansatz in der Dermatologie. Z Hautkr 71: 902–907
Pines D (1981) Skin communication: early skin disorders and their effect on transference and countertransference. Int J Psychoanal 61: 315–323
Rechenberger I (1979) Tiefenpsychologisch ausgerichtete Diagnostik und Behandlung von Hautkrankheiten. Vandenhoeck & Ruprecht, Göttingen
Schaller C, Alberti L, Pott G, Ruzicka T, Tress W (1998) Psychosomatische Störungen in der Dermatologie – Häufigkeiten und psychosomatischer Mitbehandlungsbedarf. Hautarzt 49: 276–279
Schmid-Ott G, Jäger B, Lamprecht F (1999) Psychoanalytische Methoden in der psychosomatischen Dermatologie, Z Dermatol 185: 77–81
Stangier U, Gieler U, Ehlers A (1996) Neurodermitis bewältigen. Verhaltenstherapie, Dermatologische Schulung, Autogenes Training. Springer, Berlin
Stephanos S (1983) Zur Problematik des omnipotenten Objekts – eine psychoanalytische Studie über Psoriasis. Jahrbuch der Psychoanalyse 15: 145–168
Thomä H (1980) Über die Unspezifität psychosomatischer Erkrankungen am Beispiel einer Neurodermitis mit zwanzigjähriger Katamnese. Psyche 34: 589–624
Tuke D (1884) Influence of the mind upon the body. Churchill, London

15 Psychopharmacological Therapy in Dermatology

In primary psychiatric disorders, therapy with psychopharmaceuticals should optimally be undertaken in cooperation with a specialist in psychiatry, especially if potent neuroleptics are indicated and long-term outpatient treatment is necessary. Suicidal and homicidal ideation, violent outbursts, and general situations rendering patients a risk to themselves or others, or situations in which patients are unable to provide food, clothing, and shelter for themselves contraindicate attempts to provide psychodermatologic care and are better cared for by emergency psychiatric services until stabilized. Because suicidal ideation, planning, and attempts may be triggered by antidepressant stimulation in teenagers and patients with inhibited depression, when the dermatologist is forced to medicate patients who will not accept referrals to psychiatric services, careful monitoring needs to be done and a contingency plan put in place for the eventual appearance of those symptoms, psychiatric decompensation, complications, or poor outcome. The clinician must feel proficient in evaluating the underlying, coexisting, or secondary psychiatric disorders and be comfortable prescribing and monitoring psychoactive medication. If the clinician has evidence that the patient will not go to a psychiatrist, the pros and cons of psychoactive medication need to be carefully balanced together with the patient before starting treatment with it. If the joint decision is to perform the psychopharmacologic intervention, depending on the local standard of practice, informed consent need to be signed before the medication is begun and basic vital signs and laboratory information obtained in order to evaluate the potential side effects of the medication.

Treatment of the main psychiatric symptoms underlying, coexisting, or appearing as a consequence of dermatological conditions is outlined in this chapter: delusions and thought disorders, depressive mood, anxiety, obsessive–compulsive disorders, and disorders of impulse control.

Initiation of diagnostics and therapy can in some cases only be made successfully in a liaison interview with a psychiatrist and dermatologist. Due to organizational aspects, this is often possible only in tertiary care environments (hospital).

Compliance of the patients undergoing counseling or pharmacological therapy in cooperation with a psychiatrist or prescribed by the dermatologist is, however, not a certainty in dermatology.

Combined treatment of the patient by the dermatologist and psychiatrist in the framework of a liaison service in the dermatology clinic has proven useful.

When psychiatric symptoms are part of or the major component of the skin disease in the course of a dermatosis, drug treatment is indicated, but when the patient is not motivated for consulting or liaison referral to a neurologist or psychiatrist, or if this is not available on site, the dermatologist could undertake therapy with psychopharmaceuticals.

A prerequisite is that the dermatologist has adequate knowledge and experience with psychopharmaceuticals with respect to indication, contraindication, side effects, and interactions.

Modern Psychopharmacological Therapy

The spectrum of therapy possibilities and approved medications for antipsychotic therapy, for example, is broad. The development of new modern psychopharmaceuticals has resulted in recent years in a considerable number of novel, specifically effective medications in addition to the classical neuroleptics and tricyclic antidepressants.

With the more specific interactions, the number of side effects has been reduced; despite that, the willingness of patients to undergo long-term therapy has not increased. Improvement in compliance continues to be elusive.

Therapy with classic neuroleptics (such as haloperidol) is initiated these days usually only under careful consideration of the side effect spectrum – particularly risks for tardive dyskinesia or those due to a desired side effect – or when a previously successful therapy is to be continued or reinstated.

Indication Clarification

Psychopharmacological therapy may be indicated in some cases of primary or secondary psychiatric disorders and comorbidities.

Indications for Psychopharmacological Therapy in Dermatology

1. Primary psychiatric disorders with reference to the skin: In addition to delusional disorders, these include compulsive disorders, somatoform disorders, and psychogenic itching, in which skin changes are secondary events.
2. Secondary psychiatric disorders due to dermatoses: These comprise secondary psychiatric disorders due to a cutaneous disease, in which the dermatosis is the stressor causing a psychopathological response. The symptoms develop following the model of an adjustment disorder, with depression or/and anxiety as a consequence of dealing with the dermatosis, which may make psychopharmacotherapy necessary.
3. Comorbidities: These involve juxtaposition of psychiatric disorder and dermatosis. A clear delineation between the former groups (2 and 3) is not always possible.

! Comorbidities are present if a skin disease and a psychiatric disorder coexist.

Deterioration of the skin condition may potentiate a psychiatric disorder in various ways, such as by intensifying a latent depression. On the other hand, depression may lead to exacerbation of the skin condition if skin care is neglected or compliance is impaired due to the psychiatric disorder.

The indication for psychopharmacotherapy is generally directed at the predominant symptoms of the underlying psychiatric disorder.

Clarification of Indications for Psychopharmaceuticals ("How Do I Find the Right Medication?")

- Unequivocal diagnosis of the primary disorder and secondary symptoms
- Determination of target symptoms (clear indication definition)
- Selection of the substance depending on its mode of action (desired effect)
- Consideration of undesired side effects
- Clear performance and long-term control strategy (advance information about side effects, delayed onset of action, dose titration)

Therapy with psychopharmaceuticals has some traits seen in no other area of drug therapy in medicine:

- The identical psychopharmaceutical may act differently in different patients.
- A medication from the same group may act differently in the same patient.
- The medication dose differs from patient to patient (titration).
- The selection and indications of a psychopharmaceutical may be made on the basis of the side effects profile.
- The off-label use of psychopharmaceuticals in dermatology is sometimes due to a lack of studies.

A foresighted treatment plan and patient motivation are necessary to an extent unlike in any other area, especially because the onset of effect is often evident only after several weeks. Individual titration and dose adjustment are necessary from the initial dose to the maximum and maintenance doses through to the tapering-off dose. In some cases, a medication change is required.

Main Indications and Primary Target Symptoms of the Medications

Essentially, there are symptoms of the psychiatric disorders underlying, coexisting, or generated by the dermatological condition. Decreasing the target psychiatric symptoms is what makes the prescribed psychopharmacological therapy appropriate and effective. The target symptoms are those of psychoses, anxiety disorders, depressions, compulsive disorders, and impulse control disorders (Table 15.1).

In addition, there are special cases in dermatology, such as pain and sleep disorders and particular forms of pruritus, in which the use of antihistamines with anxiolytic effects may be indicated.

Evaluating the underlying psychiatric condition and psychiatric symptoms may include information from different sources: classic history taking, including mental status; review of previous records; dermatological consultations or/and structured interviews; questionnaires; or, as mentioned above, psychiatric liaison consultation.

Dermatologic Conditions with Underlying Psychotic/Confusional Functioning

Previous records of these patients may reveal failed treatment attempts; a structured interview may suggest psychotic/confusional functioning; questionnaires and mental status may confirm the presence of delusions. Another orienting clue is the consideration of common presumptive underlying conditions of the specific dermatologic complaint. Different psychiatric conditions may underlie specific dermatological disorders (see Chap. 1); some psychiatric conditions are more frequently the cause of a particular dermatological disorder, such as the case in delusional parasitosis (DP). In the presence of an irreducible false belief of infestation, it becomes obvious that there is an underlying delusional disorder focused on the skin, leading to secondary skin manifestations. Other disorders such as dermatitis artefacta require more exploration and may less frequently have a specific correlation with an underlying psychiatric condition, functioning more as a syndrome, able to have more diverse causations. When the presence of these delusional characteristics is detected, the attempts to clarify and reduce them fail, and in the absence of a traumatic or cultural underlying explanation, the dermatologist needs to conclude that the underlying functioning is psychotic/confusional.

Table 15.1 Main indications for psychopharmaceuticals in dermatology (*SSRIs* selective serotonin reuptake inhibitors)

Psychiatric disorder	Drug group	Medication
Psychiatric diseases (delusional parasitosis, hypochondriacal delusions, and others)	Antipsychotics (neuroleptics)	1st choice: aripiprazole (Abilify), risperidone (Risperdal), quetiapine (Seroquel), olanzapine (Zyprexa)
		2nd choice: pimozide (Orap)
Depressive disorders	Antidepressants	1st choice SSRI: citalopram (Celexa, Cipramil, Cipram) fluoxetine (Prozac), sertraline (Zoloft), paroxetine (Paxil), venlafaxine (Luvox)
		2nd choice: Tricyclic antidepressants: doxepin (Sinequan, Doxal, Doxepin, Doxedyn)
Anxiety and panic disorders	Anxiolytics (tranquilizers)	Acute/transient
		1st choice: benzodiazepines (note: habituation potential)
		Chronic
		1st choice: buspirone (Buspar) (persistent anxiety)
		2nd choice: doxepin (Sinequan, Doxal, Doxepin, Doxedyn), paroxetine
		3rd choice: benzodiazepines (note: habituation potential)
Compulsive disorders	Medications with anti-compulsive disorder effect	1st choice: SSRIs: paroxetine, escitalopram, sertraline, citalopram (Celexa, Cipramil, Cipram), fluoxetine, fluvoxamine
		2nd choice: Tricyclic antidepressant: clomipramine (Anafranil)

Delusion of parasitosis, hypochondriacal delusions, body dysmorphic delusions, or other body-related delusional disorders (see Sect. 1.2) are more likely to be caused by psychotic/delusional functioning, in which the form is often monosymptomatic.

After arriving at the diagnostic certainty of the underlying psychotic condition, a number of considerations should be weighed before commencing therapy with neuroleptic medications:

- The patient's suffering
- Limitations generated in the patient's life by the disease
- Possible side effects
- The likelihood of compliance
- The existence of necessary psychosocial resources
- The patient's social and cognitive functioning

Treatment of Dermatologic Conditions with Underlying Psychotic/Delusional Functioning

Neuroleptics are medications that influence thought processing and experience. **Target symptoms** of neuroleptics are the psychotic symptoms: visual, auditory, and tactile hallucinations; delusions; paranoid ideation; ideas of reference; states of psychomotor excitation; reduction of psychotic anxiety; decreased affective intensity; and, in general, deceptive perceptions.

Neuroleptics exercise their antipsychotic effect by blocking the (D2) dopamine receptors in the mesolimbic projection (tegmentum to nucleus accumbens) and decreasing the activity of the pathway postulated to be responsible for the psychotic symptoms. First-generation antipsychotic agents, also called conventional agents, are remarkably effective in decreasing psychotic symptoms. They are also effective at blocking other postsynaptic dopamine D2 receptors widely distributed in the brain, causing numerous side effects:

- Intense extrapyramidal rigidity and excitation (akathisia) mainly by blocking the nigrostriatum pathway; an irreversible condition called tardive dyskinesia appears to be linked to the intensity of the extrapyramidal activity
- Hyperprolactinemia/galactorrhea and menstrual cycle disturbance by acting on the tuberoinfundibular pathway
- Marked worsening of the already existent apathy, withdrawal, and slow psychic functioning by acting in the mesocortical pathway, which in turn may worsen psychotic functioning.

Pimozide, a 1st-generation antipsychotic, is still used in delusional diseases in dermatology in the United States. There are two reasons for this:

- Numerous reports have been published on the use of pimozide in dermatology patients.
- Treatment costs are considerably lower than with other therapies.

The newer neuroleptics with fewer extrapyramidal motor side effects should be used in dermatology. These so-called atypical neuroleptics are characterized by the fact that their effect is more specific and produces fewer extrapyramidal and cortical withdrawal side effects than the 1st-generation or conventional neuroleptics, like those derived from butyrophenone or diphenylbutylpiperidine. They also generate markedly less tardive dyskinesia.

Currently, experience is available in dermatology with the following relevant neuroleptics: risperidone (Risperdal), olanzapine (Zyprexa), quetiapine (Seroquel), aripiprazole (Abilify), ziprasidone (Geodon), and pimozide (Orap). The neuroleptics primarily used in dermatology are listed in Table 15.2.

Risperidone (Risperdal), aripiprazole (Abilify), ziprasidone (Geodon), and quetiapine (Seroquel) are the drugs of first choice in psychiatric disorders with psychotic functioning. These atypical neuroleptics have a low and favorable side effects profile and thus better acceptance on the patient's part, and they are preferred by the authors for this reason. The lower side effects of the atypical neuroleptics are attributable to blocking both the postsynaptic dopamine D2 and the serotonin 5HT2A receptors, increasing the release of dopamine in pathways other than the mesolimbic, markedly decreasing the side effects that are so prominent in the 1st-generation neuroleptics. This is the case in the following:

- Risperidone (Risperdal)
- Quetiapine (Seroquel), which also has muscarinic alpha-1 and alpha-2 agonism
- Olanzapine (Zyprexa), in which there is in addition blocking of D1 and alpha-1 agonism as well as 5HT2C antagonism
- Aripiprazole (Abilify) has lower dopamine D2 blocking with 80% binding coupled with 5HT1A agonism
- Ziprasidone (Geodon) antagonism with serotonin 5HT2C, agonism 5HT1A.

Due to the rarity of patients with delusional diseases, there are no broad controlled studies on the newer antipsychotic drugs but only isolated case reports and empirical treatment observations in the area of dermatology.

The duration of treatment and the dose must be determined in each individual case. The duration should be at least 1 month until the onset of action, dose titration, or substance switch (in case of nonresponse). In responders, therapy should be given for 6 months and may sometimes be necessary over a period of years.

Neuroleptics permit the patient distancing from the illness. In addition, neuroleptic antihistaminics such as promethazine (Atosil) are especially indicated in psychomotor excitation and anxious agitation. Due to their often good antiallergic/antihistaminic effect, they are sometimes the choice in patients with urticaria and atopic dermatitis (Table 15.2).

The dermatological disease with underlying psychotic/confusional functioning most frequently observed in dermatology is delusion of parasitosis (DP), initially called acarophobia. The complete disappearance of DP often cannot be achieved even with adequate drug therapy. Improvement and transition of a serious DP to a less intense form can be considered therapeutic success or the goal of therapy, and can often mean clear stabilization and social integration of the patient. In DP, depending on the seriousness of the underlying psychosis, only 30–50% remission is likely.

Atypical Neuroleptics

Risperidone

Indication: Risperidone is a well-tolerated neuroleptic with a relatively low side effects profile. It can especially be successfully used in elderly patients with DP when possible heart disease and, if appropriate, electrocardiography (ECG) control are taken into account.

Before beginning therapy with risperidone, the following baseline evaluations need to be obtained:

Dose: The initial dose of risperidone (Risperdal) in dermatology is 0.5–1 mg daily with a slow dose increase every 5–7 days until a maximum dose of 4–6 mg is attained.

Side effects: The side effects include dizziness, sedation, hypotension, weight gain, constipation, abdominal pain, possible decompensation of diabetes, hyperglycemia (frequent and dose-dependent), anxiety, extrapyramidal rigidity, akathisia, hyperprolactinemia and restlessness. Risperidone can also minimally prolong the QT interval on ECG. Tachycardia and sexual dysfunction may also be seen.

Quetiapine

Indication: Therapeutic success in DP can be achieved with quetiapine (Seroquel).The use in elderly patients, including patients with brain diseases (dementia), appears particularly favorable.

Dose: Treatment is begun with 25 mg twice daily and can be increased to a dose of 150–800 mg/day.

Side effects: Fatigue, sedation, weight gain, mild anticholinergic symptoms, dizziness, hypotension, and tachycardia occur in rare cases. Dry mouth, constipation, and abdominal pain may be seen. Orthostatic dysregulation is also possible. The drug increases diabetes risk and dyslipidemia.

Olanzapine

Indication: Olanzapine (Zyprexa) is very well tolerated but is often discontinued, especially by younger patients, because of its anticholinergic effects and pronounced weight gain.

Dose: The initial dose is 5 mg/day, and further increases and titration are done to a dose range of 5–20 mg per day.

Table 15.2 Classification of neuroleptics

Low-strength neuroleptics	
– Few extrapyramidal side effects	Promethazine (Atosil)
– Strong sedative effect	Triflupromazine (Psyquil)
– Strong vegetative suppression	Levomepromazine (Neurocil)
	Thioridazine (Melleril)
	Alimemazine (Repeltin)
	Melperone (Eunerpan)
High-strength neuroleptics	
– Strong extrapyramidal side effects	Pimozide (Orap)
– Weak sedative effect	Haloperidol (Haldol)
– Little vegetative suppression	
Atypical neuroleptics	
	Quetiapine (Seroquel)
	Olanzapine (Zyprexa)
	Risperidone (Risperdal)

Table 15.3 Typical and atypical antipsychotics in dermatology (*EPS* extrapyramidal syndrome, *NMS* neuroleptic malignant syndrome)

Drug	Dose (mg/day)	Side effects					
		EPS	NMS	Metabolic syndrome	Seizures, hypotension	Cardiac	Other[b]
Olanzapine (Ziprexa)[a]	5–20	+/–	+/–	++++	+		Sedation
Risperidone (Risperidal)[a]	0.5–6	++	+/–	+++	+	Hypertension	Hyperprolactinemia, dizziness
Quetiapine (Seroquel)[a]	25–800	+/–	+/–	+++	+	+/–	Cataracts
Ziprasidone (Geodon)[a]	20–160	+	+/–	++	+	Arrhythmia	Prolonged QT
Aripiprazole (Abilify)[a]	2.5–30	+/–	+/–	+/–	+		Headache
Pimozide (Orap) (typical antipsychotic)	1–6	+++	+	–	++	Arrhythmia	Prolonged QT

[a] Atypical antipsychotics

[b] All antipsychotics have been associated with early death in the elderly

15

Side effects: Anticholinergic effects such as dry mouth, urinary impairment, dizziness, sedation, hypotension, and constipation may decompensate diabetes or decrease glucose tolerance. Very rarely, extrapyramidal rigidity, constipation, and blurred vision may occur, and there is frequently remarkable weight gain. The drug increases the risk for diabetes mellitus and dyslipidemia. Pain and abnormal gait may occur.

Aripiprazole

Indication: Aripiprazole (Abilify) is well tolerated and has minimal anticholinergic effects but is discontinued at times because of its activating effects, particularly at low doses. It is also the atypical neuroleptic associated with less weight gain.

Dose: The initial dose is 2,5 mg/day, with further increases and titration to a dose range of 15–30 mg per day. Antipsychotic effects may be present in low dosages of 5–10 mg/day, but at times side effects and activation are prominent with low dosage.

Side effects: Anticholinergic effects such as dizziness, sedation, orthostatic hypotension, nausea, occasional vomiting, extrapyramidal akathisia (rare), constipation, and insomnia may occur, and there is frequently minimal or no weight gain.

Ziprasidone

Indication: Ziprasidone (Geodon) is very well tolerated but often discontinued, especially by younger patients, because of its anticholinergic effects and weight gain.

Dose: The initial dose is 5 mg/day, with further increases and titration to a dose range of 20–160 mg orally per day in divided doses.

Side effects: Activating side effects occur with low dosage. Side effects that may occur include anticholinergic effects such as dry mouth, nausea, asthenia, skin rash, dizziness, sedation, hypotension, constipation, decompensation of diabetes, decreased glucose tolerance, extrapyramidal rigidity (very rare), and blurred vision. Remarkable weight gain frequently occurs.

Serious rare side effects of atypical neuroleptics include tardive dyskinesias, neuroleptic malignant syndrome, seizures, hyperosmolar coma, diabetic ketoacidosis, and increased risk of cerebrovascular accident (CVA) and death in the elderly.

Neuroleptic malignant syndrome is a rare side effect (incidence 0.2%) and is more frequent with high doses or rapid titration:

- Hyperthermia (>38°C)
- Change in mental status
- Diaphoresis
- Muscle rigidity
- Tachycardia

Baseline and follow-up are required for patients receiving atypical neuroleptics:

- Weight: initially and monthly; follow every 3 months
- Height
- Body mass index: calculate monthly (overweight >25)
- Blood pressure (hypertension >140/90 mmHg): follow every 3 months and more frequently in the elderly
- Document family history of obesity, dyslipidemia, diabetes
- Measure waist at umbilical level
- Laboratory exams:
- Fasting glucose (>100 prediabetic, >125 diabetic): check every 3 months
- Lipid profile with triglycerides: monitor and treat abnormalities every 6 months
- Prolactin level (with risperidone): consider switching if abnormal

Typical Neuroleptics: Pimozide

Indication: Pimozide (Orap) has been used in the United States as the drug of first choice in monosymptomatic hypochondriacal psychosis with paranoid symptoms. The original indication was schizophrenia.

Dose: The initial dose of 1 mg daily should be increased over 4–5-day intervals until a dose of 4–6 mg/day is attained. Higher doses are also administered in individual cases. The duration of therapy should be 5–6 months.

Side effects: The side effects spectrum is characterized by sedation, blurred vision, constipation, dry mouth, sedation, hypotension, Parkinsonian rigidity, akathisia, tardive dyskinesia (5% per year of treated patients), tardive dystonia, extrapyramidal disorders, and occasionally fatigue, insomnia, or anxiety disorders. Negative symptoms (neuroleptic-induced deficit syndrome), prolactin elevation, amenorrhea, and sexual dysfunction may also be seen.

Serious side effects include the following:

- Neuroleptic malignant syndrome (rare)
- Seizures (rare)
- Dose-dependent QT prolongation
- Dose-dependent ventricular arrhythmias and sudden death
- Increased risk of CVA and death in the elderly

Individual case reports have been published on the sudden death of patients with chronic schizophrenia treated with high doses of pimozide, due to possible cardiotoxic side effects. These side effects have not been described for low-dose therapy.

Other Neuroleptics

Other older neuroleptics such as haloperidol (Haldol), melperon (Eunerpan), and thioridazin (Melleril) are rarely used within the context of dermatology and will not be discussed further.

Depressive Disorders

A general indication for the use of antidepressants/psychopharmaceuticals is recommended to the dermatologist if, during the course of the dermatosis, depressive symptoms are part of or a dominant feature of the skin disease (Fig. 15.1).

Depressive symptomatology can be detected with standard instruments, self-assessment questionnaires, and classic history and mental status examinations.

In several dermatologic conditions, mood disorders can be present. Depressive episodes may be part of several mood disorders, and distinguishing the mood disorders to which the depressive episode belongs allows the clinician to implement the appropriate treatment decision. Following the DSM-IV-TR, truly depressive disorders (i.e., major depressive disorder, dysthymic disorder, and depressive disorder not otherwise specified) are distinguished from bipolar disorders by the fact that the patient has no history of ever having had a manic, mixed, or hypomanic episode, allowing a more liberal treatment with antidepressants. Major depressive episodes can also be present in bipolar disorders (i.e., bipolar I disorder, bipolar II disorder, cyclothymic disorder, and bipolar disorder not otherwise specified). In these cases, treatment with antidepressants can precipitate a manic or hypomanic episode. Therefore, mood stabilizers are the main pharmacological medication, whereas antidepressants need to be used with extreme caution.

In the general medical practice as well as in dermatology, the appropriate use of antidepressants for truly depressive disorders without manic/hypomanic episodes and for mood disorders due to a general medical condition is widely accepted.

A good orienting example is the diagnostic criteria for a typical major depressive episode in the DSM-IV-TR. These criteria include the following:

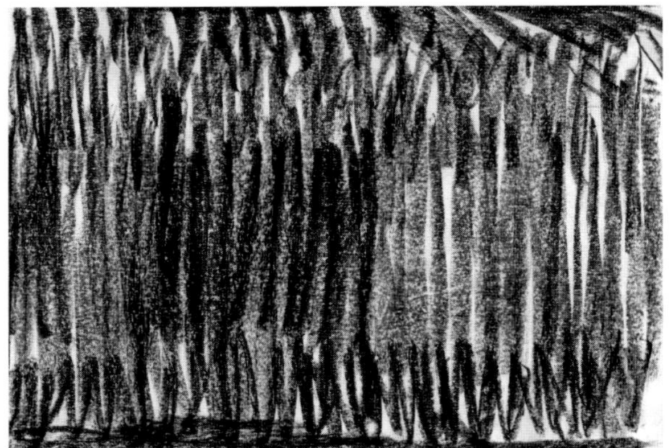

Fig 15.1 Depression in art therapy

A. Five (or more) of the following symptoms present during the same 2-week period and representing a change from previous functioning; at least one of the symptoms is either (1) depressed mood or (2) loss of interest or pleasure.
   - Depressed mood most of the day, nearly every day, as indicated by either subjective report (e.g., feels sad or empty) or observation made by others (e.g., appears tearful). Note: In children and adolescents, can be irritable mood.
   - Markedly diminished interest or pleasure in all, or almost all, activities most of the day, nearly every day (as indicated by either subjective account or observation made by others).
   - Significant weight gain or weight loss when not dieting (e.g., a change of more than 5% of body weight in a month), or decrease or increase in appetite nearly every day. Note: In children, consider failure to make expected weight gains.
   - Insomnia or hypersomnia nearly every day.
   - Psychomotor agitation or retardation nearly every day (observable by others, not merely subjective feelings of restlessness or being slowed down).
   - Fatigue or loss of energy nearly every day.
   - Feelings of worthlessness or excessive or inappropriate guilt (which may be delusional) nearly every day (not merely self-reproach or guilt about being sick).
   - Diminished ability to think or concentrate, or indecisiveness, nearly every day (either by subjective account or as observed by others).
   - Recurrent thoughts of death (not just fear of dying), recurrent suicidal ideation without a specific plan, or a suicide attempt or a specific plan for committing suicide.

Note: This does not include symptoms that are clearly due to a general medical condition, or mood-incongruent delusions or hallucinations.

B. The symptoms do not meet criteria for a mixed episode.
C. The symptoms cause clinically significant distress or impairment in social, occupational, or other important areas of functioning.
D. The symptoms are not due to the direct physiological effects of a substance (e.g., a drug of abuse, a medication) or a general medical condition (e.g., hypothyroidism).
E. The symptoms are not better accounted for by bereavement; that is, after the loss of a loved one, the symptoms persist for longer than 2 months or are characterized by marked functional impairment, morbid preoccupation with worthlessness, suicidal ideation, psychotic symptoms, or psychomotor retardation.

Another way to orient the diagnosis is by using a self-assessment questionnaire such as the Mood Disorder Questionnaire, which, if the individual affirmatively answers seven out of 13 questions, establishes the likelihood of bipolar disorder I or II. Scales applied by the practitioner have the advantage of being able to be applied several times during treatment (e.g., Hamilton Depression Scale) and thereby can measure the progression of the antidepressant medication.

15

Dermatological Conditions with Possible Underlying, Concurrent, or Reactive Depressive Episodes

The spectrum comprises a number of dermatoses, with an underlying depressive disorder as a comorbidity or as an adjustment to the dermatological disease.

- Atopic dermatitis
- Prurigo diseases
- Psoriasis
- Alopecia areata
- Chronic urticaria
- Trichotillomania
- Skin-picking syndrome (neurotic excoriations)
- Compulsive disorders with reference to the skin
- Somatoform disorders
- Hypochondriacal disorders
- Body dysmorphic disorders
- Cutaneous dysesthesias
- Idiopathic forms of pruritus

The main groups of medications for treatment of a depressive disorder differ according to their pharmacological properties and principles of action.

The following belong to the main group of antidepressants:
- **Selective serotonin reuptake inhibitors (SSRIs)**
- **Dopaminergic, noradrenergic reuptake inhibitors**
- **Tricyclic antidepressants**
- **Monoaminoxidase (MAO) inhibitors**

Antidepressants increase the concentration of serotonin and interact usually in the synaptic cleft with the serotonergic and noradrenergic system, which plays a decisive role in not only depression but also in anxiety and compulsive disorders.

The classic tricyclic antidepressants amitriptyline, imipramine, and desipramine are rarely used in dermatology (with the exception of postherpetic neuralgia) because of their anticholinergic or extrapyramidal side effects.

In the treatment of depression, prescription of SSRIs and, only rarely, tricyclic antidepressants (such as doxepin) is currently the treatment of choice.

The *target symptom* of the antidepressant is primarily a mood-lightening effect, as well as relief of anxiety, a calming, drive-increasing, or drive-suppressing effect, and a decrease in compulsive disorders.

Moreover, three different complexes of depressive target symptoms can be differentiated:
- Anxious agitated symptoms
- Psychomotor-inhibited disorder
- Vital impaired mood and somatic disorder

Up to 6 weeks may elapse before a mood-lightening effect is observed. The danger of suicide is increased if drive increases before the mood change is effected. The patient can then perhaps muster the energy to attempt suicide, which he or she could not do earlier because of apathy. Extreme caution is required here.

Compulsive disorders and other primary psychiatric dermatoses may also be included in the expanded main indications for antidepressants.

Indications for Antidepressants in Primary Psychiatric Disorders when Depression is Underlying or Concurrent

- Delusional parasitosis with underlying depression
- Compulsive disorder with underlying depression
- Dermatitis artefacta (trichotillomania, acne excoriée)
- Impairment of impulse control
- Psychogenic pruritus/dysesthesias/pain syndrome
- Somatoform disorders with depression
- Somatization disorders with depression
- Body dysmorphic disorders

Unlike the desired effect, the onset of side effects is immediate. Xerostomia, impaired sexual function, weight gain, and fatigue, as well as restlessness (even akathisia) and anxiety disorder are reported as the most frequent reasons for discontinuing medication. The therapeutic withdrawal of medication is by having the patient slowly taper off.

If the target symptoms and indication for therapy with antidepressants are clear, the following aspects of psychopharmacotherapy must be heeded in the second step.

General Notes on Therapy with Antidepressants

After indication for therapy of primary antidepressant target symptomatics, the antidepressant must be selected, taking into account side effects with respect to sedation and stimulation, keeping possible interactions with sexual function in mind.
- For patients with mixed patterns of depression, agitation, and anxiety, doxepin (Sinequan) may be the first choice, followed by paroxetine (Paxil, Paxil CR), escitalopram (Lexapro), or venlafaxine (Efectin, Efexir, Effexor, Effexor XL, Effexor XR).
- The patient's compliance in adhering to antidepressant therapy is often difficult and can be improved by cautious dose increases. The dose can be increased every 4 days until therapeutic response or until the individually effective dose is attained.
- Halving the dose and increasing the dose slowly by half of the initial dose every 3–5 days should be done, especially in the elderly and children.
- Overall, antidepressant initial therapy is administered for 2–3 weeks before an optimal therapeutic dose range is found. Maximal-dose therapy should be administered for 6 weeks before efficacy is rated (or the substance changed).

- The duration of therapy for the first appearance of disease is 6–9 months on average and
- 5 years for the first relapse,
- Lifelong with a second relapse.

Side effects
- A single dose may be administered if insomnia or sedation occurs as a side effect. If insomnia occurs under medication, the dose should be taken in the morning. If the dominant side effect is fatigue, the entire dose should be taken in the evening.
- A switch to non-SSRIs should be made in erectile dysfunction.
- *Note*: A combination with antihistamines can lead to serious arrhythmia.
- Substance switch: If there is no adequate improvement in symptoms after 4–6 weeks or if pronounced side effects have occurred, a different substance group should be selected as an alternative.

Selective Serotonin Reuptake Inhibitors

Selective serotonin reuptake inhibitors (SSRIs) are among the newer antidepressants and correspond in efficacy to the tricyclic antidepressants but have fewer side effects. They are used in the treatment of compulsive disorders in addition to treatment of depression.

SSRIs are well tolerated, including by elderly patients. The side effects of the SSRIs are primarily constipation, nausea, headache, restlessness, and insomnias. Unlike with the tricyclic antidepressants, patients tend to lose weight when on SSRI therapy.

In dermatology, good efficacy can usually be attained with low doses (Table 15.4).

Indication. SSRIs are the therapy of first choice, the most often administered, and the most effective group in depressive disorders as well as in dermatology. They should also be the therapy of first choice for compulsive disorders.

SSRIs comprise the largest group of nontricyclic antidepressants and all have a similarly good effect. The selection of the right SSRI depends on the desired side effect and thereby primarily on the ratio of agitation to lack of drive. Three groups can be differentiated:

- Less agitation/more lack of drive
  - Therapy option: stimulation ++
  - First choice: escitalopram (Lexapro), fluoxetine (Prozac)
- Agitation equals lack of drive
  - Therapy option: little sedation, little increase of drive
  - First choice: sertraline (Zoloft)
- More agitation/less lack of drive
  - Therapy option: sedation ++
  - First choice: paroxetine (Paxil)

Side effects. SSRIs are generally much better tolerated than tricyclic antidepressants are. States of restlessness, nervousness, and insomnia may occur as side effects. Some patients complain of nausea, diarrhea, and an increase in anxiety symptoms. SSRIs can also lead to erectile dysfunction; in this case, the antidepressant group should be changed, for example to non-SSRIs, or to supplementary therapy with peripherally active substances such as the phosphodiesterase inhibitors sildenafil and vardenafil.

Fluoxetine

Indication: Depression, compulsive disorder

Dose: Fluoxetine should be started at a dose of 10 mg daily, followed by slow adequate dose finding. A higher dose is often necessary in compulsive disorders. Fluoxetine leads more often than the other SSRIs to anxiety disorders and insomnia.

Paroxetine

Indication: Depression, compulsive disorder, panic, generalized anxiety disorder, and sociophobia, as well as posttraumatic stress disorders. Paroxetine is well tolerated.

Dose: The dose in depression is 20 mg/day; in compulsive disorders it is often 50 mg/day.

Sertraline

Indication: Depression

Dose: Sertraline (daily dose 25–200 mg) increases activity less than fluoxetine does and is less sedating than paroxetine.

Escitalopram

Indication: Depression, panic disorder, interferon alpha-induced depression (malignant melanoma). Escitalopram (Lexapro) is especially effective for concurrency of a depressive disorder and a panic disorder.

Dose: The dose is 10–30 mg daily.

Fluvoxamine

Indication: Depressive disorders and compulsive disorders. Fluvoxamin (Luvox) has also been extensively studied in depression, compulsive disorders, and body

15

dysmorphic disorders. Fluvoxamin is used rather rarely in Germany.

Dose: The dose is 50–300 mg per day.

Non-SSRIs

A group of antidepressants comparable with respect to indication and efficacy to the SSRIs are the non-SSRIs, a heterogeneous group of medications that may lead the way in the future because of their more specific mode of action.

The main advantage may lie in a better side effects spectrum with respect to lack of impairment of sexual function. However, the sometimes pronounced weight gain may be a disadvantage.

Venlafaxine (Effexor) is a selective serotonin/noradrenalin reuptake inhibitor (SNRI) in this group, which is nonanticholinergic and nonsedating (Table 15.4).

Venlafaxine

Indication: Venlafaxine (Efectin, Efexir, Effexor, Effexor XL, Effexor XR, Trevilor) is an antidepressant for treatment of depression and accompanying anxiety disorders and agitation. Apart from doxepin (Sinequan, Doxal, Doxepin, Doxedyn), a therapy attempt can be made with venlafaxine as second choice, with good efficacy in patients with such mixed disorders. Venlafaxine is one of the newest serotonin antagonists and noradrenalin reuptake inhibitors and has an antidepressant effect comparable to the SSRIs.

Table 15.4 Pharmacotherapy with antidepressants

Mechanism of action	Drug	Dose mg/day	Side effects
Selective serotonin reuptake inhibitors (SSRIs)	Citalopram (Celexa)	10–60	Anxiety, irritability, increased suicide rates, akathisia, sexual dysfunction, hypomania/mania, agitation, weight gain
	Escitalopram (Lexapro)	10–30	
	Fluoxetine (Prozac)	10–60	
	Fluvoxamine (Luvox)	50–300	
	Paroxetine (Paxil)	20–60	
	Sertraline (Zoloft)	25–200	
Norepinephrine–serotonin reuptake inhibitors	Venlafaxine (Effexor)	37.5–225	Hypertension, tachycardia, anxiety
	Duloxetine (Cymbalta)	20–60	
Norepinephrine–dopamine reuptake inhibitors	Bupropion (Wellbutrin)	100–450	Seizures; avoid in patients with convulsive history or eating disorders
Tricyclics	Amitriptyline (Elavil)	25–300	Arrhythmias, hypertension, orthostatic hypotension, dry mouth, constipation, sexual dysfunction; avoid in glaucoma
	Nortriptyline (Aventyl)	50–150	
	Clomipramine (Anafranil)	75–250	
	Doxepin (Sinequan)	25–200	
Presynaptic α2,5HT2c/5HT3 antagonist	Mirtazapine (Remeron)	15–45	Agranulocytosis, weight gain, dizziness

Note: The combination of SSRIs and antihistamines may cause serious arrhythmias

Dose: The dose should begin at 37.5 mg or one-half tablet and can be increased at 3-day intervals to 150–225 mg/day.

Side effects: Venlafaxin has a favorable side effect spectrum. Most frequent are nervousness, hypertension, and insomnia. Impaired sexual function reportedly occurs in only 10% of treated patients. Concurrent administration with MAO inhibitors is contraindicated.

Other Non-SSRI Antidepressants

Mirtazapin

Mirtazapin (Remeron) is a modern tetracyclic antidepressant (NaSSA) with a favorable side effect spectrum. In doses of 15–45 mg, weight gain, somnolence, dizziness, edema, or headache occur as side effects. Single case reports show good efficacy in patients with glossodynia. In general, it appears to be the antidepressant of choice in depression with the presence of significant physical pain.

Bupropion (Wellbutrin, Wellbutrin XL, Wellbutrin SR, Zyban; not approved for depression in Germany)

Indication: Nicotine addiction (Germany), depression (United States)

Bupropion also has an antidepressant effect comparable to that of the SSRIs, but it is approved in Germany only in the slow-release form (Zyban 150 mg slow-release) for the treatment of nicotine addiction. In cases of impaired sexual function, bupropion can be an alternative therapy to SSRIs.

As an antidepressant, the initial dose is 100 mg twice a day, gradually increasing to a total daily dose of 300 mg. The maximum dose is 450 mg.

Side effects: Insomnia and agitation are the most frequent; tremors, dry mouth, and impaired sexual function occur rarely. Early during therapy it may trigger epileptic convulsions.

Duloxetine (Cymbalta)

Serotonin and norepinephrine reuptake inhibitor; increases serotonin, norepinephrine, noradrenaline, and dopamine.

Indication: Duloxetine 20–60 mg/day has an antidepressant effect comparable to that of the SSRIs and SNRIs, and it also decreases anxiety and chronic pain.

Side effects: Side effects include nausea, diarrhea, insomnia, decrease appetite, sexual dysfunction, sweating, increased blood pressure, induction of hypomania (rare), and suicidal ideation, attempts, and consummation (rare).

Tricyclic Antidepressants

Currently, tricyclic antidepressants are only rarely used in the therapy of depression (Table 15.4).

Doxepin

Indication: Depression, pruritus, anxiety

Doxepin (Sinequan, Doxal, Doxepin, Doxedyn) has a broad indication spectrum: endogenous, psychogenic, or somatogenic depression with anxious, agitated presentation as well as functional organ complaints resulting from masked depressions, chronic states of pain, and also withdrawal symptoms from sedatives, alcohol, and drugs.

In dermatology, it is suitable for use especially because of its antihistaminergic effect, which is both sedative and antipruritic, making it an effective treatment in pronounced pruritus (Fig. 15.2). This may be given, for example, in lichen simplex chronicus in association with a depressive disorder or in cholinergic urticaria because of the intensive H1 antihistamine effect. Doxepin is capable of successfully breaking through the itching–scratching and itching–depression cycles as well as an existing pain–depression cycle in depressive patients.

Doxepin (Sinequan, Doxal, Doxepin, Doxedyn): Indications in Dermatology

- Frequent indications
  - Prurigo (doxepin is the ideal drug for depressive patients with prurigo)
  - Dermatoses with significant itching (pruritus sine materia)
  - Breaking through the itching–scratching and pain–depression cycles
- Other possible indications
  - Skin-picking syndrome (neurotic excoriations), disorders of impulse control
  - Compulsive disorders
  - Anxious-agitated complaint patterns
  - Functional organ complaints
  - Somatization disorders

In agitated depression, the sedation may be a desired side effect in defining the indication.

15

Dose: The dose should begin with 25–50 mg in the evening and then be titrated at 5–7-day intervals to a higher dose up to the target dose of 100–200 mg/day. The antidepressant effect is not usually achieved until after 2 weeks, and the therapeutic effect can only then be rated. However, the onset of antipruritic effect is immediate.

The blood levels of doxepin may fluctuate greatly from patient to patient; if possible, levels should be measured to ensure that they are therapeutic.

Side effects: Sedation, malaise, orthostatic hypotension, weight gain, and anticholinergic side effects such as dry mouth may occur and sometimes lead to discontinuation by the patient.

Particular attention must be paid to a possible cardiac repolarization impairment. An ECG should be performed prior to therapy to control prolonged QT intervals and also later to record arrhythmias under doxepin.

The dermatologist should not undertake doxepin therapy if the patient has a history of manic-depressive disorders, but should use an alternative medication or request a liaison consult. There is a risk of suicide and overdosing.

Other Tricyclic Antidepressants (Amitriptyline, Imipramine, Desipramine Group)

The tricyclic antidepressants amitriptyline (suppressant effect in agitated depression, pain disorders, itching anxiety), imipramine (neutral depression-relieving, compulsive disorder), and desipramine (psychomotor activation in inhibited depression) are now only rarely used in dermatology.

Amitriptyline (Elavil, Tryptanol, Endep, Elatrol, Tryptizol, Trepiline, Laroxyl) may be indicated in chronic pain disorders (postherpetic neuralgias).

Amitriptyline

Indication: Depression, pain disorders.

Amitriptylin (Elavil) is used for treating depression and chronic pain. In dermatology, it is suitable for use in cutaneous pain syndromes such as glossodynia and postherpetic neuralgia as well as other cutaneous sensory complaints including burning, stabbing, biting, or tingling.

Dose: The dose should begin with 25 mg in the evening and then be titrated upward to a target dose of 150 mg/day.

Side effects: Sedation, orthostatic hypotension, anticholinergic effects, dry mouth, and gastrointestinal symptoms have been cited as side effects.

Note: Extrapyramidal side effects and suicidal tendencies must be evaluated when the inhibition is removed.

Compulsive Disorders

SSRIs are especially used in compulsive disorders (Table 15.5).

Good efficacy has been reported with fluoxetine, sertraline, paroxetine, fluvoxamine, and escitaprolam.

Indication: The indication and selection of the specific medication in compulsive disorders depends on the desired side effect spectrum of the drug. Particularly good efficacy has been described for SSRIs, in addition to depression and compulsive disorders, dermatitis paraartefacta with impaired impulse control (trichotillomania, acne excoriée) and other factitious disorders with transition to compulsive symptomatics. SSRIs are also very effective in body dysmorphic disorders.

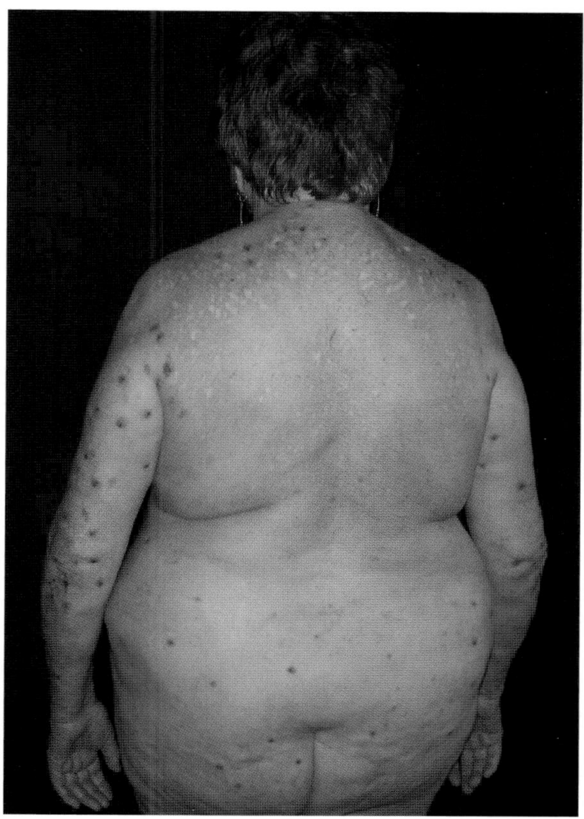

Fig 15.2 Prurigo and depression

Table 15.5 Psychopharmacotherapy of compulsive disorders in dermatology (*SSRI* selective serotonin reuptake inhibitor)

Psychiatric disorder	Medications
Compulsive disorders	1st choice: SSRI – paroxetine (Seroxat), sertraline (Gladem, Zoloft), escitalopram (Lexapro), citalopram (Celexa, Cipramil, Cipram), fluoxetine (Prozac, Fluctin), fluvoxamine (Fevarin)
	2nd choice: Tricyclic antidepressants – clomipramine (Anafranil)

Dose: A higher SSRI dose is sometimes necessary than in therapy of depression alone (see above).

Duration of treatment: The treatment should last at least 4–8 weeks until improvement in symptoms can be rated, and a different preparation should be selected only after 6 weeks. The total time of treatment to the first withdrawal test should be planned for 6–12 months.

Side effects: The side effects in compulsive disorders correspond to those when used as antidepressants. The definition of indication should take desired side effects into account.

Anxiety and Panic Disorders

General note: Anxiety disorders are characterized by excessive worry, tension, agitation, and restlessness, which may be treated by psychotherapy, pharmacotherapy, or combination therapy of psychotherapy with psychopharmaceuticals.

Tranquilizers (Lat. *tranquilare,* to soothe) are medications that, in their target symptoms, relieve anxiety and tension and also have sedative and sleep-promoting effects.

When used as an anxiolytic, the other properties are considered desired side effects (sedation) or undesired side effects (concentration impairment).

The transition from anxiolytic to hypnotic (sedative) is usually fluid and dose dependent and also depends on half-life. The speed at which an active metabolite becomes available is decisive for the profile of action.

The tranquilizers primarily include substances in the groups of benzodiazepines, nonbenzodiazepines (buspirone), plant-based sedatives, and low-strength neuroleptics.

In defining the indication for therapy of anxiety disorders, differentiation must be made in the first place between transient, brief, stress-related anxiety disorders and chronic anxiety disorders (Sect. 3.3.2).

"How do I find the right medication?"
First, chronic anxiety disorder must be distinguished from a transient anxiety disorder (lasting up to a few weeks) or an acute panic attack in defining the indication for drug treatment.

In selecting the psychopharmaceutical, the habituation potential must be taken into account if long-term therapy is planned (Table 15.6).

Benzodiazepines

Benzodiazepines are used in anxiety disorder – both generalized anxiety disorders as well as acute anxiety disorders and panic disorders. Whether the effect of the benzodiazepine is anxiolytic, sedating, or sleep-inducing depends largely on the dose administered. Diazepam is a good lipid-soluble medication that is quickly absorbed and thus can develop its efficacy rapidly in acute anxiety disorder.

The benzodiazepines are differentiated on the basis of their efficacy (potency) and half-life:

- Short-acting benzodiazepines:
  - Midazolam (Versed)
- Middle-acting benzodiazepines:
  - Lorazepam (Ativan)
  - Alprazolam (Xanax)
- Long-acting benzodiazepines:
  - Diazepam (Valium)
  - Flurazepam (Dalmadorm)

Benzodiazepines with longer half-lives should be used especially in persistent states of excitation in order to prevent recurrence between doses. Benzodiazepines with shorter half-lives are primarily used for sleep disorders.

Table 15.6 Pharmacotherapy for anxiety (*HL* half-life)

Medication	Drug group/HL	Indications	Dosage	Side effects
Buspirone (Buspar)	Nonbenzodiazepine	Chronic anxiety	5–30 mg/day	Giddiness
	HL 2–3 h	Inner restlessness		Headache
	Late onset of action after 2–4 weeks	States of tension		Nervousness
				Impaired concentration
				No sedation
				No impairment of sexual function
				No habituation potential
Alprazolam (Tafil, Xanax)	Middle-length benzodiazepine	Acute and chronic states of tension, excitation, and anxiety	1–2 mg/day initial dose	Insomnia
	HL 10–14 h	Additionally, low antidepressant efficacy	3–4 times 0.125–0.25 mg/day	Sedation
				Impaired concentration
				Habituation potential
				Use up to 4 weeks; withdrawal by tapering
Lorazepam (Ativan)	Middle-length benzodiazepines	Short-term treatment of anxiety, tension, excitation, and sleep impairments, especially in the presence of other somatic diseases	1–5 mg/day	Fatigue
	HL 12–15 h			Languorousness
				Impotence
		Sedation prior to diagnostic and operative procedures		Tremors
				Impaired orgasm
				In epileptics, the convulsion threshold may be lowered after withdrawal
Diazepam (Faustan, Valium)	Long-acting benzodiazepines	Acute and chronic states of anxiety, tension, and excitation	5–20 mg/day	Fatigue
	HL 20–40 h		Dose to be kept as low and duration of therapy as short as possible	Languorousness
		Amnestic effect prior to surgery		Hangover effects
		Muscle cramps		Tolerance development
		Status epilepticus		Habituation potential

Advantages: There is rapid effect and quick sedation, especially when given intravenously.
Disadvantage: Long-term therapy leads to withdrawal symptoms, addiction, and tolerance development.

Side effects: When benzodiazepines are withdrawn, real withdrawal symptoms may occur, with primarily vegetative symptoms up to convulsions and psychotic episodes. These must be distinguished from the rebound phenomenon (restlessness, anxiety, insomnia). Due to a tolerance development with reduced efficacy at the same dose, there may be a recurrence of the initial symptoms that originally led to the medication's use.

Other side effects are erectile dysfunction, reduced libido, impaired concentration, inability to drive, alcohol intolerance, and paradoxical excitation, especially in the elderly with brain-organic diseases.

Alprazolam

Indication: Anxiety disorder; states of tension and excitation, such as in acute stress-dependent hyperhidrosis; need for a middle-acting benzodiazepine with a half-life of 10–14 h. Alprazolam often produces an antidepressive effect.

Dose: Alprazolam (Xanax) 1–2 mg/day. For dermatological patients with generalized anxiety disorders, lower initial doses are often sufficient.

Side effects: Due to the addiction potential, use should be limited to 3–4 weeks. Alprazolam and chlorazepam are used most often in dermatology in the United States. Attention must be paid to the fact that the medications are also taken by drug addicts and have an addiction potential.

Diazepam

Indication: Rapid efficacy in immediate treatment of acute anxiety or panic disorders, especially in intravenous administration. Diazepam (Valium) has a half-life of 20–40 h and thus also has good efficacy in chronic anxiety and states of excitation.

Dose: Diazepam 5–20 mg/day.

Side effects: Because of the addiction potential, use should be limited to 3–4 weeks.

Nonbenzodiazepines

Buspiron

Indication: If drug therapy should be required in treatment of anxiety disorder for more than 4–6 weeks, nonbenzodiazepines should be used, for which buspirone (Buspar) is the first choice. This is a partial serotonin 5-HT receptor agonist and D2 blocker, which permits safe long-term therapy with sufficient anxiolytic effect and little sedative effect.

Advantage: Hardly any withdrawal symptoms or habituation
Disadvantage: Late onset of effect (acute stress may already be over and dealt with)

It must be remembered that buspirone shows a therapeutic effect only after 2 weeks. This is a problem in the case of acute anxiety symptoms.

Dose: The buspirone dose of 5 mg should be administered three times daily, and a maximum of 60 mg/day (mean dose 30 mg/day) should not be exceeded.

Side effects: Usually there are only mild side effects such as headache and nausea.

Alternatives

The following alternatives can be considered for therapy of chronic anxiety:

1. Doxepin for treatment of chronic anxiety disorders, whereby usually 50 mg or less per day is administered. Doxepin is nearly as effective as diazepam but without the corresponding side effect spectrum.
2. Paroxetine (Seroxat) can be used as another attempt, at a dose of 20–50 mg/day.
3. Doxepin (Sinequan, Doxal, Doxepin, Doxedyn) should be preferred for patients with mixed presentations of anxiety and depression, or a therapy attempt can be made with venlafaxine (Trevilor).

As an alternative to buspirone, doxepin and paroxetine can be used in anxiety disorders.

Special Group: Beta Blockers

Beta-receptor blockers do not belong to psychopharmaceuticals in the actual sense, but they show very good efficacy in vegetative symptoms of psychiatric disorders, especially anxiety disorders. Their advantage lies in a lack of central nervous system (CNS) side effects such as impaired concentration and sedation.

Flushing and sweating are among the special indications in dermatology, along with other vegetative symptoms that require internal-medical clarification, including tachycardia, palpitations, dizziness, tension headache and migraine, hypertensive crises, hyperventilation and respiratory distress, feeling of constriction in the chest, tremors, muscular tics, feeling of weakness, and nausea and vomiting.

Special use can also be justified in so-called stage fright. Beta-receptor blockers such as propranolol or oxprenolol may be helpful in situational anxiety (such as fear of examination). Often, 10–20 mg propranolol prior to the feared event is sufficient.

Caution is required in known heart disease, asthma, and allergies (wasp sting allergy); these conditions are thus possible contraindications, and side effects, including erectile dysfunction and reduced reaction capacity, must be taken into account.

Hypnotics

In some cases, insomnias are predominant in the complaint symptoms of depressive or anxiety disorders. In certain patient groups, hypnotics may show sufficiently good therapeutic success. The habituation potential must be kept in mind.

Hypnotics from the group of nonbenzodiazepines, such as zolpidem, should be used as therapy of first choice.

The hypnotics of second choice are mostly benzodiazepines with a short half-life in order to induce sleep but avoid drowsiness the following morning. Brotizolam, temazepam, nitrazepam, and lormetazepam, which should be used only for short times, belong to this group (Table 15.7).

Table 15.7 Hypnotics (*HL* half-life)

Medication	Properties	Indications	Dosage	Side effects
Zolpidem (Stilnox, Ambien)	Nonbenzodiazepine	Short-term treatment of insomnias (trouble falling asleep)	8 mg/day	Fatigue
	Different agonist of the GABA receptors			Reduced reaction capacity
	HL 2–3 h			Low addiction potential
				Rebound and tolerance development
Brotizolam (Lendormin)	Short-acting benzodiazepine	Trouble falling asleep and sleeping through the night	0.125–0.25 mg/day	Fatigue
	HL 4–9 h			Languorousness
				Impaired concentration
				Interaction with alcohol
				Tolerance and addiction
Lormetazepam (Noctamid)	Short- to middle-acting benzodiazepine	Impaired sleep with frequent waking periods and trouble falling asleep again	1 mg/day	See brotizolam
	HL 8–12 h			

Antihistamines with Central Effect

Skin diseases are very often accompanied by significant pruritus. Therapy with antihistamines follows a stepwise plan, whereby treatment usually begins with nonsedating antihistamines, and sedating antihistamines are administered later.

Stepwise Plan for Antihistamines

- Step 1: Nonsedating antihistamines (cetirizine, loratadine, fexofenadine)
- Step 2: Sedating antihistamines (clemastine, hydroxyzine)
- Step 3: Psychopharmaceuticals
  - Antihistamines with CNS effect (promethazine)
  - Tricyclic antidepressants (doxepin)

Table 15.8 Antihistamines with central effect

Medication	Dosage	Indications	Side effects
Hydroxyzine (Atarax)	25–75 mg/day, preferably evenings in two to three doses	Itching in urticaria and atopic dermatitis with states of anxiety, tension, and restlessness	Arrhythmias
		Sleep disorders	Reduced reaction capacity
			Sedation
Promethazine (Atosil, Prothazin)	Initial dose 25 mg/day	Allergic diseases	Sedation
	Maximum dose 200 mg/day	Restlessness	Reduced reaction capacity
		Excitation	Anticholinergic effect
		Substitute medication in stubborn pruritus	Danger of thrombosis
			Malignant neuroleptic syndrome
Tricyclic antidepressants			
Doxepin (Sinequan, Doxal, Doxepin, Doxedyn)	Initial dose 25–50 mg/day	Antidepressant effect	Dry mouth
		Antihistaminic effect	Malaise
		Pain disorders	Tremors
	Maximum dose 100–200 mg/day		Sedation
			Sweating
			Obstipation
Opipramol (Insidon)	50–150 mg/day	Anxiety	Dry mouth
		Tension	Malaise
		Depressive mood	Tremors
		Vegetative organ complaints	Sedation
			Sweating
			Obstipation

Nonsedating (cetirizine, loratadine, fexofenadine) and sedating (clemastine, hydroxyzine) antihistamines are unsuccessful in some cases of persistent pruritus. Pruritus has a mental component and can be elicited or exacerbated by stress. Thus, there may be a central genesis/triggering of pruritus that responds better or only to psychopharmaceuticals.

Low strength neuroleptics also develop a good central antipruriginous effect and can thus be promising in incontrollable pruritus in the corresponding indication.

The use of antihistamines with CNS effect or of tricyclic antidepressants is indicated if the target symptoms are central-nervous-related itching combined with psychomotor restlessness.

Antihistamines with neuroleptic effect (antiallergic neuroleptics) and some other tricyclic antidepressants show good efficacy in therapy-resistant central pruritus (Table 15.8).

Hydroxyzine

Indication: The main indication for hydroxyzine (Atarax) is itching in urticaria and atopic dermatitis when nonsedating antihistamines show inadequate improvement in symptoms. Hydroxyzine (sedating antihistamine) is especially effective in anxiety, tension, and states of restlessness and can be successfully used in the evening to treat insomnia. During the day, a combination with centrally active antihistamines is used to reduce the side effects. In cases of insomnia and nocturnal itching, hydroxyzine is the drug of first choice and should be administered in the evening.

Dose: 25–75 mg/day in two to three doses, especially in the evening.

Side effects: Reduced reaction capacity, sedation, and arrhythmias are among the frequent side effects.

Promethazine

Indication: Promethazine (Atosil, Prothazin) is an antiallergic neuroleptic and is the substitution medication as drug of second choice in stubborn pruritus. It is especially suitable in allergic diseases with restlessness and states of excitation.

Dose: The initial dose is 25 mg daily, and the maximum dose is 200 mg/day.

Side effects: Predominant are sedation and limitation of reaction capacity. In addition, anticholinergic side effects, a danger of thrombosis, and the malignant neuroleptic syndrome must also be watched for.

Doxepin

Indication: The tricyclic antidepressant doxepin (see above) gives the best results in pruritus, depression, anxiety, and cholinergic urticaria with depression and also in prurigo diseases. Moreover, the itching–scratching or itching–depression cycle can often be successfully broken. The affinity of doxepin for histamine H1 receptors in vitro is 56 times greater than that of hydroxyzine and 775 times greater than that of diphenhydramine.

Formerly, amitriptyline and pimozide (second choice) were successfully used in these indications.

Other Antihistamines

For restless and irritable patients with depression and itching administration of opripamol (in Germany) has been found useful.

Ondansetron (Zofran) is a serotonin receptor antagonist for the treatment of nausea and vomiting, especially in connection with chemotherapy. Recent studies show that ondansetron in a dose of 8–12 mg/day orally brings good improvement in pruritic symptoms of patients with atopic dermatitis (Zenker et al. 2003).

The good therapeutic success of UVA1 and SUP phototherapy in therapy-resistant pruritus should also be mentioned here.

Reference

Zenker S, Schuh T, Degitz K (2003) Behandlung von Pruritus als Symptom von Hauterkrankungen mit dem Serotonin-Rezeptorandayonist Ondansetron. JDDG 1: 705–710

Further Reading

Benkert O, Hippius H (1996) Psychiatrische PharmakoTherapy, 6. Aufl. Springer, Berlin

Buchheim P (1997) PsychoTherapy und Psychopharmaceuticals. Schattauer, Stuttgart

Gupta MA, Gupta AK, Haberman HF (1986) Psychotropic drugs in dermatology. A review and guidelines for use. J Am Acad Dermatol 14(4): 633–645

Hoegl L, Hillert A, Fichter M (1996) Psychopharmacological Therapy und Hauterkrankungen. Psyche 22: 513–516

Koblenzer CS (2001) The use of psychotropic drugs in dermatology. Dermatol Psychosom 2: 167–176

Koo JY, Ng TC (2002) Psychotropic and neurotropic agents in dermatology: unapproved uses, dosages, or indications. Clin Dermatol 20(5): 582–594

Lee E, Murase J, Koo J, Lee CS (2003) Psychopharmacology in dermatological practice: a review and update. Dermatol Psychosom 4: 131–140

Meiss F, Fischer M, Marsch WC (2003) Gabapentin in der Behandlung der Glossodynie. JDDG (Suppl 1): 95

Orfanos C, Garbe C (2002) Therapy der Hautkrankheiten, 2. Aufl. Springer, Berlin

Phillips KA, Najjar F (2003) An open-label study of citalopram in body dysmorphic disorder. J Clin Psychiatry 64(6): 715–720

Phillips KA, Albertini RS, Rasmussen SA (2002) A randomized placebo-controlled trial of fluoxetine in body dysmorphic disorder. Arch Gen Psychiatry 59(4): 381–388

16

SAD Light Therapy, Vagal Stimulation, and Magnetic Stimulation

16.1 Light Treatment of Seasonal Affective Depression

The use of light therapy has proven beneficial, especially for the special form of seasonal affective depression (SAD) during the winter months. SAD light therapy with white light is considered an effective form of treating SAD. SAD light therapy has a spectrum in the range of visible light (Fig. 16.1).

SAD light therapy (Kripke 1998; Meesters et al. 1999; Partonen and Lonnqvist 1998) biomedically replaces the missing sunlight (Humpel et al. 1992) during the brief periods with limited daylight in the winter months. Light therapy is performed, depending on the type of equipment, for 30 min at up to 10,000 lux in the morning hours (Fig. 16.2).

The mechanism of action is assumed to be stimulation of the eyes, which possibly leads to regulation of the sleeping–waking rhythm. Nerve stimulation by photons could explain the antidepressant effect. The light produced by the SAD lamp, which has a spectrum similar to daylight, is absorbed by the retina in the eye and stimulates the brain to secrete serotonin and melatonin.

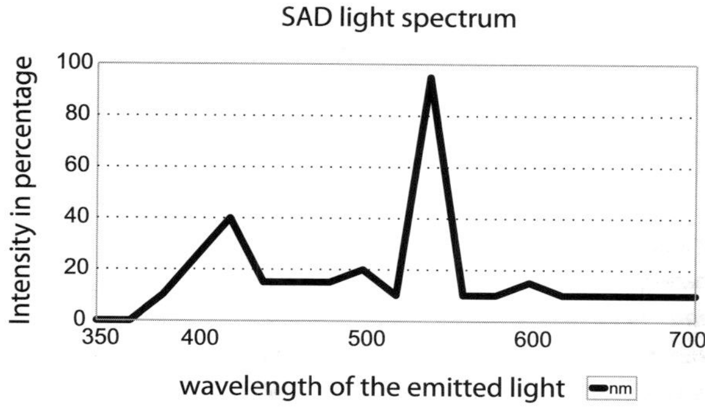

Fig. 16.1 Light spectrum for use for seasonal affective depression (*y*-axis: intensity in percentage; *x*-axis: wavelength of the emitted light)

Fig. 16.2 Light therapy room for patients with seasonal winter depression

16.2 Treating Depression with Vagus Nerve Stimulation

Left vagal nerve stimulation is an outpatient procedure in which an electrode is surgically wrapped around the left branch of the vagus nerve (the right branch innervates the heart). A pulse generator linked to the electrode is placed subcutaneously in the clavicular region.

The procedure was approved for the treatment of resistant epilepsy more than a decade ago, and in 2003 the U.S. Food and Drug Administration (FDA) approved the procedure for unipolar and bipolar depressive episodes of at least moderate severity with a duration of at least 2 years, or two previous major depressive episodes, or inadequate response to at least four treatment trials; insurance carriers may have different requirements for funding the procedure. The presence of psychotic symptoms is exclusionary.

The results of the initial multisite evaluation on patients with marked chronicity – with more than half of them having been treated at one point with electroconvulsive therapy (ECT) – showed one-third with marked improvement, one-third with some improvement, and the remaining third with no change or reporting worsening.

Although no deaths had been attributed to the procedure or to the use of stimulation as of 2003, some of the side effects reported in a study prior to FDA approval included hoarseness, cough, voice alteration, chest pain, earaches, and nausea. Some of these side effects can be decreased by changing the stimulation rate. After 2 years, a marked decrease in side effects has been reported.

16

16.3 Transcranial Magnetic Stimulation

Transcranial magnetic stimulation (TMS) is a noninvasive method for brain stimulation that was introduced in the mid-1980s. By the placement of a small coil over the scalp and application of an alternating current, a magnetic field passing through the brain is generated. The technique was initially used to investigate nerve conduction because of its ability to generate muscular-evoked potential. Because of the low side effects compared with ECT, and particularly the fact that it does not require general anesthesia and does not induce memory loss, multiple studies were begun to explore the possibility of using the technique to replace ECT. Some studies show some success in major depression. The stimulation of the left prefrontal cortex has been associated with antidepressant properties.

The FDA has approved multiple TMS devices for research purposes. Currently, no device has received FDA approval for TMS of the brain as a therapeutic procedure. At this time, one device has been approved in Israel and Canada as a treatment for depression.

The procedure can also be considered a possible alternative to antidepressant medications when these need to be avoided for medical reasons or when concerns of the risk of precipitating a manic/hypomanic episode with an antidepressant are present.

References

Humpel C, Neudorfer C, Philipp W, Steiner HJ, Haring C, Schmid KW, Schwitzer J, Saria A (1992) Effects of bright artificial light on monoamines and neuropeptides in eight different brain regions compared in a pigmented and nonpigmented rat strain. J Neurosci Res 32: 605–612

Kripke DF (1998) Light treatment for nonseasonal depression: speed, efficacy, and combined treatment. J Affect Disord 49: 109–117

Meesters Y, Beersma DG, Bouhuys AL, van den Hoofdakker RH (1999) Prophylactic treatment of seasonal affective disorder (SAD) by using light visors: bright white or infrared light? Biol Psychiatry 46: 239–246

Partonen T, Lonnqvist J (1998) Seasonal affective disorder. Lancet 352: 1369–1374

Further Reading

Fitzgerald PB, Benitez J, de Castella A et al (2006) A randomized, controlled trial of sequential bilateral repetitive transcranial magnetic stimulation for treatment-resistant depression. Am J Psychiatry 163(1): 88–94

George MS, Nahas Z, Borckardt JJ, et al (2007) Vagus nerve stimulation for the treatment of depression and other neuropsychiatric disorders. Expert Rev Neurother 7(1): 63–74

George MS, Rush AJ, Marangell LB, et al (2005) A one-year comparison of vagus nerve stimulation with treatment as usual for treatment-resistant depression. Biol Psychiatry 58(5): 364–373

Grunhaus L, Schreiber S, Dolberg OT et al (2003) A randomized controlled comparison of electroconvulsive therapy and repetitive transcranial magnetic stimulation in severe and resistant nonpsychotic major depression. Biol Psychiatry 53(4): 324–331

Rush AJ, Marangell LB, Sackeim HA, et al (2005a) Vagus nerve stimulation for treatment-resistant depression: a randomized, controlled acute phase trial. Biol Psychiatry58(5): 347–354

Rush AJ, Sackeim HA, Marangell LB, et al (2005b) Effects of 12 months of vagus nerve stimulation in treatment-resistant depression: a naturalistic study. Biol Psychiatry 58(5): 355–363

The Difficult or Impossible-To-Treat Problem Patient

17

One of the greatest challenges for a dermatologist is the patient who is difficult or even impossible to treat under somatic aspects.

Usually, a primary underlying emotional disorder, such as acarophobia, artefacts, body dysmorphic disorder, or dermatoses with secondary profit from disease, is clearly and readily recognizable, even in the routine dermatological practice. Therapy of the emotional disorder is thus predominant right from the start, even though there is often no motivation on the patient's part.

Latent problems, which become apparent later in the course of dermatological treatment, are much more challenging to approach and also result in costly and excessively time-consuming consultations.

The foundation is usually a lack of insight into the disease and a lack of compliance. This frequently occurs because of denial, repression, or other defense mechanisms, including dissociative phenomena. The result is that adequate somatic therapy can hardly be performed.

This often presents the dermatologist with an unsolvable problem and can lead to feelings of helplessness or even rage and annoyance in the treating physician – representing countertransference. The underlying causes in difficult or impossible-to-treat patients are usually latent problematic maladjustments and unconscious conflicts that result in impediments in the therapeutic situation. The characteristic and most frequently encountered problems that particularly occur in dermatology can be summarized as follows.

Problematic Maladjustments and Conflicts in Skin Patients

- Overattribution
- Rigid one-sided causality
- Overidentification with the skin
- Inner proximity-distance conflict

Overattribution: The cause of all negative experiences in life is ascribed to the skin disease. This is a relief from a psychoanalytic point of view, which postulates that confrontation with one's own personality and inner conflicts can be avoided.

Rigid or one-sided causal attribution: The disease has only one cause for the patient, for example, an allergy. This understanding of disease enables relief – usually only for a limited time – because as long as there is hope of a cure, there is no need to concern oneself with the chronicity of the disease.

Overidentification with the skin: The patient sees himself as a person with a skin disease in all areas of life, living through the disease and not with it, as it exerts the decisive influence on the individual's life.

In dermatology patients, an *inner proximity–distance conflict*, which is subjectively hard to resolve, is often relevant (Detig 1989): On the one hand, there is need for proximity to others, but on the other hand, the patient is afraid of the proximity.

The Doctor–Patient Relationship

If emotional transference conflicts predominate in the dermatological visit or if the doctor is chosen as the arena for acting out a conflict-laden thematic (relationship conflict), the patient is usually difficult.

Difficult patients can present in the following ways in the doctor–patient relationship in daily practice (Gieler and Augustin 2000):

- The aggressive patient, who is dissatisfied, makes excessive demands (exaggerated demand behavior), and exerts pressure
- The exploitative patient, who uses the doctor to attain advantages (such as early retirement and secondary profit from disease)
- The dependent patient, who shows no active coping with the disease
- The emotionally remarkable patient, who is restless, depressive, moody, and nervous
- The "expert killer," with an unclear or missing diagnosis, who offers no compliance, has negative expectations about treatment, and reports frequent discontinuation of therapy ("doctor shopping")

Depressive patients tend to enrage the doctor by their derogatory comments. A maximum variant of the pathological patient–doctor relationship is the "expert-killer syndrome."

Expert Killers and Doctor Shopping

17

The term "expert-killer syndrome" is used and observed primarily in the psychosomatics of chronic states of pain, such as fibromyalgia syndrome.

The expert-killer syndrome is characterized clinically by the triad of diffuse complaint symptoms with a number of examinations or operations, lack of diagnosis, and a pathological doctor–patient relationship.

> **Diagnostic Criteria of "Expert-Killer Syndrome"**
>
> - Diffuse complaint symptoms with numerous clinic visits and ancillary tests or operations
> - Lack of diagnosis
> - Pathological doctor–patient relationship

Typically, the patient has frequently terminated therapy and frequently changed physicians; thus, the term "doctor shopping" can appropriately be applied. Characteristically, the previous doctors are described to the new "expert" as poor and incompetent (patient quote: "He only tried things out"). The new doctors are put under the ambitious pressure of a real challenge (patient quote: "You are my last hope"), but the patient's pathological expectations cannot be fulfilled.

The doctor–patient relationship is characterized by an initial exaggerated idealization of the physician, which soon turns to distrustful rejection and termination of the relationship. The trigger is often a narcissistic insult to the patient. All of the doctor's efforts are usually doomed to failure from the beginning. In general, the interactions described remain unconscious for both parties in the purely somatic setting.

Procedures in Difficult Doctor–Patient Relationships

Resolution of the cited conflicts and mechanisms in the patient are often barely possible for the dermatologist, especially under time pressure. The dermatologist's top priorities are perception of the situation, a reduction of measures to only what is medically appropriate, and a sparing biopsychosocial approach.

Introduction of a combination therapy with dermatological basic therapy, strengthening of coping strategies, and provision of adequate information and knowledge about the disease (psychoeducation) have proven beneficial. In psychosomatic dermatology, establishing or improving the patient's motivation with respect to a psychosomatic understanding of illness plays an outstanding role, since only in the very rarest cases is this motivation as strong as the patient's willingness to undergo somatic treatment.

Avoidable Medical Treatment Errors

To a large extent, doctors' errors in dealing with and interviewing psychosomatically difficult problem patients are a taboo topic in training, postgraduate, and continued education, as well as in daily practice. Fortunately, the somatic physician is usually forgiven for making them.

However, medical factors that are detrimental treatment errors need to be avoided and biopsychosocial aspects must also be taken into account in the doctor–patient relationship.

> **Typical Avoidable Medical Treatment Errors**
>
> - Somatization of emotional problems
> - Confrontation too early

- Insistence on rapid improvement
- Suggestion of positive points of view
- Incorrect interviewing
  - Blaming and reproaching
  - Appeals ("pull yourself together") and "patent cures"
  - Attempts to convince

Beware of decisions made in the depressive phase.

These treatment errors often arise under time pressure or due to a purely biosomatic causality approach, and they may contribute in the long run to somatization and chronification of emotional disorders.

Even when expanded psychosocial factors are taken into account, no uncritical suggestion of a positive point of view should be made, nor the patient talked into psychotherapy. Writing a referral to a psychologist is usually not enough in this context and is seldom used by the patient.

Compliance

It is assumed that about 50% of all patients are inadequately compliant or not compliant at all. Up to 20% of patients do not fill their prescriptions, and up to half of the remaining patients use the medication incorrectly (Urquhart 1994). In dermatology, the highest medication noncompliance is in psoriasis, with 30–66% noncompliance; acne, with 32–51% noncompliance; and atopic dermatitis, with up to 68% noncompliance (Poli et al. 2001; Krejci-Manwaring et al. 2007). Differentiation is made between primary and secondary forms of noncompliance.

Primary noncompliance indicates that the patient does not have the prescription filled. Secondary noncompliance includes incorrect administration or dosage errors, as well as unintentional nonadministration and forgetfulness.

The causes differ greatly from patient to patient. According to lay hypotheses, there is fear of side effects (Sect. 3.3.2). Information deficits or administration instructions that are too difficult and complicated can also lead to noncompliance. Compliance improvement thus comprises not only taking medications as directed, adhering to dietary rules, weaning from pleasure-giving toxins, and keeping consultation appointments, but also communicating through the structured interview. Communication with the patient must reflect his or her subjective needs and concepts. It is mandatory that the patient understand the diagnosis and therapy concept through simple and easy-to-remember information.

In order to improve compliance, the doctor should initially provide only the most important information about the therapy. Three items are enough:

1. How do I use it?
2. How often do I use it?
3. What should I do if I have a problem?

It is very helpful to have patients repeat all instructions in their own words and let them ask questions. But in addition, the doctor should promote nonverbal contact (eye contact!) and use the patient's own language. If there is any doubt, the instructions must be repeated several times for the patient.

Improvement in compliance in the doctor–patient communication plays a central role in the successful therapy of numerous dermatoses, such as acne (Draelos 1995).

References

Detig CH (1989) Hautkrank: Unberührbarkeit aus Abwehr? Psychodynamische Prozesse zwischen Nähe und Distanz. Vandenhoeck & Ruprecht, Göttingen

Draelos ZK (1995) Patient compliance: enhancing clinician abilities and strategies. J Am Acad Dermatol 32: 42–48

Gieler U, Augustin M (2000) Der Problempatient in der Hautarztpraxis. In: Plettenberg A, Meigel WN, Moll I (Hrsg) Dermatologie an der Schwelle zum neuen Jahrtausend. Aktueller Stand von Klinik und Forschung. Springer, Berlin, S 725–730

Krejci-Manwaring J, Tusa MG, Carroll C, Camacho F, Kaur M, Carr D, Fleischer AB Jr, Balkrishnan R, Feldman SR (2007) Stealth monitoring of adherence to topical medication: adherence is very poor in children with atopic dermatitis. J Am Acad Dermatol 56: 211–216

Poli F, Dreno B, Verschoore M (2001) An epidemiological study of acne in female adults: results of a survey conducted in France. J Eur Acad Dermatol Venereol 15: 541–545

Urquhart J (1994) Role of patient compliance in clinical pharmacokinetics. A review of recent research. Clin Pharmacokinet 27: 202–215

Further Reading

Beck D (1977) Das Koryphäen-Killer-Syndrom. Dtsch Med Wochenschr 102: 303–307

Green LW, Mullen PD, Friedman RB (1991) Epidemiological and community approaches to patient compliance. In: Cramer JA, Spilker B (eds) Patient compliance in medical practice and clinical trials. Raven, New York, pp 373–386

The Helpless Dermatologist

The physician could be caught in the polarity between a highly respected, interesting, and sometimes widely varied profession on the one hand and, on the other hand, working to the limits of exhaustion, responding to increasing legal bureaucratization, and experiencing professional alienation. Moreover, if the patients have high or even increasing demands while resources are dwindling, inadequate care sometimes results. There are also increasing numbers of difficult patients with serious personality disorders and patients with artefacts or body dysmorphic disorders. In these cases, problems of transference and countertransference are often encountered. Additionally, on many occasions the required services are not reimbursed by insurance companies, and physicians find themselves dispensing intense and laborious services for free. The frequent need of psychodermatological services by uninsured patients certainly generates an increased burden on the physician and the medical establishment.

The often untiring commitment—sometimes in addition to regular working hours and on weekends—can lead to serious disorientation, sensory crises, or exhaustion and depression. In the latter, one's own analysis and coping with stress are gradually given less space, including less time for reflection, since the demands from outside (e.g., constant availability, consultation willingness, and decisional capacity) are becoming increasingly intense.

Physicians increasingly report that the high stress affects their family life. The ability to adequately cope with stress becomes more and more difficult, and added to this situation are irregular meals, lack of exercise, sleep deprivation, anxiety disorders, or even medication and alcohol abuse, as well as increasing family conflicts.

Dermatologists' mental health levels have been found to average lower than their physical health levels (Jurkat 2006), with the physical and mental health levels being higher in female dermatologists than in their male colleagues. In comparison to other medical specialists, dermatologists differ only slightly in their health-related quality of life. Therefore, it may be advisable to implement preventive measures concerning their comparatively low mental health status, especially for males.

One possibility for breaking the circle is the Balint group, which may be relieving and emotionally supportive and may even enable one to overcome conflicts after establishing a trusting relationship with other colleagues. Restructuring of general working hours and establishing increasingly satisfactory doctor–patient relationships may help physicians move from a problem fixation to a solution orientation.

References

Jurkat HB, Cramer M, Reimer C, Kupfer J, Gieler U (2007) Health-related quality of life in dermatologists compared to other physicians. Hautarzt 58(1): 38–47

18 The Dermatologist's Personal Challenges Within the Institutional Framework: Developing the Psychodermatologic Practice

Institutions can be understood as complex transactional spaces in which multiple purposes, missions, and personal interests need to be balanced and satisfied concurrently. These include the patients' need for care; the economic needs for the service, administration, and infrastructure to function; and the practitioners' needs for learning, training, and professional development, to name a few. First we will look at how these pressures are accommodated within institutions, and then we will track some of the components of the individual process of adjusting to the practice. Finally, we will discuss ways to provide support to those delivering the care.

Institutions take shape and develop according to (1) the moment and psychosocial context of their creation, (2) influenced by their funding and (3) by how the staff and institution mature (4) in response to how research and evaluations weigh and qualify the results of the clinical interventions, and also (5) by responding to the psychological comfort, reward, and security experienced by the team of practitioners and patients.

1. Psychodermatologic services are created or maintained for a variety of reasons. For example, they may be the interest of a foundation or university, the product of a government decision or a reflection of pressures by a consumer association, or the result of a professional group to organize specific services and deliver appropriate services to patients with special needs in a busy dermatology clinic. The context of the institution's creation will often not only influence its mission but may determine its hierarchical structure as well as the availability, allocation, and use of resources.
2. Funding is an important determinant that shapes the structure of the clinic, the population to be served, and the quality and scope of services provided. These factors strongly permeate the institution, influencing the structure and modalities of care delivery. The differences in the functioning of psychodermatological clinics vary according to whether they rely on a prepaid health maintenance organization (HMO), funding from research grants, budget allocations, or the modalities of billing the insurance services covering the patients. These economic dimensions regulate multiple characteristics, including variations in the existence of services and the acceptance of therapeutic approaches. The funding will obviously regulate the type of coverage, the portion allocated for primary prevention, the existence of all types of extended psychosocial services, the extent of working hours, and, at times, even the scientific orientation of research, psychoeducation, and information services.
3. The maturation of the clinic and staff and the accumulation of research and experience lead to development of an "institutional memory" as well as an operational memory concretized in refining and establishing cost-effective procedures; manualization; facilitating the training of residents, postdoctoral fellows, and new staff; and integration of a multidisciplinary team capable of mutually enriching and potentiating the capabilities and knowledge of the staff, particularly the integration of psychodermatological procedures not only in diagnosis but also through the interventions. Another reshaping force is the tension created among modalities centered on deliv-

ering services versus obtaining research data. Finally, a multipersonal process of theoretical coherence takes place, providing the "orientation" to the clinic and widening the door for the selection, training, and integration of new professionals and midlevel providers. Of particular relevance is the presence of trust and interest for the development of personal individual growth projects in synchronization with the global set of goals in the institutional culture.

4. It is hoped that success will generate a strong drive to grow in the direction causing it; this is often the case in clinical and research work. But finding and evaluating the results of the clinical, research, or administrative interventions requires a steep investment. Conducting follow-up agreements, making home visits, monitoring patients' compliance to treatments, evaluating remissions in patients not currently attending, monitoring patient satisfaction, and evaluating each step of the referral/follow-up are examples of the expensive interventions needed to evaluate results and find the positive ones as well as the causes for failures.
5. The institutional milieu is difficult to describe but easy to feel. One of the most powerful factors is the character and comfort of the relations with "friendly" or "competitive" peers, inviting and enjoying institutional participation. The institutional milieu can be supportive and forgiving and encourage a focus on the tasks at hand, or it can be rigid and unwelcoming and focus on personality rather than on contributions to the common goals. The peer relationships often reflect the relationships with coordinators. How much the line staff feels that their functions are valued and their communications attended to and that they are considered valuable people is often reflected in peer relations.

   These are some of the ingredients regulating the institutional culture, milieu, or group character and are the main generator of the feelings of psychological safety experienced by those working in the clinic or department. Bion differentiated "work" groups that are mainly interested in the task at hand as being more cohesive, with a tendency to accommodate and contain their members working together. Groups with more primitive functioning are more interested in testing the capability of the coordinators, expecting too much from them, and often are not a good place for the participants to feel contained.

   Last but not least, psychological safety and comfort are better experienced when the physical environment is conducive to the task and welfare of the person working there, and hence has a human nature, light, space, privacy, and the basic tools for operation. The psychological safety and comfort of the staff surely contribute in part to the experience conveyed to the patient.

On the one hand, obtaining fulfillment by delivering care to the psychodermatological patient has many challenges related to the difficulties of giving care to highly disturbed patients. On the other hand, integrating to institutional life has many challenges, too. From the perspective of the individual practitioner, the process of integrating to a psychodermatologic practice includes integration of the following: (1) aspects of the dermatologist's own inner world and needs, (2) ability to tolerate the chaos, confusion, and massive projections of the patient, 3) ability to join, deal with, and become satisfied in the process of quenching the patient's clinical needs within the support, complexities, and constraints of institutional life, and 4) training in critical areas.

1. The choice of a medical career may have foundations in personal altruistic needs, attempts to improve the lives of others, or some grandiosity; there are also often personal problems that the practitioner is trying to address from his or her own past. These circumstances are the sources of the practitioner's strengths and weaknesses. Very often, the practitioner hopes to find growth, enjoyment, and pleasure in professional life. Because of these important expectations related to the practitioner's present and past, confronting a reality that is markedly different and includes more difficulties than were expected may be challenging and can lead to some degree of disappointment. Finding himself or herself with much less power to heal than what was expected may impair the caregiver's satisfaction, and the shortcoming may be compounded by the challenges of adjusting to a working environment, peers, and supervisors. All of these obstacles may conspire against the clinician's achievement of the stable, contained state required to diagnose and in turn care for and contain highly disturbed patients.
2. The patient consulting for a psychodermatologic condition brings baggage loaded with the more challenging psychiatric conditions, without the needed awareness of them. The psychotic/confusional functioning of the patient with delusional parasitosis is compounded by the patient's difficulties in approaching his or her psychiatric delusional condition as such. The patient comes to enlist the dermatologist to take care of a condition that does not truly exist,

creating in the dermatologist a context in which he or she needs to be the expert on finding and exterminating an inexistent plague. Often there is a preexisting antagonistic relation with the dermatologist, who is perceived as someone who will not believe the patient's delusional construction, someone with whom to have conflict and bitterness even before the chief complaints are elicited for the first time. The lack of reality of the situation and the difficulty in creating a trustful and sincere doctor–patient relationship makes the psychodermatologist perceive himself or herself inside a psychotic world without tools for emerging. At the same time, the dermatologist perceives the patient's suffering and intense need for help but realizes that the patient is requesting help without wanting to dispel the delusions. The process of detecting the demand of services from the patients and including them in a path leading to the abandonment of delusional thinking is the ultimate challenge for constructing a progressively trustful doctor–patient relationship.

3. Joining: The construction of an appropriate encounter involves postponing personal weakness on the side of the practitioner and the client to engage in a relationship that is mutually beneficial. The development of an alliance and a cooperative association for decreasing the patient's suffering is the cornerstone of the joining and the constitution of a clinical relationship. The maintenance of the alliance is facilitated by genuine interest in the patient's perceptions, no matter how distorted they are.
   A good alliance and association will reflect understanding and will include attentive listening, often with "mirroring," to clarify the understanding of what is elicited by the patient, including the understanding of signs, symptoms, and personal situations. "Mirroring" or "pacing" basically consists of adopting or matching the other person's (in this case, the patient's) language, posturing, gestures, body language, and even breathing rhythm. This behavior on the part of the health provider has been proven to increase doctor–patient rapport. Paying attention to the patient's hopes, needs, and wants can be the basis for meaningful dialogue and agreements. A realistic dialogue to the degree that is appropriate to maintain a solid alliance and providing a map of resources and procedures to orient the patient to community and in-house resources fully consistent with the institutional model of service delivery can also enhance the alliance. A good encounter and alliance will facilitate the patient's affective investment, attention, and compliance; will contribute to his or her feeling of receiving good care; and also will help the practitioner in his or her own process of discovering how to become satisfied in professional practice.
4. Professional growth may be the result of increasing expertise in different areas, including the following:
   Contextualization of the psychodermatologic consultation and diagnostic process, including, when meaningful, the immediate context of the patient's life, work relations, family relations, finances, particular personal circumstances, material and affective losses, aging, familial vital cycle, and so on. Having a narrow focus is not the best approach to psychodermatology, considering that the stressors from any source can trigger anxiety and worsen underlying psychopathology.

- Training in the use and interpretation of diagnostic tools, structured interviews, questionnaires, and family and community interventions.
- Training in how to deal with the decompensating patient; psychosis; homicidal and suicidal ideation, plans, or attempts; violent outbursts in the clinical situation; and other rare crises.

Developing expertise in using a structured interview will markedly facilitate not only the diagnostic process regarding underlying psychiatric conditions but also the use of appropriate interventions with the patient during treatment.

A given is that psychodermatologists are often under stress because of the inherent difficulties in relating with the patients, their own personal lives, and the institutional life.

An important aspect of the integration between the institutional and the individual domains is the process of delivering appropriate care to the practitioner – taking care of those giving care to the patients. It can take different shapes in different institutional cultures. How to transform traumatic incidents and failures in wisdom is one of the institutional challenges.

Ways to support the weight of the pain and responsibility in the face of poor outcomes include the following:

- Share the clinical and administrative responsibilities in hiring, firing, and decision making.
- Invest time and resources in retracing and examining the work in clinical meetings and process groups, where personal and group dissatisfaction can be contained and dealt with.
- Reinforce and ensure the staff's psychological safety.
- Acknowledge failed clinical interventions and procedures.

Liaison Consultancy

19

The psychosomatic liaison service is regarded as central to psychosomatic consultancy in dermatology. It implies the regular cooperation between psychological, psychotherapeutic, and somatic therapists in a consolidated and efficient manner (Pasquini et al. 1997; Wise 2000).

The liaison psychosomatic doctor is a psychotherapist who is firmly incorporated into the somatic treatment team.

The liaison psychosomatic doctor is a member of the medical treatment team whose activity is routinely included in the workings of the dermatology department. The thematic foci of this liaison are diagnoses of psychosomatic disorders and advice to treating physicians and caregivers regarding appropriate therapeutics of such disorders. The liaison model lowers the inhibition threshold between organic and psychological medicine and achieves a seamless unison for everyday dermatological practice. Integrated care brings a clear advantage over external consulting service or referrals.

The diagnostic interviews are performed by a dermatologist with a subspecialty in psychotherapy or in cooperation with a psychologist in the treatment rooms of the dermatologist's practice or the dermatology clinic. If needed, a psychiatrist is also brought in, especially in primary emotional disorders or delusional diseases.

The physician working as the hospital liaison consultant has special knowledge and abilities in the diagnostic and therapeutic area of psychosomatics. He or she is able to perform complex differential diagnoses and therapies, even in difficult and multimorbid patients.

The 50–60-min psychologically oriented interviews are documented in a case report form. The questionnaires on coping with skin diseases (*Marburger Hautfragebogen*, MHF; Stangier et al. 1997) and the SCL-90-R (symptom checklist) can be used for the basis of diagnosis as psychological instruments in the liaison consultancy (Franke 1995). Additional psychological testing instruments for self-rating and rating by others are used in the event of further suspected diagnoses.

After the patient interview, a suspected diagnosis is made based on the clinical interview. Assessment of the psychological test instruments is then made and serves to check the diagnosis, compare the severity for course observations, and check therapy within the framework of the psychosomatic consultancy.

Special attention must be paid in the psychosomatic liaison consultancy to the criteria that determine psychological problems at the organ level. Among these are relationships between the time of first manifestation, duration of existence, possible symbolic language of the skin, and perceptions of emotions. Moreover, somatic, psychosomatic, and sociocultural aspects can be quickly and adequately incorporated into therapy in an integrative liaison consultancy (Herzog and Hartmann 1990; Rees 1983).

Advantages of liaison consultancy are its flexibility and rapid establishment of personal contact in diagnostics and treatment, overcoming the usually high threshold of fear among patients.

The liaison consultancy has a screening function and acts especially as a diagnostic instrument, checking motivation and, if appropriate, coordinating the initiation of adequate psychotherapy (Pontzen 1994; Schleberger-Dein et al. 1994). The goal is the conception of an overall interdisciplinary treatment plan that incorporates various areas of expertise.

Advantages of Liaison Consultancy

- Management of problem patients
- Flexibility and rapid establishment of contact
- Overcoming of threshold fears
- Ability to deal with irritations
- Diagnostics of emotional disorders
- Disclosure of illness-eliciting events (life events)
- Inclusion of sociocultural living habits
- Reduction of omitted diagnoses
- Indication for psychotherapy
- Explanation of complex facts and therapy concepts
- Motivation for psychotherapy
- Initiation of adequate psychotherapy
- Quality assurance
- Prevention

Recommendations for treatment are discussed with the patient, and another appointment is made to check motivation if appropriate. This includes initiation of adequate deep-psychological, analytical, or behavior-therapeutic psychotherapy (Rosenbaum and Ayllon 1981; Schmid-Ott et al. 1999).

In addition, the doctor in the liaison consultancy can take into account and support the aims of the psychotherapist, especially when somatic therapy is performed in parallel and when the dermatoses recur during the course of treatment.

References

Franke G (1995) Die Symptom-Checkliste von Derogatis – Deutsche Version – Manual. Beltz, Weinheim

Herzog T, Hartmann A (1990) Psychiatrische, psychosomatische und medizinpsychologische Konsiliar- und Liaisontätigkeit in der BRD. Nervenarzt 61: 281–293

Pasquini M, Bitetti D, Decaminada F, Pasquini P (1997) Insecure attachment and psychosomatic skin disease. Ann Ist Super Sanita 33: 605–608

Pontzen W (1994) Psychosomatischer Konsiliar- und Liaisondienst. Psychotherapeut 39: 322–326

Rees L (1983) The development of psychosomatic medicine during the past 25 years. J Psychosom Res 27: 157–164

Rosenbaum MS, Ayllon T (1981) The behavioral treatment of neurodermatitis through habit-reversal. Behav Res Ther 19: 313–318

Schleberger-Dein U, Stuhr U, Haag A (1994) Die psychosomatisch-psychosoziale Bedarfs- und Versorgungssituation im Akutkrankenhaus – Ergebnisse einer Befragung internistischer Stationsärzte und -ärztinnen. Psychother Psychosom Med Psychol 44: 99–107

Schmid-Ott G, Jäger B, Lamprecht F (1999) Psychoanalytische Methoden in der psychosomatischen Dermatologie. Z Dermatol 185: 77–81

Stangier U, Ehlers A, Gieler U (1997) Der Marburger Hautfragebogen. In: Manual zum Fragebogen zur Bewältigung von Hautkrankheiten. Hogrefe, Göttingen

Wise TN (2000) Consultation liaison psychiatry and psychosomatics: strange bedfellows. Psychother Psychosom 69: 181–183

Further Reading

Geyer M (1989) Methodik des psychotherapeutischen Einzelgesprächs. Barth, Leipzig

20 New Management in Psychosomatic Dermatology

The dermatologist is the decisive manager of the patient with respect to adequate diagnostics and initiation of therapy in psychosomatic dermatology (Lange et al. 1999; Simmich et al. 1998).

Psychotherapy for Dermatologic Patients

Psychotherapy is weighted and used in clinical practice to different degrees according to training and the doctor's own strengths. It is employed in the following forms:

- Psychotherapy in the context of basic psychosomatic care in the dermatology office
- Psychotherapy in a temporally and organizationally distinct manner alongside the dermatology office
- Psychotherapy of dermatologic patients in the office of a specialist psychotherapist
- Psychotherapy in psychosomatic or behavior therapy outpatient departments
- Psychotherapy in the course of consultative and liaison psychosomatics in dermatology departments
- Psychotherapy as an integral component of educational programs for chronic inflammatory skin diseases in the office or outpatient rehabilitation clinic
- Psychotherapy in the context of dermatologic rehabilitation
- Psychotherapy in the context of psychosomatic rehabilitation (in appropriate clinics, departments, wards)
- Psychotherapy in the acute psychosomatic inpatient clinical setting
- Psychotherapy of dermatologic patients in the psychiatric office or clinic
- Psychotherapy of dermatologic patients in university outpatient and inpatient departments of dermatology

Within the mentioned contexts, varying methodological and theoretical concepts of psychotherapy are applied for psychotherapy for dermatologic patients. The importance of different indications for individualized care depending on the problem and conflict situation in the individual case must be studied in more detail in the future.

Outpatient Practice Models

Numerous measures for health promotion basically focus on the doctor's practice. Prevention, quality assurance, and prophylactic measures in health care succeed only when psychosocial aspects are taken into consideration (Mittag 1991).

The practice of psychosomatics is characterized these days by medical psychosomatic primary care on the one hand and the specific activities of the psychotherapeutic specialist on the other (Chap. 18).

Here, various practice models exist side by side within the dermatological practice. Psychosocial aspects of the disease and treatment processes should be given more relevance, paying more attention to the doctor–patient relationship.

In the doctor–patient relationship, the tenability of the cooperation depends particularly on communication. If trust is weak, the therapy team suffers, and problems with compliance arise.

Inhospital Psychosomatic Therapy Concepts

Inhospital therapy in psychosomatic dermatology ranges from psychosomatic primary care in the acute clinic to inhospital psychosomatic long-term therapy with a dermatological focus, including rehabilitation facilities. The dermatological day hospital, which includes psychosomatic aspects, closes a gap in psychosomatic dermatology.

In a dermatological clinic, instituting a psychosomatic liaison consultancy has proven beneficial as a first step. The liaison consultancy (Chap. 19) of dermatologist and psychotherapist, psychologist, or psychiatrist in the dermatological clinic is a central building block for diagnostics and therapy in emotional and also sociocultural problem areas and can bring clear focus to the decision-making process for further procedures. It is especially helpful if the liaison doctor constructs a regional network of communication structures between outpatient and inpatient psychotherapeutic therapists over the years.

Additionally, depending on the training and availability of personnel, more intensive programs can be conducted with individual or group psychotherapy, relaxation procedures, social training to cope with everyday hassles, and creative group procedures.

Inpatient concepts comprise intensive team-treatment models, which usually include individual and group therapy, relaxation procedures, social training, body-awareness therapies, and creative therapy and are supplemented by team conferences (Table 20.1). Although currently found in Europe, no psychodermatological in-patient service is currently available in the United States.

Individual and group therapies are especially found in facilities with a psychosomatic focus.

Individual therapies. Deep-psychologically-oriented individual therapies lasting for various times can be held up to three times a week and individual patient foci dealt with intensively. During individual therapy, serious crises may occur in the framework of blocked and repressed conflicts that become conscious. The therapist must professionally cushion and direct these (Chap. 13, 14).

Topic-centered group therapy. Topic-centered group therapy is one approach for group therapy. The participants first have to agree on a common topic (for example, "What is harassing me?"). This procedure may lead initially to embarrassed silence, so the group leader has to take the initiative in maintaining the discussion.

Because chronically dermatologically ill persons suffer from similar detriments due to their diseases, it is also recommended that current problems be addressed in the group. Relaxation techniques to reduce tension and control stimulation may accompany group therapy.

Social training. Social training and group experiences, such as visits to public events or exhibitions, especially for patients with a tendency toward withdrawal, sociophobias, or depressive disorders, are a first step toward change and emerging from isolation.

Everyday coping. Problems of the skin disease in everyday living can be very effectively addressed in group discussions, especially during inhospital treatment, in day clinics, and during rehabilitation measures.

Included in this are management and feasibility of complicated care procedures at home and strengthening of learned multimodal body care. Another focus in ev-

Table 20.1 Four pillars of inhospital therapy in psychosomatic dermatology

Psychotherapy	Real life level	Creative level	Body level
Deep-psychological individual therapy Behavior therapy Group therapy including topic-centered group therapy	Social training Everyday coping Treatment schooling (external therapy)	Creative processes: painting, pottery-making, music	Movement therapy Concentrative movement therapy Breathing therapy Autogenic training Muscle relaxation
Psychotherapist Psychologist Specialist for psychotherapeutic medicine Psychiatrist	Nurses Doctors	Gestalt, music, art therapist	Movement and ergotherapy
Team conferences			

20

eryday coping is found in general factors of coping with the disease. Topic-centered everyday coping can very often promote access to biopsychosocial treatment concepts and be the cornerstone of individual motivation for more detailed indicated therapies. Depending on the facility, a decision should be made whether everyday coping can be assisted by caregivers.

Creative therapy. Painting is one of the most frequently applied creative therapies. First a topic is assigned, such as "How do I feel in my skin?" or "self-portrait" or "family picture," and then the pictures are discussed in the group. Very often, the easily interpretable unconscious content of the pictures enables direct access to current conflicts. This, however, may lead to serious crises, which should be immediately addressed by a psychotherapist. Creative therapies are thus embedded in an intensive supplementary procedure within the inhospital psychotherapeutic treatment concepts.

Body-awareness therapies. Body-awareness therapies such as concentrative movement therapy have gained popularity recently to enable patients to have better emotional access to their skin. There is often a dissociative feeling toward the skin within the framework of the disease or an emotional relationship that has been lost but which can be improved with body-awareness therapy. The procedure has a high acceptance level.

Relaxation procedures. Relaxation procedures are mostly used as an accompanying measure in dermatology. Stabilization of symptoms can be achieved, especially in restlessness, insomnia, and excitation and also in pruritus. The use of relaxation techniques in combination with education has proven beneficial in patients with atopic dermatitis. Usually the various procedures can be applied successfully with no great risk (see Chap. 14 on relaxation therapy).

Psychosomatic Day Clinic

The dermatological day clinic that includes psychosomatic aspects closes a gap in care that has existed for years in psychosomatic dermatology. A particular advantage of the dermatological day clinic is the flexible management of problem patients, whereby threshold fears with respect to the biopsychosocial disorder can be rapidly overcome.

Care in the day clinic is available on weekdays. Intensive local therapy takes place, and the patient is also given support for self-help, learning individual aspects of his or her skin disease, skin treatment, and skin care procedures. One focus in the day clinic is on the psychosocial aspects of the skin disease during a liaison consultation and topic-centered group therapy particularly oriented to coping with the disease.

Deep-psychological diagnostics of emotional disorders and, if appropriate, indication for psychotherapy are part of the program. In addition, there is psychoeducation designed for the individual patient, including everyday coping and strengthening of coping with the disease and includes the possibility for focal therapy. The patient also learns relaxation techniques.

Based on the day clinic concept, new experiences can be continued at home, since contact with private surroundings remains intact.

References

Lange S, Zschocke I, Langhardt S, Amon U, Augustin M (1999) Effekte kombinierter therapeutischer Maßnahmen bei Patienten mit Psoriasis und atopischer Dermatitis. Hautarzt 50: 791–797

Mittag H (1991) AIDS prevention and sexual liberalization in Great Britain. Soc Sci Med 32(7): 783–791

Simmich T, Tränckner I, Gieler U (1998) Integrative Kurzzeitpsychotherapie bei Hauterkrankungen. Hautarzt 49: 203–208

A Look into the Future

21

In the coming years, one can certainly look forward to interesting research results, especially in the area of psychoneuroimmunology, which will reveal new aspects of the biopsychosocial interactions between the skin and the psyche.

Communication between the brain and the peripheral organs is accomplished by means of various nerve and hormone signals (Fig. 21.1).

There is a very close association between the central nervous system and the skin. They are formed during embryogenesis from a common blastodermic layer, the ectoderm. Messenger substances, especially the neuropeptides and neurotransmitters, form one central connector (Figs. 21.2, 21.3).

Intensive research on biopsychosocial aspects will be able to contribute in the future to decisive advances in the understanding of disease, disease prevention, and quality improvement in dermatology and medicine as a whole. Emotional stress influences the body's defense mechanisms. Body and soul – psyche and immune system – communicate with one another via messenger substances. Identification of these messenger substances is a central task in basic research in psychosomatics, but it must be assumed that there is more than one "missing link."

Direct line. The nerve cells of the skin do not end, as was long assumed, in the lowest layer of the skin (basal membrane). Very fine nerve fibers branch out, reaching the superficial layers of the skin as well as innervating mast cells and Langerhans cells, among others. Some of these cells play a central role in inflammatory processes as well as in the genesis of pruritus. All evidence indicates that emotions such as anxiety, rage, and joy are "transferred" through this pathway toward the skin. Several studies have already shown that stress-related changes do in fact occur in immune cells.

Communication within the body. The cells themselves communicate via so-called messenger substances. These are, for example, neuropeptides, which a cell releases to elicit certain reactions in the neighboring cells.

There is evidence that various neuronal messenger substances that control the growth of nerve cells are upregulated under stress and are increased in inflammatory reactions in the skin.

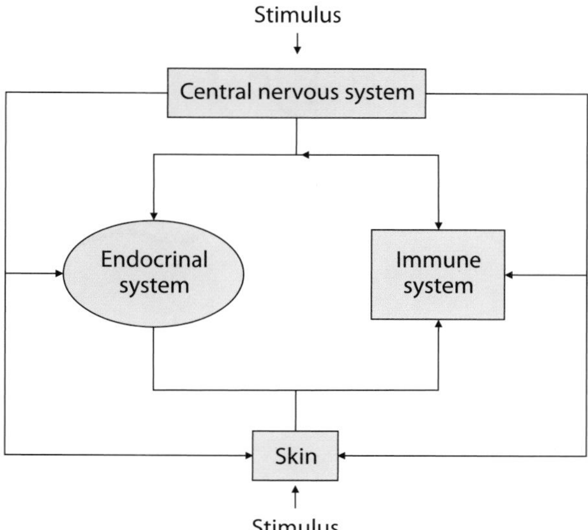

Fig. 21.1 Communication between central nervous system and skin [from Uexküll T von (1995) Psychosomatische Medizin, 5. Aufl. Urban & Schwarzenberg, München]

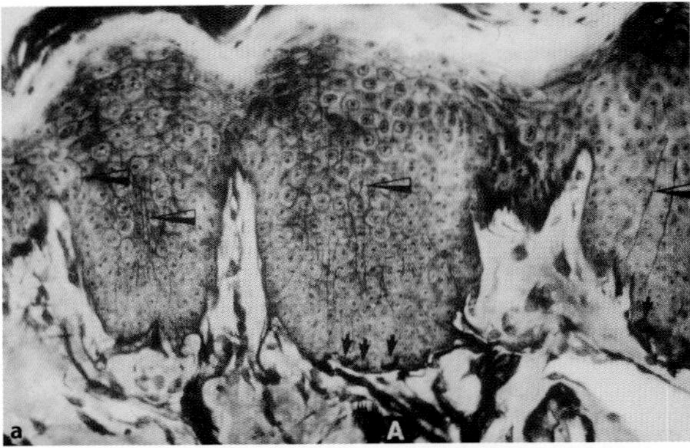

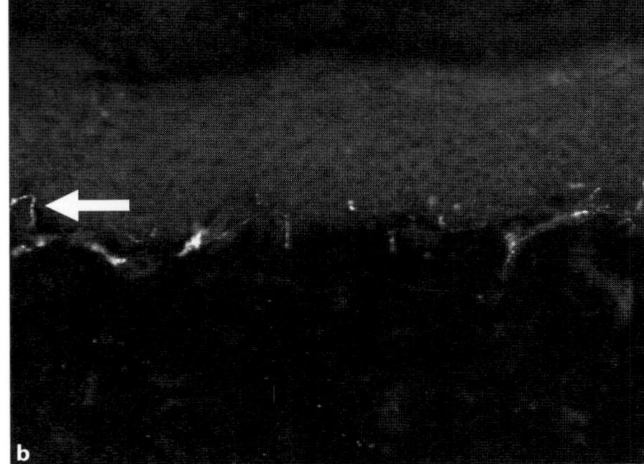

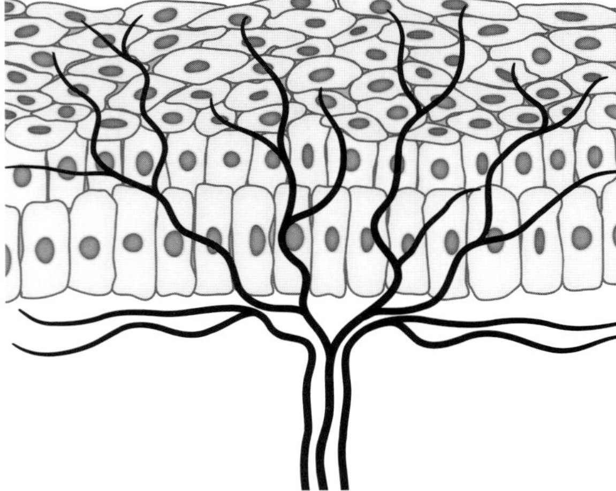

Fig. 21.2a–c Nerve endings in the skin

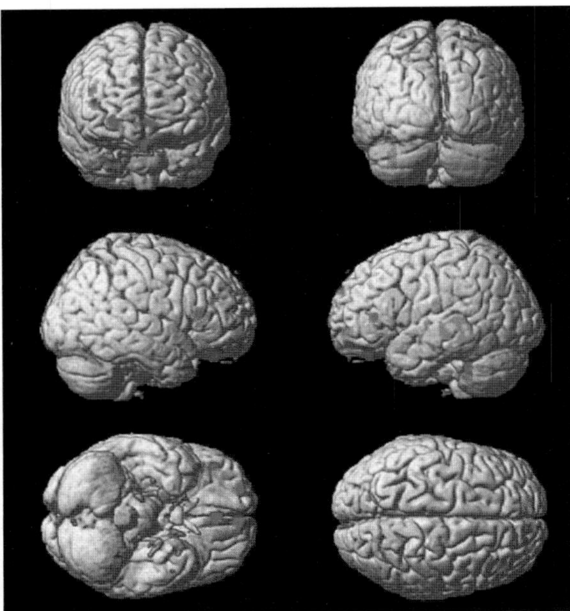

Fig. 21.3 Nuclear medical diagnostic procedure with imaging of metabolic processes (single photon emission computed tomography and positron emission tomography)

Pruritus following psychosocial stress. Pruritus is particularly associated with mental processes and can be elicited or potentiated by stress.

For some people, the psyche apparently plays a greater role than in others. However, surveys show, for example, that approximately 70% of patients suffering from atopic eczema report that emotional stress augments their symptoms.

Filter for therapy candidates. As an example, patients with atopic dermatitis do not represent a uniform population. Within this disease are patients who exhibit an externally provoked form of the disease, being particularly susceptible to environmental allergens such as house dust, pollen, or foods. The psyche may not have a great influence in the clinical evolution of these patients. In those patients who do not have an enhanced allergy susceptibility, emotional stress probably plays a significant role. The goal of the psychodermatologist is, among other things, to detect this latter group using the appropriate methodology. Psychological training, education, and psychotherapy have a particularly significant ameliorating effect in these patients.

Tailor-made medications. In the future, when the immunological mechanisms and messenger substances and the interactions that trigger an eczema episode are known, the chain of inflammatory processes could be interrupted by tailor-made medications. A patient's tormenting itching could also be more specifically controlled. Current antihistamines sometimes function poorly in atopic patients because other substances (such as acetylcholine) are coresponsible for the pruritic skin. If this can be confirmed, special acetylcholine blockers could be developed to halt episodes of pruritus in atopic dermatitis. At the moment, we have only individual mosaic tiles from the big puzzle.

But we're making progress.

Part V

Appendix

Books on Psychosomatic Dermatology

A1

Ader R (2006) Psychoneuroimmunology, 4th edn. Academic Press, New York

Alt C (1988) Symptomwahrnehmung, Symptomerleben, Körpererleben und Kontaktverhalten bei Jugendlichen mit Akne. Roderer, Regensburg

Anzieu D (1989) The skin ego. Yale University Press, New Haven

Benthien C (1999) Haut Literaturgeschichte—Körperbilder—Grenzdiskurse. Rowohlt Taschenbuchverlag, Reinbek bei Hamburg

Bion WR (1961) Experiences in groups. Tavistock Publications, London

Bosse K, Hünecke P (1976) Psychodynamik und Soziodynamik bei Hautkranken. Verlag für Medizinische Psychologie im Verlag Vandenhoeck & Ruprecht, Göttingen

Brosig B, Gieler U (2004) Die Haut als psychische Hülle. Psychosozialverlag, Gießen

Burg G, Geiges ML (2001) Die Haut, in der wir leben—Zu Markt getragen und zur Schau gestellt. Rüffer & Rub, Zürich

Coles R, Seville R, Gieler U, Stangier U (1989) Skin diseases. In: Paulley JW (ed) Psychological management for psychosomatic disorders. Springer, Berlin

Detig-Kohler C (2002) Hautnah—Im psychoanalytischen Dialog mit Hautkrankheiten. Psychosozialverlag, Gießen

Favazza AR (1996) Bodies under siege: self-mutilation and body modification in culture and psychiatry. Johns Hopkins University Press, Baltimore

Feinmann C (1999) The mouth, the face and the mind. Oxford University Press, Oxford

Gieler U (1992) Akne und Psyche. In: Friederich HC (Hrsg) Praxis der Akne-Therapie. Wissenschaftliche Verlagsgesellschaft, Stuttgart

Gieler U (1994) Psychosomatische Hauterkrankungen im Alter. In: Platt F, Friederich HC (Hrsg) Handbuch der Gerontologie, Bd 9. Fischer, Stuttgart

Gieler U, Bosse K (1996) Seelische Faktoren bei Hautkrankheiten—Beiträge zur psychosomatischen Dermatologie. Huber, Bern

Gieler U, Stangier U, Brähler E (1993) Hauterkrankungen in psychologischer Sicht. Hofgrefe, Göttingen

Gupta M (2005) Psychocutaneous disease. Dermatology clinics. Saunders, Philadelphia

Harth W, Gieler U (2006) Psychosomatische Dermatologie. Lehrbuch und Bildatlas. Springer Medizinbuchverlag, Heidelberg, S 1–330

Harth W (2007) Leitlinie Psychosomatische Dermatologie (Psychodermatologie). In: Korting HC, Callies R, Reusch M, Schlaeger M, Sterry W (Hrsg) Dermatologische Qualitätssicherung Leitlinien und Empfehlungen, 5. Aufl. ABW Wissenschaftsverlag, Berlin, S 411–428

Harth W (2008) Psychodermatologie und Kosmetologie. In: Worret WI, Gehring W (Hrsg) Kosmetische Dermatologie, 2. Aufl. Springer Verlag, Berlin, S 31–40

Kapfhammer G (2001) Psychotherapie der Somatisierungsstörungen—Krankheitsmodelle und Therapiepraxis—störungsspezifisch und schulenübergreifend. Thieme, Stuttgart

Kernberg O (1984) Severe personality disorders. Yale University Press, New Haven

Koblenzer CS (1987) Psychocutaneous disease. Grune & Stratton, Orlando

Koo J, Lee CS (2003) Psychocutaneous medicine. Dekker, New York

Kratzer P (2000) Neurodermitis und Mutter-Kind-Interaktion. Waxmann, Münster

Michel KM, Karsunke I, Spengler T (1997) Kursbuch 129 Ekel und Allergie. Rowohlt, Berlin

Montagu A (1980) Körperkontakt, 2. Aufl. Klett-Cotta, Stuttgart

Musalek M (1991) Der Dermatozoenwahn. Thieme, Stuttgart

Niebel G (1995) Verhaltensmedizin der chronischen Hautkrankheit—Interdisziplinäre Perspektiven der atopischen Dermatitis und ihrer Behandlung. Huber, Bern

Panconesi E (1984) Stress and skin diseases—psychosomatic dermatology. In: Parisch LC (ed) Clinics in dermatology 2(4). Lippincott, Philadelphia

Petermann F (1997) Asthma und Allergie, 2. Aufl. Hofgrefe, Göttingen

Phillips K (2005) The broken mirror: understanding and treating body dysmorphic disorder. Oxford University Press, New York

Rajagopalan R, Sherertz E, Anderson RT (1998) Care of skin diseases—life quality and economic impact. Dekker, New York

Rechenberger I (1976) Tiefenpsychologisch ausgerichtete Diagnostik und Behandlung von Hautkrankheiten. Verlag für Medizinische Psychologie im Verlag Vandenhoeck & Ruprecht, Göttingen

Schubert HJ (1989) Psychosoziale Faktoren bei Hauterkrankungen. Verlag für Medizinische Psychologie im Verlag Vandenhoeck & Ruprecht, Göttingen

Seikowski K (1999) Haut und Psyche—Medizinisch-psychologische Problemfelder in der Dermatologie. Westdeutscher Verlag, Opladen/Wiesbaden

Stangier U, Gieler U, Ehlers A (1996) Neurodermitis bewältigen. Springer, Berlin

Stangier U (2002) Hautkrankheiten und Körperdysmorphe Störung. Hogrefe, Göttingen

Updike J (1990) Selbst-Bewußtsein. Rowohlt, Reinbek bei Hamburg

Walker C, Papadopoulos L (2005) Psychodermatology. Cambridge University Press, New York

Weyh FF (1999) Die ferne Haut—Wider die Berührungsangst, 1. Aufl. Aufbau-Verlag, Berlin

Selected Books on Atopic Dermatitis

Gieler U, Schulte A, Rehbock C (1998) Kinder und Neurodermitis—Fragen und Antworten, 1. Aufl. Kilian, Marburg

Niebel G (1998) Diagnose Neurodermitis—wenn die Haut juckt, muß man nicht hilflos bleiben. Hansisches Verlagskontor, Lübeck

Scheewe S, Warschburger P, Clausen K, Skusa-Freeman B, Petermann F (1997) Neurodermitis-Verhaltenstrainings für Kinder, Jugendliche und ihre Eltern. Quintessenz Verlag MMV, München

Szczepanski R, Schon M, Lob-Corzilius T (2000) Neurodermitis: Das juckt uns nicht! 2. Aufl. Thieme, Stuttgart

Contact Links

A 2

Dermatology Organizations in Germany, Europe, and the United States

- American Academy of Dermatology
  http://www.aad.org/
- European Academy of Dermatology
  http://www.eadv.org/
- Website der Deutschen Dermatologischen Gesellschaft
  http://www.derma.de/
- American Social Health Association
  http://www.ashastd.org
- American Society for Dermatologic Surgery
  http://www.asds-net.org
- Skin Cancer Foundation
  http://www.skincancer.org
- American Society for Dermatologic Surgery (ASDS)
  http://www.aboutskinsurgery.com
- The Society for Pediatric Dermatology
  http://www.pedsderm.net
- The Genetic Alliance
  http://www.geneticalliance.org
- European Society for Dermatology and Psychiatry
  http://www.psychodermatology.info
- Arbeitskreis Psychosomatische Dermatologie Sektion der DDG
  http://www.akpsychderm.de
- Berufsverband Dermatologie
  http://www.uptoderm.de/public/index.html

Psychology Organizations

- Ärztliche Gesellschaft für Psychotherapie AÄGP
  http://www.aaegp.de/wissenbeirat/fachgesellschaften.html
- DKPM – Deutsches Kollegium für Psychosomatische Medizin
  http://www.dkpm.de/
- Deutsche Gesellschaft für Psychoanalyse, Psychotherapie, Psychosomatik und Tiefenpsychologie (DGPT) e. V.
  http://www.dgpt.de/
- Deutsche Gesellschaft für Psychotherapeutische Medizin e. V.
  http://www.dgpm.de/
- Deutsche Ärztliche Gesellschaft für Verhaltenstherapie (DÄVT)
  http://www.daevt.de
- Deutsche Balint-Gesellschaft e.V. (DBG)
  http://www.balintgesellschaft.de
- Other Psychology Organizations in Germany:
  http://www.dysmorphophobie.de
  http://www.psychotherapiesuche.de
  http://www.psychotherapeuten-liste.de
  http://www.kompetenznetzwerk-depression.de

Professional Publications

- "Dermatology + Psychosomatics"
  http://www.karger.com/journals/dps/dps_jh.htm
- Dermatology Image Atlas, Johns Hopkins University
  http://dermatlas.med.jhmi.edu/derm/
- DOIA Dermatologie-Atlas
  http://dermis.multimedica.de/
- Leitlinien
  http://www.AWMF-Leitlinien.de
- Bundeszentrale für gesundheitliche Aufklärung
  http://www.bzga.de

Self-Help Groups in Germany and the United States

- National Self-Help Clearinghouse
  http://www.selfhelpweb.org
- American Social Health Association
  http://www.ashastd.org

- National Alopecia Areata Foundation
  http://www.naaf.org
- Cicatricial Alopecia Research Foundation
  http://www.carfintl.org/faq.html
- Children's Alopecia Project
  http://www.childrensalopeciaproject.org
- AcneNet
  www.skincarephysicians.com/acnenet/index.html
- Aging SkinNet
  http://www.skincarephysicians.com/agingskinnet/index.html
  http://www.skincarephysicians.com/eczemanet/index.html
- National Eczema Association
  http://www.nationaleczema.org
- Foundation for Ichthyosis & Related Skin Types
  http://www.scalyskin.org
- National Rosacea Society
  http://www.rosacea.org
- Scleroderma Foundation
  1-800-722-4673 ext. 10
- Skin Cancer Foundation
  http://www.skincancer.org
- National Vitiligo Foundation
  e-mail: info@vnfl.org
- National Coalition for Cancer Survivorship
  http://www.cansearch.org
- Vascular Birthmark Foundation
  http://www.birthmark.org/
- EczemaNet
  http://www.skincarephysicians.com/eczemanet/index.html
- International Pemphigus Foundation
  http://www.pemphigus.org
- National Psoriasis Foundation
  http://www.psoriasis.org
- PsoriasisNet
  http://www.skincarephysicians.com/psoriasisnet/index.html
- Vitiligo Support International
  http://www.VitiligoSupport.org
- National Rosacea Society
  http://www.rosacea.org
- Skin Picking
  http://www.stoppickingonme.com/
  http://www.stoppicking.com/PsycTech/Program/StopPicking/Public/HomePage.aspx
  http://www.homestead.com/westsuffolkpsych/SkinPicking.html
- Psoriasis Forum
  http://www.psoriasis-forum-berlin.de/

NAKOS – Nationale Kontakt- und Informationsstelle zur Anregung und Unterstützung von Selbsthilfegruppen
Wilmersdorfer Str. 39
1062 Berlin, Germany
Tel.: +49-30-31018960
Fax: +49-30-31018970
E-mail: selbsthilfe@nakos.de
http://www.nakos.de

Akne Forum e. V.
Postfach 611218
22457 Hamburg, Germany
Fax +49-40-5504931
E-mail: Dr.Kunze@akne-forum.de
http://www.akne-forum.de

Alopecia Areata Deutschland (AAD) e. V.
Postfach 100 145
47701 Krefeld, Germany
Tel./Fax: +49-2151-786006
E-mail: alopecie@aol.com
http://www.kreisrunderhaarausfall.de

Interessengemeinschaft Epidermolysis Bullosa (IEB) e. V.
Lahn-Eder-Str. 41
35216 Biedenkopf, Germany
Tel.: +49-6461-87015
Fax: +49-6461-989627
E-mail: ieb@ieb-debra.de
http://www.ieb-debra.de

Deutscher Neurodermitis Bund e. V.
Spaldingstr. 210
20097 Hamburg, Germany
Tel.: +49-40-2308-10, -94
Fax: +49-40-231008
E-mail: info@dnb-ev.de or dnb-ev@t-online.de
http://www.dnb-ev.de

Deutscher Psoriasis Bund e. V.
Seewartenstr. 10
20459 Hamburg, Germany
Tel.: +49-40-223399-0
Fax: +49-40-223399-22
E-mail: info@psoriasis-bund.de
http://www.psoriasis-bund.de

Selbsthilfe Ichthyose e. V.
Lauterbacher Str. 11
36323 Grebenau, Germany
Tel.: +49-6646-918675
Fax: +49-6646-918677
E-mail: selbsthilfe-ichthyose@t-online.de
http://www.ichthyose.de

Kontakt- und Informationsforum für Selbstverletzungen
http://www.hp2.rotelinien.de

Sklerodermie
Am Wollhaus 2
74072 Heilbronn, Germany
Tel: +49-7131-3902425
Fax: +49-7131-3902426
E-mail: sklerodermie@t-online.de
http://www.sklerodermie-sh.de

Urticaria Gesellschaft e. V.
Schiffenberger Weg 55
35394 Gießen, Germany
Tel.: +49-641-7960666
Fax: +49-641-7960667
E-mail: Urtikaria.Gesellschaft@urtikaria.de
http://www.urtikaria.de

Deutscher Vitiligo Verein e. V.
Friedensallee 27
25436 Tornesch, Germany
Tel.: +49-4122-960090 or 040-578690
Fax: +49-4122-960091
E-mail: info@vitiligo-verein.de
http://www.vitiligo-verein.de

Tulpe e. V. – Verein zur Betreuung und Hilfe von Hals-, Kopf- und Gesichtsversehrten
Amselweg 4
68766 Hockenheim, Germany
Tel.: +49-6205-208921
Fax: +49-6205-208920
E-mail: info@tulpe.org
http://www.tulpe.org
http://www.gesichtsversehrte.de

Verband für Unabhängige Gesundheitsberatung (UGB) e. V.
Sandusweg 3
35435 Wettenberg/Gießen, Germany
Tel.: +49-641-80896-0
Fax: +49-641-80896-50
E-mail: info@ugb.de
http://www.ugb.de

Hospitals for Psychodermatology

- Klinik für Psychosomatik und Psychotherapie der Justus-Liebig-Universität Gießen; Ludwigstraße 76; 35392 Gießen, Germany; Tel.: +49-641-99-45631 (psychosomatic dermatology: Prof. Dr. med. U. Gieler)
- Rothaarklinik Bad Berleburg, Abt. Dermatologie (chief physician: Dr. J. Wehrmann); Am Spielacker 5; 57319 Bad Berleburg, Germany; Tel.: +49-2751-831-239 or 8310 (psychodynamic orientation)
- Roseneck Klinik, Dermatology Department (department head: Dr. A. Hillert); Am Roseneck 6; 83209 Prien, Germany; Tel.: +49-8051-682210 (behavior therapy orientation)
- Klinik Wersbacher Mühle; Wersbach 20; 42799 Leichlingen, Germany (dermatology: Dr. Pawlak); Tel.: +49-2174-3980 (psychoanalytically oriented clinic)
- Martin-Luther-Universität Halle-Wittenberg, Clinic and Polyclinic for Skin Diseases, Ernst-Kromayer-Straße 5/6, 06097 Halle, Germany; Tel.: +49-345-557-3947/3970 (Prof. C.M. Taube)
- Vivantes Klinikum Berlin, Clinic for Dermatology and Phlebology, Landsberger Allee 49, 102495 Berlin/Friedrichshain, Germany; Tel.: +49-30-130-21308 (private consultant: W. Harth)
- Integrative Dermatology Center, Psychocutaneous Diseases, University of Rochester, Rochester, NY, USA; Tel.: +1-585-275-3872 (directors: Francisco Tausk, MD, dermatology, and Andrea Sandoz, MD, psychiatry)
- Psychocutaneous Clinic, University of Wisconsin, Madison, WI, USA; Tel.: +1-608-265-7670 (director: Ladan Mostaghimi)

ICD-10 Classification

A3.1 ICD Diagnosis Key for Psychosomatic Dermatology

Psychosomatic Skin Diseases

(in which emotional factors play an important role in the etiology)

Diagnosis	F-key	Key
	Psychosomatic psychiatry	Dermatology
Acne vulgaris	F 54	L 70.0
Alopecia areata	F 54	L 63.0
Balanitis simplex	F 54	N 51.2
Hypertrichosis	F 54	L 68.0
Hirsutism	F 54	L 68.0
Hyperhidrosis	F 54	R 61.0
Contact dermatitis	F 54	L 25.0
Atopic dermatitis	F 54	L 20.0
Perioral dermatitis	F 54	L 71.0
Prurigo nodularis	F 54	L 28.1
Prurigo simplex subacuta	F 54	L28.2
Psoriasis vulgaris	F 54	L 40.0
Rhinitis allergica	F 54	I 30.1

Psychosomatic Skin Diseases

(continued)

Diagnosis	F-key	Key
	Psychosomatic psychiatry	Dermatology
Seasonal rhinitis allergica	F 54	I 30.2
Perennial rhinitis allergica	F 54	I 30.3
Stomatitis aphthosa	F 54	K 12.0
Urticaria	F 54	L 50.0
Urticaria cholinergica	F 54	L 50.5
Urticaria factitia	F 54	L 50.3
Vitiligo	F 54	L 80.0

Psychiatric Diseases that Relate to the Skin

Diagnosis	F-key	Key
	Psychosomatic psychiatry	Dermatology
Acarophobia (delusion of parasitosis)	F 22.0	
Acarophobia (organic hallucinosis)	F 06.0	
Dysmorphophobia (delusional)	F 22.8	
Folie à deux	F 24.0	
Glossodynia	F 22.0	K 14.6
Hair tearing (as stereotype)	F 98.4	
Syphilis delusion (paranoid psychosis)	F 22.0	

Somatoform Skin Diseases

(in which the somatic finding does not explain the subjectively experienced complaint)

Diagnosis	F-key	Key
	Psychosomatic psychiatry	Dermatology
Alopecia androgenetica	F 45.9	L 64.9
Dysmorphophobia, body dysmorphic disorder	F 45.2	
Glossodynia	F 45.4	K 14.6
Pruritus sine materia	F 45.8	
Somatoform disorder (dysesthesias of the skin)	F 45.4	
Telogenic effluvium	F 45.9	L 65.0

Artificial Skin Diseases (factitions disorders)

(elicited by manipulation of the skin)

Diagnosis	F-key	Key
	Psychosomatic psychiatry	Dermatology
Acne excoriée	F 68.1	L 70.5
Artificial disorder general	F 68.1	L 98.1
Autoerythrocytic purpura (Gardner–Diamond syndrome)	F 68.1	
Cheilitis factitia crustosa	F 68.1	
Thumb sucking	F 98.8, F 68.1	
Dermatitis factitia	F 68.1	L 98.1
Lichen simplex chronicus vidal (neurodermatitis circumscripta)	F 68.1	L 28.0
Münchhausen syndrome	F 68.1	
Münchhausen by proxy	F 74.8	
Nail biting	F 98.8, F 68.1	
Pseudoknuckle pads	M 72.1	
Malingering/simulation	Z 76.5	
Trichotillomania	F 63.3, F 68.1	
Cheek and lip biting	F 68.1	K 13.1

Sexual Function Disorders

Diagnosis	F-key	Key
	Psychosomatic psychiatry	Dermatology
Dyspareunia (nonorganic)	F 52.6	
Erection disorder psychogenic	F 52.2	
Pruritus vulvae	F 52.9	L 29.2
Vulvovaginitis candidomycetica	F 52.9	B 37.3

Glossary

A 4

- **Adjustment disorders**: Impaired adjustment process after life changes, usually with anxiety, depression, and social withdrawal
- **Agoraphobia**: Fear of open places, which may occur in connection with crowds and public places
- **Ambivalence**: Concurrent presence of various contradictory feelings and ambitions
- **Anancastic personality disorder**: Corresponds to compulsive personality disorder with the main trait being a rigid pattern of perfectionism in both thinking and acting
- **Anxiety**: Feeling of threat and danger accompanied by physical vegetative symptoms such as sweating, tremors, dry mouth, palpitations, and respiratory distress
- **Comorbidity**: The concurrent presence of an emotional disorder and a skin disease
- **Compliance**: Patient's willingness to cooperate in diagnostic and therapeutic measures (such as taking medications)
- **Compulsive acts**: Acts that are usually experienced as tormenting and insuppressible, such as hand washing and control of orderliness, which arise due to some compulsive fear
- **Compulsive disorders**: These comprise compulsive thoughts or compulsive acts that may occur in various combinations
- **Compulsive thoughts**: Recurrent, invasive, and inappropriate thoughts or fantasies that cause anxiety and great uneasiness
- **Conversion**: An (unresolved) emotional conflict becomes physical symptoms that sometimes have a symbolically expressed context (for example, genital pruritus)
- **Coping strategies**: Emotional coping strategies/ways to cope with disease
- **Countertransference**: Totality of all reactions of the doctor or psychotherapist on the patient, including the projections resulting from the transference
- **Cyclothymia**: Persistent mood instability with numerous episodes of mild depression and mild euphoria
- **Defense**: Unconscious mode of behavior to protect against impermissible urges, desires, or emotional conflicts and thus reduce anxiety. Defense mechanisms comprise repression, projection, sublimation, splitting, and others
- **Delusional disorder**: Pathological and false assessments of reality that are experienced as subjective certainty, sometimes with complex ideation constructs. Various forms exist: hypochondriacal delusions, delusions of parasitosis, jealousy delusions, love delusions, guilt delusions, and others
- **Dissociative disorder**: Partial or complete decoupling (dissociation) of emotional and physical functions and loss of the normal integrative functions of memory, consciousness, sensation, and control of bodily functions. Unpleasant feelings are usually blocked
- **Dysthymia**: Chronic persistent, mild depressive mood
- **Empathy**: Sensitive procedure and understanding
- **Hallucinations**: Delusional perceptions without corresponding external stimuli, which the patient believes to be actual sensory impressions (such as tactile, acoustic, olfactory hallucinations)
- **Histrionic**: Corresponds to the modern term "hysteric"

- **Hypochondria**: Objectively unfounded impairment of one's own health, associated with excessive self-observation and preoccupation with and fear of suffering from a serious illness
- **Life events**: Critical events in life that may be psychoreactive elicitors of illness and which are reported by the patient as events in advance of the disease (changes in lifestyle, uprooting)
- **Narcissism**: The state of being in love with oneself
- **Neuroleptic syndrome (malignant)**: Serious consequence of therapy with neuroleptics, characterized by muscle rigidity, hyperthermia, and stupor, as well as elevation of creatine kinase, transaminase, and leukocytes. Therapy includes dopamine agonists and, if necessary, electroconvulsive treatment
- **Neuroleptics**: Antipsychotics with suppressive effect on psychomotor excitability, sensory hallucinations, and delusional disorder, which influence structures of thinking and experiencing
- **Neuroticism**: An emotional disposition with a tendency to excessive worry and anxiety, as well as emotional lability with nervousness, hypersensitivity, anxiety, and excitability
- **Panic disorder**: Sudden episodes of fear with intensive vegetative symptoms
- **Personality disorder**: Deep-rooted and largely consistent behavior pattern that clearly differs from that of the majority of the population and is accompanied by impaired social functioning (emotionally unstable personality, anancastic personality disorder)
- **Phobia**: Specific fear of objects or situations (spiders, places)
- **Posttraumatic stress disorder**: Delayed, persistent emotional reaction to an extreme threat, whereby inescapable memories, emotional or social withdrawal, and vegetative hyperexcitability recur over and over
- **Schizophrenia**: Emotional disorder with multifaceted pattern of delusions, hallucinations, impaired thinking, ego disorders, affect disorders, and psychomotor disorders
- **Somatoform disorder**: Persistent and repeated occurrence of physical symptoms for which no organic cause can be identified
- **SORC**: Acronym for **s**timulus, **o**rganism-variable, **r**eaction (potentiation), and **c**onsequence. The SORC schema is the central foundation of behavior analysis of problematic behavior and consequential therapeutic concepts and alternative behaviors
- **SSRIs**: Selective serotonin reuptake inhibitors, including fluoxetine and paroxetine. This group of antidepressants has hardly any anticholinergic side effects
- **Supportive psychotherapy**: The supportive application of psychoanalytic principles to overcome or relieve an acute emotional decompensation. With this procedure, however, insight and recognition are not primarily supported or maturation steps initiated. Strengthening of the stable and intact personality traits are especially used to support the overcoming of difficulties. In addition, supportive interventions such as calming, instruction, and consultation are applied
- **Tranquilizers**: Psychopharmaceuticals with anxiety-relieving, tension-relieving, sedating, and sleep-promoting effects
- **Transference**: The projections of early childhood love, hate, or other desires that occur during deep-psychological interviews are transferred by the patient to the doctor or psychologist

Subject Index